Alice

Alice
THE MAKING OF A WOMAN DOCTOR 1914–1974

Fay Hercock

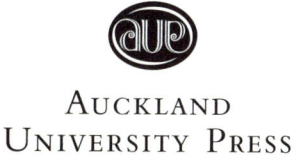

AUCKLAND
UNIVERSITY PRESS

First published 1999

Auckland University Press
University of Auckland
Private Bag 92019
Auckland
New Zealand

© Fay Hercock, 1999

This book is copyright. Apart from fair dealing for the purpose of private study, research, criticism or review, as permitted under the Copyright Act, no part may be reproduced by any process without the prior permission of the publisher.

ISBN 1 86940 206 5

Publication is assisted by the Historical Branch of the Department of Internal Affairs

Front cover photograph: *NZ Herald*
Back cover photograph: courtesy Christine Moorhouse

Printed by GP Print, Wellington

CONTENTS

Abbreviations | vi
Acknowledgements | vii
Introduction | 1
1 Becoming a Doctor | 5
2 Work and War | 23
3 Marriage | 41
4 Circles are Broken | 60
5 Full Use of Her Talents | 78
6 The Specialist | 97
7 Education for Life | 115
8 Taking a Stand | 134
9 Going to the Needy | 152
10 Widening Horizons | 170
11 New Feminism: New Medicine | 188
12 Reproductive Politics | 207
13 The Quality of Life | 226
Notes | 244
Bibliography | 270
Index | 278

ABBREVIATIONS

AKMWA	Auckland Branch, Medical Women's Association
ALRANZ	Abortion Law Reform Association of New Zealand
APC	Appeal for Population Control
BMA	British Medical Association
DCH	Diploma in Child Health (England)
DGH	Director-General of Health (New Zealand)
ECAFE	Economic Commission for Asia and the Far East
FGC	Family Guidance Centre
FPA	Family Planning Association (Britain)
FRACP	Fellow of the Royal Australasian College of Physicians
FRCP	Fellow of the Royal College of Physicians (London)
ICAVS	International Project of the Association for Voluntary Sterilisation
IPPF	International Planned Parenthood Federation
JRMO	Junior Resident Medical Officer
LFFCS	Lady Fergusson Family Counselling Service
MANZ	Medical Association of New Zealand
MRACP	Member of the Royal Australasian College of Physicians
MRCP	Member of the Royal College of Physicians (London)
MWA	Medical Women's Association
NCC	National Council of Churches
NCW	National Council of Women
NZBMA	British Medical Association New Zealand Branch
NZFPA	New Zealand Family Planning Association
NZMA	New Zealand Medical Association
NZMWA	New Zealand Medical Women's Association
RCSS	Royal Commission on Social Security
RMO	Resident Medical Officer
SEAOR	South-east Asian and Oceania Region, IPPF
SPUC	Society for the Protection of the Unborn Child
UN	United Nations
UNICEF	United Nations Children's Fund
WAAC	Women's Auxiliary Army Corps
WCC	World Council of Churches
WHO	World Health Organisation
WNSC	Women's National Service Corps
WONAAC	Women's National Abortion Action Campaign
YWCA	Young Women's Christian Association

ACKNOWLEDGEMENTS

In telling this story the contributions of others have been particularly important. The idea of a biography had its origins when Phoebe Meikle, educationalist, editor and a contemporary of Alice, approached Faulkner Bush shortly after Alice's death with the suggestion that her papers should be conserved towards this end. Over the next several years Faulkner put together what I have named the Alice and Faulkner Bush Papers. In doing so he was unsparing, not only in the time and effort he devoted to this task but in releasing particularly intimate and personal material. At the same time Phoebe, aided by volunteers, assembled the impressive array of clippings, correspondence, interviews and question slips that I have named the Meikle Collection.

By the late 1980s, when struggles with finance, intensified by failing health, had made it impossible for her to carry on, Phoebe handed all this material over to me. My own research extended the sources to more formal collections, photographs held privately or in various archives around the country and further interviews with old and new informants. The spirit of generosity demonstrated by those involved, too many of whom, unfortunately, have not lived to see the project completed, is proof of the extensive legacy of goodwill left by Alice herself. Not all who contributed have been noted in the text but each has been equally important in helping to make this book a reality. At the same time, responsibility for any misjudgments, errors or omissions must rest solely on my own shoulders.

The great stumbling block for all those who pursue a long-term project, finance, has been overcome by donations from many sources. Phoebe received particular help from the New Zealand Literary Fund, Mrs Betty Holt and an anonymous 'Well-Wisher', but she valued just as highly the smaller amounts given by so many individuals who felt Alice's story should be told. Nevertheless, it was not nearly enough, and when all else failed Phoebe fell back on her own resources, becoming her own principal source of funding. The establishment, since that time, of the Historical Branch of the Department of Internal Affairs, and the funding it makes available to historians working in the community for research, writing and publishing, have saved me from the same fate, and for this, and their patient support, I thank them. I express my gratitude also for the smaller, but no less helpful, contributions I received from the Centre for the Study of Auckland History and Society, and the Auckland Medical Research Foundation on behalf of the Sir Douglas Robb Memorial Fund.

In common with all those who use libraries and archives, I have relied very much on the staffs or individuals who care for the public and private collections I consulted in search of primary material and photographs. Just as important has been the contribution of postgraduate research from universities in the form of theses and long essays. I have been particularly fortunate in the continuing support of my friends in the Department of History, University of Auckland, who have sustained me in various ways long after I left that institution. There have been many in this category, but I must especially thank Judith Bassett, supervisor of the thesis with which I began this work and an unflagging supporter in subsequent years, and Professors Raewyn Dalziel and Barry Reay, who sacrificed their own precious time to read and comment on my preliminary drafts. Those working in history outside academia have also provided help in specialist areas, and in this regard I would like to thank in particular Diana Stuart Masters, who has shared her knowledge and sources in the field of local medical history.

Once again, Auckland University Press has provided for me the essential professional editing and publishing services on which authors rely. The long-term support of Elizabeth Caffin, the sympathetic editing skills of Anna Rogers and the practical efforts of Katrina Duncan all deserve special mention.

Last, but certainly not least, I would like to thank Alice's sisters Patricia Rogers and Aileen Odell, her brother Allenby and his wife Isabel, and especially her son Peter and her daughter Christine. The experience of public examination of the life of someone close comes to very few, and the unusual demands biography can make on surviving family members are not always appreciated by the general public. Alice's family has shared memories of a life they valued and granted access to photographs they have preserved. Above all, by permitting publication of the personal material first made available by their father, Peter and Christine have generously allowed Alice and Faulkner to speak for themselves.

Fay Hercock
Auckland
January 1999

Introduction

This is an account of the life and experiences of a New Zealand woman doctor, Alice Mary Bush, who graduated from Otago Medical School in 1937 and, after a short period in general practice during the Second World War, became a specialist allergist and paediatrician. By the time of her death in 1974 she had achieved the highest honours of her profession: fellowships of both the Australasian and Royal Colleges of Physicians. Her fulltime and successful medical career immediately sets Alice apart from her contemporaries, but two further factors place her outside the usual experiences of a woman of her time: first, the high public profile she enjoyed, and second, the fact that she maintained an active professional lifestyle while a married woman and a mother.

Alice was an exceptional person and one of the purposes of this book is to trace the influences that contributed to her worldly success. She herself had definite ideas about the development of the mature personality. Although she did not deny the importance of 'nature', inherited traits present at birth, she was more concerned with 'nurture', particularly the experiences of childhood. Her own early years contain many identifiable sources of her later attitudes and concerns, but these provide only a starting point. Characteristics already in place by the time she entered medical school would be further developed and directed by her experiences after graduation, when a wider range of theories and values, personal and professional relationships, came her way. These acted upon Alice's already firmly established sense of social responsibility and propelled her into her public role. She became involved in important debates, many of which are still continuing. These included the place of the doctor in society, the provision of health services, attitudes to emotional and mental health and personal and family relationships, the role of women, changing attitudes to sexuality, reproductive rights, the international population debate and the provision of education in all these spheres. Central to this involvement was her adoption of a philosophy of individual and social improvement that focused on these issues. Because this was an emerging movement when she first encountered it in the early 1940s, her attachment cannot be neatly attributed to a single event, text or person. Rather, it was a case of mutual development over the ensuing decade, as Alice simultaneously struggled to construct her own life, professionally and privately, into a coherent whole. By the end of the 1950s, when these new ideas had reached a crucial stage in gaining wider acceptability, they had become the mainspring of her life, so that she became a champion of the groups that were promoting them.

Though, while Alice's life was extraordinary, she also shared the experiences common to her sex. She was a daughter, wife and mother and accorded the same importance to these roles as did other women of her time. A privileged background would not exempt her from personal tragedies. Her adult years spanned the introduction of the welfare state, the Second World War, the inhibited 1950s, the revolutionary 1960s, and part of the liberated 1970s. Like everyone else, she had to face these changes and adjust to them. But it was only late in her life that women's rights became a public issue. This meant that though Alice benefited from the old feminist gains, which made a medical education accessible to her, she began practice believing that marriage and children would take priority over any career ambitions. It was only her openness to new ideas and the greater professional opportunities made available by the wartime exodus of medical men which led her to feel that she might, indeed should, 'have it all'. As a result, Alice became a rare phenomenon in mid-20th-century New Zealand society: a recognised female public figure who supported women both in their domestic role and in their search for something more. Poised between two major periods of feminist consciousness, she had no contemporary theory to sustain her. Rather, she found in old and emerging ideas elements that she could use to authorise her unusual lifestyle.

The path was not always smooth, but Alice ultimately achieved strong family support in her personal world. No similar compromise was possible in her professional world, which required a total commitment that few women with family responsibilities could accommodate; there Alice was forced to fit into existing structures. This was not selling out to a man's world; her experience was vastly different from that of her male colleagues. Some of the stresses to which she was subjected are discernible in her papers, but others are revealed only in the memories of her fellow women doctors and there are probably many more for which there are no records at all. Although Alice was usually surrounded by people, hers must often have been a lonely working life. Not only was she subject to the twin pressures of family and profession, but she also championed causes that many of her male counterparts treated flippantly or even despised. Moreover when, towards the end of her life, woman's rights did become a publicly debated issue, Alice found herself out of step with its radical tendencies. Although she had used ideology pragmatically, she had largely remained faithful to an evolutionary individualism based on 19th-century liberalism, while the cutting edge of 1960s feminism took its authority from the revolutionary mass protest movements of the time and the New Left. The resulting conflict added to other tensions for Alice over these years as she saw medicine taking a direction of which she did not approve and faced her own failing health. Her crowded last years were, at times, less than happy.

Even in her darkest hours, though, Alice was sustained by her belief that there was an ultimate good worth pursuing. This is perhaps best expressed in a letter that she wrote to her son, Peter, in 1968.

> There is good & bad. Seeking after good will lead to happiness. What you do that is bad, however much the pleasure of the moment, will be an erosion of the foundations of your happiness. . . . I believe that the pleasant things of this life were meant to be enjoyed, good food, good company, alcohol, good sights & sounds & feelings – including sex – but these alone are not enough for happiness which comes only from the pursuit of the ultimate good. You will hear many definitions of this as you go through life, and the one that is valid for you is the one that you choose for yourself. It is something that requires thought, but it is urgent that you work it out, else you go through life without a compass.[1]

Alice worked out her 'good' and found her 'compass'. Not everybody shared her views but very few, even those most strenuously opposed to her, could fail to respect the strength of her commitment and recognise the humanitarianism that underlay it. Although determined, she was essentially a compassionate woman whose journey through life was adventurous and unique.

CHAPTER I

Becoming a Doctor

I can remember as a medical student feeling so happy that I didn't know what to do.[1]

Alice was born on 7 August 1914,[2] the second child and eldest daughter of Joseph and Marjorie Stanton of Auckland. Her older brother, Warwick, was just 19 months her senior, Patricia a year younger. Another son, Allenby, and then Aileen were added to the family in 1918 and 1923. They were comfortably middle class, second-generation New Zealanders. Alice's father was an up and coming lawyer; her mother's family, the McMasters, had for many years run a quality drapery shop in Queen Street, the premier retail area of the city. At the time of Alice's birth, Joseph and Marjorie were living in Herne Bay,[3] a pleasant harbourside suburb. Their lifestyle was ordered and secure. A nursery-housemaid and a cook lived in, and a cleaning woman and gardener were employed on a casual basis. The children were loved, but not indulged. As they matured, the girls were expected to help in the house and the boys in the garden or with the family car. They respected their parents and their parents respected them. Joseph and Marjorie never smacked their children and forbade the nursery-housemaid to do so.[4] It was a happy early environment and one that undoubtedly had a profound influence on Alice. As a 25-year-old house surgeon she would write,

> For years, I have lived mostly away from home, and yet it still means to me as much as when I was at school. It is not just a convenient place to spend holidays, but it is my *home* from which for long periods I am exiled and to which I always long to return. The family ties are very strong.[5]

For the rest of her life she would remain wedded to the ideal of love and security as the basis for the successful upbringing of children and would believe that these qualities were most likely to be present in the family home of a mutually loving couple.[6] She probably first discovered that this was not the natural lot of every child as she found out more about her own father's early years.

Economic and social standing, even emotional security, were relatively recent elements in Joseph Stanton's experience. The fourth of six children born to a storeman, Alfred Stanton,[7] Joseph had been motherless from the age of seven after his mother, Fanny, had died of typhoid fever in 1891.[8] How the family managed over the next few years is uncertain. The late 19th-century state provided no assistance for widowers, and charitable aid was parsimonious and its guardians judgmental. Extended families could usually offer only temporary solutions. Perhaps partly in the hope of providing a more stable environment for his children, Alfred remarried five years after Fanny's death,[9] but for Joseph the result was further emotional trauma because he and his stepmother did not get on.[10] His personal unhappiness may well have provided the spur for an avid pursuit of independence and economic security over the next decade. After three years at Auckland Grammar School as a Rawlings Scholar, he continued his studies for matriculation at night school while working by day in a saddler's shop. By 1900 he was employed as a clerk in the office of a leading solicitor, Thomas Cotter, and attending law lectures at Auckland University College in the evenings. He graduated in 1907.

Over the same years the Stanton family religion, Methodism, provided Joseph with a culture that sustained his worldly aspirations. He was a member of Pitt Street, Auckland's leading Methodist church, where he regularly attended class meetings and was 'an enthusiastic helper' in the Sunday school.[11] The church attracted a circle of businessmen who moved together socially and shared a philosophy that balanced material self-improvement with Christian morality. This was also the era of the temperance movement and, although no hard evidence is available, it is very unlikely that the young Joseph Stanton did not at least support this campaign. Although he drank in moderation in later life, he was believed to have been a total abstainer as a youth and the movement's theoretical basis, with its emphasis on the power of individuals to change the course of their lives through their own will and effort, would undoubtedly have appealed to him. Its wider application, that the whole of society could benefit from such individual reformation, would have particular appeal for his eldest daughter.

The church also provided Joseph with a wife. The McMasters were leading members of the congregation, and Marjorie's father, Thomas, was prominent in church affairs and served on several Methodist committees. He could afford to educate all his children well. Marjorie attended arts lectures at Auckland University College, and involvement with the Student Christian Movement there, Joseph as president and Marjorie as secretary, provided further opportunities for them to spend time together.[12] Although Marjorie did not graduate, she worked sporadically as a mathematics teacher in private schools until January 1911 when she and Joseph were married.[13] It was the perfect match of its day: Marjorie, socially confident and warm, made an ideal wife for a rising professional man, while Joseph, with his personal probity and worldly ambition, provided the emotional and financial stability on which a woman, indeed a family, could depend.

With his marriage, Joseph's transformation from working class boy to middle class man was complete. His future concerns would more closely reflect the activities of Thomas McMaster than those of his own father, whose entire energies had been taken up in simply trying to keep his family together. Joseph worked hard in his professional life, and it flourished. Following the death of Thomas Cotter, he took over the practice and Cotter's post as city solicitor. He later absorbed another legal firm and by the early 1920s had taken two partners. He had also paid £2,050 for over an acre of land in prestigious Mountain Road, Epsom, on which he built a solid two-storeyed home, Denestone.[14] The house contained a large nursery for the children, and the extensive grounds were landscaped to include a tennis court. In 1925 Marjorie purchased a beach house at Waiake on the North Shore, now known as Torbay but popularly referred to at that time as Deep Creek.[15] Situated where beach met creek, complete with tennis court and boathouse, for over 40 years it provided the setting for holidays and gatherings of the extended family and friends. Joseph was now a leading citizen of Auckland, listed in *Who's Who* as city solicitor, a member of the board of governors of the Auckland Grammar School and of the Auckland District Repatriation Board, and honorary solicitor to the Auckland Patriotic Association. During 1926, the children were cared for by various relations while their parents embarked on an extended tour of England, Scotland and the Continent.

This was, by any measure, an impressive rise in financial and social standing for the son of a struggling working class family. Her father's achievements deeply impressed Alice, and as a young woman she found no reason to question his beliefs or standards. His progress in life confirmed for her the possibilities for even the disadvantaged individual within existing political and social structures. She saw his professional success as the very model of what might be produced by committed pursuit of educational opportunity combined with the Protestant work ethic. To Alice, his voluntary work for the various causes he favoured seemed to provide the ideal balance between individual interests and those of society, between personal ambition and Christian charity. She summarised her feelings in May 1940, after observing Joseph listening to a wartime radio address by Prime Minister Peter Fraser.

> Daddy was very grave. I think that he is just beginning to realise the possibility of things really breaking up, & because he has been so sure of things the realisation is doubly hard. . . . I'm proud of him. I think he is the main reason for my clinging to many of the principles of the present system. He started from the bottom with no advantages & now that he is near the top there is no arrogance about him, material things mean much to him & yet he has been generous almost to a fault in business transactions & a lot of his time and energy are spent on works that bring no remuneration . . . . as I watched him this evening unutterably sad at the thought that many of the things that have been almost a religion with him are likely to pass away I just wished that I could protect him from too much hardship.[16]

This letter was written at a time when Alice was becoming more aware of just how much she, and her brothers and sisters, had been protected by their parents. The Stanton children mixed in the limited circles and attended the private schools favoured by Auckland's social élite. Alice and her sisters were first sent to Hill Top School, conducted in the family home of the headmistress, Phyllis Boult, and within walking distance of Denestone. Because of the school's small size, Hill Top girls were given very close to individual tuition. In 1927, when Alice was in her last year, 41 pupils aged from five to 14 years were taught by five women with various levels of formal qualification and involvement.[17] Miss Boult did not aim to prepare children from a privileged background for a future life of leisure. The approach to work was serious, the atmosphere disciplined despite the homely setting. 'Young people, you are superficial and lacking in concentration,' she would admonish her pupils when their attention wandered. 'Left to you, what will happen to the world?'[18] The school's motto, frequently alluded to, was 'Perseverando', for sports the somewhat more prosaic 'Play the Game'. Alice spent seven years at Hill Top, imbibing English literature and grammar, elementary mathematics, geography, painting, French, handwork and physical education, along with the smell of fresh hops from the brewery next door. The girls in her year were entered for the Proficiency examination, the first time the school had offered candidates. All passed with high marks and those who, like Alice, went on to the Diocesan School for Girls, a much larger Anglican girls' school in Epsom, impressed staff and students there with their solid scholastic grounding.[19]

Alice began her secondary education at Diocesan in 1928 and remained there for four years. As a senior student, she became involved in committees, sports teams, amateur dramatics and editing the school magazine. She was also appointed a house and school prefect. Apart from the fact that she matriculated in 1930, her academic achievements remain publicly unrecorded. The school's headmistress at the time, Miss H.K. Sandford, disapproved of competitive stimulus in learning. School prizes were abolished and the money directed to building up the school library, which she believed to be inadequate for pupils wishing to proceed to university.[20] These were unusually liberal views for the time and perhaps the reason for Miss Sandford's short tenure.

How much they affected Alice is hard to tell. The affairs of Diocesan did not feature strongly in her later life, whereas Miss Boult and Hill Top retained her affectionate attention until her death. In the late 1950s Alice and her father put considerable effort into moves to keep the school going when it hovered on the brink of closure. For a short time after Alice's death, Hill Top, relocated at Blockhouse Bay, was renamed Stanton Junior College, apparently in gratitude for this support.[21] In 1944, when considering the educational needs of her first child, something that Alice took very seriously, she explained her preference for Hill Top to her husband in academic terms: 'perhaps if Hill Top is still going she could there acquire the love of learning and form good thinking habits, after that I guess it wouldn't matter where she went to school. I think it's the first 5 yrs. that matter.'[22]

The school's approach to preparing individuals for their place in society must, however, have been very attractive to her. In 1951 its aims were identified by Miss Boult, who remained its headmistress until the early 1960s, as

> ... helping the child to build up a balanced personality; to teach her to live equably with other people; to bear her share of responsibility in life; to have a spirit of service; to learn the joy of work; to practise self discipline, to be just, enthusiastic, hard-working, conscientious, happy and self-controlled.[23]

This was just the same blend of internalised self-discipline and the 'joy of work', individual responsibility and social service, which Methodism preached and to which Alice was strongly committed in her adult life. Miss Boult might also have been writing the prescription for what most people would regard as the makings of a good doctor.

It appears from reminiscences of Alice's contemporaries that these influences were already bearing fruit during her schooldays.[24] They remembered her as an equable, co-operative girl, eager to participate in activities and willing to take on responsibility. She also appears to have possessed the happy knack of being able to get on with her work when others larked about without being regarded as a killjoy. Yet Alice herself recalled far less self-assurance. 'I was never what you'd call popular, as a girl,' she was to write in 1945, 'I think I must have been rather dull, socially.'[25] Photographs taken when she was at Diocesan show her as sturdy in build, though not above average in height, with a delicate facial bone structure and regular features promising mature beauty rather than attention-grabbing youthful prettiness. In the official portrait of the school hockey team, taken in 1931 when she was in her mid-teens, she faces the camera directly, her gaze steady, her mouth good-humoured, arms clasped behind her back, fitting perfectly into the group. Only in one detail is her appearance slightly awry. One point of her large white blouse collar protrudes over her serge gym slip, while the other is tucked neatly away. This is the only indication that, beneath that smooth middle class exterior, an element of nonconformity might be lurking, but even this small lapse is shared by two others in the group. All the indications are that this was a girl comfortable with the values of her family and unlikely to question the structures within which she had been brought up, even though she had reached youthful maturity at the peak of the Depression years.

Economically, the Stantons survived the Depression reasonably well. Although there was undoubtedly a little belt-tightening, the family was still able to cope with the costs of private or tertiary education for five children and the maintenance of two properties. A later, short, spell of financial stringency during 1940 was described by Alice at the time as 'bad, very bad, worse than any of the years in the slump'.[26] The early 1930s were, in fact, the years in which Joseph and Marjorie launched their progeny into full membership of Auckland society. Although they themselves retained their Methodist connection, the children became Anglicans. Alice and Patricia were confirmed in the Diocesan chapel in 1930.[27] In June 1932 Alice, dressed in a gown of ivory chiffon velvet, with pink flowers on one shoulder, made her formal debut at Government House.[28] The Depression experience was not politically radicalising – rather the reverse. In 1935, in his only recorded political involvement, Joseph moved not left but right, supporting the proposed parliamentary candidacy of Sir Alexander Herdman, 'the 66 year-old arch conservative'.[29] Even the editor of the staid Auckland morning paper, the *New Zealand Herald*, felt support given to this candidate, emanating principally from the Northern Club, of which he was president, was misplaced.[30]

The most painful episode for Alice and her family over these years was an intensely personal one. In August 1931 Alice's older brother, Warwick, died of exposure during a tramping trip to National Park in the central North Island. Despite continued searching, his body was not recovered until the middle of September.[31] Friends and family were devastated. Fellow students at Auckland University College subscribed to search expenses and

James Bertram, a contemporary, wrote a lyrical obituary for *Craccum*, the student paper, headed by a quotation from A.E. Housman's 'On an athlete dying young'.[32] Large crowds attended the funeral at Denestone and in 1933 a brass memorial tablet was fixed to a rock, marking the spot where Warwick's body had been found.[33] This protracted and public bereavement was undoubtedly particularly difficult for Alice. Warwick, she and Patricia, born in consecutive years, had formed a unit within the family. They had grown up together and, as young adults, were still close. They went as a group to the private dances held by their friends, circumstances in which a good-looking, considerate, older brother was a priceless asset to a young woman unsure of herself on the social scene. Alice and Warwick shared similar values and were intellectual equals. Both were planning professional careers.

How does a young woman, 17 years old, deal with the sudden death of a beloved brother? For the first time Alice encountered pain and loss that neither her family's love, nor their financial and social standing, could ease. Yet, even as a teenager, Alice was never lost in self-pity and, as her personal experiences broadened, so would her concerns and her questions. Two years after Warwick's death she wrote,

> ... it's only in the last couple of years that I have realised how much pain & suffering there is in the world & I know I can't hope to escape it. I sometimes think I have already had more than my share of good things, but I don't think it does to lie down to it so I'm determined to enjoy life in spite of pain. I sometimes think it's almost easier to get over one's own troubles than it is over other people's. ...
>
> What is the meaning of pain, physical & mental? Why are some people struck down just on the threshold of life, like Warwick was? ... there is a man [who is] ... well over 80 & is now losing his mind & yet lingers on. Why should all this be?[34]

This is the first evidence of what was to become a preoccupation for Alice: how best to achieve 'quality of life'. For her parents, Warwick's death was also a major crisis. They had lost everything they could wish for in an eldest son. Marjorie had not been well for some time and now, to their dismay, the children watched Joseph's health deteriorate visibly, as if in response to his son's death. Their concern was increased the following year when an exploratory operation revealed the presence of bowel cancer, necessitating further surgery. It was during this period of intense family stress that Alice began her training in medicine.

Alice has left no record of why she wanted to become a doctor, only that she 'couldn't remember a time' when she didn't want to be one.[35] There does not seem to have been an immediate role model. Marjorie's brother, Archie, was a doctor but Alice's personal contact with him was very limited since he had lived and practised in England since the First World War. Girls' secondary schools did not actively encourage pupils towards ambitious career choices, particularly those involving science subjects.[36] The *Diocesan High School Chronicle* notes 14 old girls attending university at this time, but only Alice was taking a medical degree. There is no evidence that personal experience of the social and economic deprivation of the Depression inspired her future career decision and by the time Warwick died she was already preparing for her medical intermediate year, so that tragedy can be discounted as a primary motivator. The most likely explanation lies in the religious culture and the middle class nature of the Stantons' family life, which would regard the practice of medicine, even for women, as both favourable and accessible. Women doctors of the 1930s lay in a direct line of descent from middle class 19th-century feminists who wished to take the feminine virtues that sustained women's domestic role into the wider world. This is most obviously demonstrated by the motto of their international association, 'Matris Animo Curant', which translates as 'They care in a motherly spirit'.[37] The medical profession had unwittingly reduced the ideological tension of women moving into predominantly masculine territory by representing itself in traditionally feminine apolitical and nurturing terms. The idea that women had a 'natural' talent for medicine was both pervasive, and limiting, for most of Alice's professional life. Hercus and Bell, in their 1964 history of the Otago Medical School, defined women as

> ... natural, instinctive doctors, with a strong bias to the simpler remedies; not for them complex carbon ring derivatives. The well-known tribute "a ministering angel thou", obviously refers to their zeal in administering such comforts as paregoric, ipecacuanha wine, Gregory's powder, rose-hip syrup, mustard plasters and caster oil – that enemy to internal rest. We marvel that with such a long record in unqualified practice their entry into formal medicine was so long delayed.[38]

Alice supported the idea that women had a valuable gender role to play in medicine, observing in an address made quite late in her life that

> There is a large field of medicine in which therapeutic success is quite independent of the sex of the doctor, but in a significant number of cases relief of distress is possible only when a very special relationship can be established between patient and doctor. Some patients need a father figure, some need a mother figure to guide them through their difficulties. In the ideal medical service both should be available.[39]

On the same occasion she used religion as the authority for women taking on such a role, referring to the parable of the talents and the need to account to God for the gift of life.

> All of us hope for our children a life of service which will earn for them the precious praise "Well done thou good and faithful servant". Will this be bestowed on the woman who endowed with the talent to heal the bodies and minds of thousands has used these talents only in a small family circle?[40]

These sentiments reflected her family's Methodist background, in which individual self-improvement and service to others were seen as mutually supportive, or as Alice herself put it in 1968, 'one's duty to oneself to develop to the full the talents one has, and one's duty to others to be kind'.[41] These elements also composed the classical career combination for women doctors: they tended to be to the forefront in any charitable enterprise, particularly those concerning women and children, or they were employed in quasi-charitable roles, such as the School Medical Service.

Even so, for most of Alice's life the proportion of women doctors remained very small because the ideology that said women's 'natural' qualities fitted them for the medical profession also placed economic and educational barriers in their way. Although the doors of the country's medical school had always been open to female students, only 92 women had qualified between 1896 and 1931. Medical training was a particularly long and expensive undertaking, and even in middle class families that valued education cost was a factor. It made good sense to outlay substantial sums of money to provide a future breadwinner with remunerative qualifications, but the same argument did not necessarily apply to a daughter at a time when few middle class women worked outside the home after marriage, and most women married.⁴² Moreover, Alice entered medical school when Joseph's health was causing serious concern. This must have given both him and his daughter pause when considering a significant financial undertaking covering at least five or six years. Although the Stantons were liberal parents for their time, respecting their offspring as individuals and encouraging them to make their own decisions, they also insisted that they take responsibility for themselves.⁴³ Apparently Alice and her father came to an agreement. She would have her chance at medicine, but she would repay the costs involved. In April 1940, during her first months in private practice, Alice referred to their final settlement.

> My training cost £535, including board, and the following arrangement has been made. I make no further payments now, but if Daddy dies before I do, then I shall receive £300 less from his estate than I otherwise would have. All very complicated, but he seems to think that is fair, so now if things remain normal I have no obligations, except, of course if anything drastic happened to Daddy's business . . . then I should, of course, do the right thing.⁴⁴

The next hurdle was academic: passing the medical intermediate examination. Again, this raised particular problems for young women. Some candidates regarded it as an advantage to travel to Dunedin for their intermediate year in order to take the examination at the University of Otago, where the teaching of physics was considered superior and the papers were set and marked.⁴⁵ This meant leaving home when around 17 years of age, a prospect not likely to appeal to parents of daughters in the early 1930s. Alice attended Auckland University College for this year. Women candidates faced a further handicap because the examination was composed entirely of sciences.⁴⁶ Girls' schools had found it difficult to offer a full science and mathematics programme since homecraft and child care had been included as compulsory subjects in the state school syllabus. The move had been undertaken in an attempt to curb a falling national birth rate by elevating the status of domestic duties under the category of 'Home Science'.⁴⁷ Although women students were allowed to substitute a matriculation pass in home science for one in chemistry,⁴⁸ such a course was inadequate for tertiary scientific study. This must have been obvious to both Alice's parents and the staff at Diocesan School, since she was one of a very small group who received coaching in science, including physics, from the mathematics teacher in her final year. Alice's marks for her medical intermediate examination seem to justify such precautions. Although she gained a respectable 69 per cent in biology and organic chemistry, she had more difficulty with the comparatively esoteric inorganic chemistry and physics, in which she received 53 per cent and 52 per cent respectively.[49]

Only now was Alice ready to begin her career at medical school. Her parents had given her the opportunity to prove herself and the money to sustain her while she was a student, but this had been achieved only after much thought, discussion, negotiation and application. The more ephemeral aspects of her family's contribution to her eventual professional success are discernible in the first primary evidence that comes from Alice herself, a letter written to a friend in 1933, her first year in Dunedin. In it Alice moves from a personal tragedy, the sudden deaths of close relatives of two fellow students which had recalled Warwick's death, to question the larger scheme of things, and her place within it.

> ... the knowledge that I crave most of all is the knowledge of human nature, that I may understand and help other people.
>
> I wish I could satisfy myself as to the meaning of things. I cling to an unreasoned conviction that life is not chaos but order, but I'm absolutely unable to place the pieces in the pattern....
>
> And yet there is happiness in the world, & beauty that I am sure was meant to be enjoyed. I got a little parcel from home yesterday, it contained a bracelet & necklet of pearls and filigree silver, a beautiful thing ... is it wrong to love pretty things like that? I know many people have not enough to eat & yet I can accept something that is entirely for adornment, & yet I don't think I could bring myself to sell those useless things and give the money to the poor, or perhaps I could if I thought it was really required of me .... I wish I could be sure within myself what is right & what is wrong ....
>
> I wonder if I'm really living yet, or is it just a negative sort of existence, avoiding mostly the things that are wrong but not actively setting out to do the things that are right?

Alice described the contents of this letter as 'the thoughts that make up my life almost as much as my actions do'. By its conclusion its contents had become so intimate and important to her that she turned the last sheet of notepaper on its side and wrote: 'My dear Mother & Daddy, This is a letter that I started to Meg, but I decided to send it to you instead. Please don't laugh at it. With all my love, Alice.'[50]

Alice's letter is redolent of the soul-searching and self-examination associated with Nonconformism. Although she was now formally an Anglican, it was the older family values that continued to dominate her thinking. The fact that only 6 per cent of practitioners registering in the 1930s came from Methodist families makes this a significant source,[51] apart from her gender, of Alice's future 'difference' within her profession. The joy and fulfilment she could find in applying herself to her work were to prove important to Alice's career, but it is the final sentence, linking 'really living' with 'actively setting out to do the things that are right', which was to prove most significant, the foundation of a life based on the belief that thoughts and theories were valueless unless acted upon. Alice, writing on the eve of her 19th birthday, considered herself 'still only a child'. In fact she was now a young woman, stepping into a world beyond the family, although at Otago Medical School she would find little that would challenge her conservative values.

Numbers at the school had been increasing following a recession in the late 1920s, and during most of Alice's years there it was the largest faculty in the university.[52] Although its members served on the student executive and took part in major university occasions such as the capping carnival, concerts and amateur dramatics, they formed a discrete group within the larger community. Their separateness was partly physical. They spent most of their time in the medical school buildings and the hospital, located two blocks from the main campus, only occasionally sharing classes with students from other professional schools.[53] But they were also bonded by a sense of professional destiny. A contemporary recalled,

> I think most of the people who became medical students had a sense of vocation, saw themselves as budding doctors. Doctors were accorded a special place in society, and they felt they had to live up to it. I think it was as simple as that.[54]

In their formal class photographs the male students stand, suited and tied, barely distinguishable from the teaching staff. The impression is one of confident conservatism. Only those few with links to the Student Christian Movement, where more radical views were exchanged, would became actively concerned with such major issues of the 1930s as pacifism, unemployment and alternative economic and political theories, even at an intellectual level.[55] For most, the Depression simply fuelled personal ambition, providing an impetus to work harder because an extra year could make the difference between a medical career or ending up 'back on the farm or somewhere'.[56]

Alice appears to have had no links with the Student Christian Movement and nor was she immediately exposed to the alternative viewpoints that life in a student hostel might have provided. She began her student years boarding with a maternal aunt who was married to Richard Lawson, the university's professor of education. The household, which also included the Lawsons' daughter Ida, an arts student, and Ida's cousin Tom, studying dentistry, was sometimes light-heartedly referred to as 'Lawson's College', but for Alice it was very close to living in her own home. She was a conscientious and successful student who would climb the stairs in the evenings to study in her room, armed with a hot-water bottle and thick socks to stave off the cold, which she felt acutely.[57] To her medical school contemporaries she seemed pleasant, intelligent, poised in social situations and unprovokingly conservative in her views.[58] Some were struck by the attractive air of 'keenness'[59] that she demonstrated in her 1933 letter.

> I have 'Varsity for at least another four years after this one. I sometimes get terribly impatient to think it must be so long before I even start, but I love the work, though it's pretty stiff at times, & if all the years fly by as the last 2 have done the end will come almost too soon. I went to the Medical Ball with Tony the other night & he was envying someone who was nearly through. I said I was glad to be at the beginning rather than at the end, but that was only half true, I'm longing to be at the end, but I'm determined to enjoy the intermediate stages to the full.[60]

Class photographs suggest that, like most young women between the ages of 18 and 22, Alice gained a measure of personal confidence during her Dunedin days, gradually relaxing an early, serious, persona and allowing her essentially warm nature to emerge. In 1934 she looks a regular blue-stocking, hair in a bun, dressed in a severe grey suit complete with shirt and tie. In contrast, the only other two women students wear soft dresses. By 1936 Alice is more in tune with them, wearing a dressy suit in a light-coloured fabric with a blouse featuring large pearl buttons and a decorative trim. She was also more engaged in the social life of the university, living in St Margaret's Hostel, and fulfilling the roles of Lady Vice-president of the Students' Association and Chairman of the Women Students' Club. She had already been secretary of both the Women Students' Club and the Medical Debating Society.[61]

Three other women, Nan Berry, Margaret Jackson and Beatrice Nelson, completed the medical course with Alice that year, in a class of over 60 men. Since almost all the staff were also men,[62] it was hardly surprising that articles in the *Digest*, the medical school magazine, constantly referred to practitioners and students of the medical profession in masculine terms. Apart from an article by Arthur Porritt on Soviet Russia (where 'medicine . . . is at present as a science at a very low ebb'), which referred to women doctors as comprising 65 to 75 per cent of that country's low-paid, low-status practitioners, women featured as patients or frazzled students in need of Ovaltine 'to nourish and build up the nerves'.[63] Their presence loomed largest in the occasional gossip columns, which reported engagements and marriages of graduates in appropriate literary style under such headings as 'Behold we Libel' and 'Heart Shots'.[64] Clearly, this was a man's world into which women would just have to fit. Male classmates initially accorded them a polite tolerance which, by graduation, warmed into respect, even affectionate camaraderie. Their shared experience did not remove the men's assumptions of gender difference, but it did reduce them in comparison with attitudes to women from other faculties. A male contemporary recalled

> a very wholesome and warm friendship and comradeship, in all the trials and experiences we went through together.
>
> When it seemed they might appreciate support, in potentially embarrassing situations, I can recall very few instances of their being left in the lurch; and the rare occasions where a lecturer or examiner was insensitive in his approach aroused marked resentment. . . .
>
> Women students of other faculties were seen as women first and students afterwards, I think.[65]

On a practical level, however, the university experience for a woman in medicine was rather more particular than this recollection might suggest.

In lectures the women in Alice's year habitually sat together at the front bench, a practice that may have reached the status of a convention, since Eleanor Baker recalled doing the same thing at the turn of the century.[66] As was usual at the time, they had their own common room where they could take a tea tray collected from the canteen attached to the men's common room. Most mornings they preferred to cross the street to a corner shop, where they could buy a snack.[67] In the dissecting room the women shared a table at the direction of the lecturer,[68] a move that may have been seen as sensitive in view of the undoubted trauma both men and women experienced when introduced to that initially unnerving experience. Senior staff occasionally entertained small groups of male students to dinner at their club. Since women were barred from such establishments, alternative functions in staff homes or in hotel dining rooms were arranged for female students. Women did not attend the annual medical students' dinner, where it was generally accepted the men wanted to 'let their hair down'.[69] Because many of these arrangements directly reflected accepted social relations between the sexes, Alice had no problem accommodating both her femininity and her medical training.

> . . . in the medical school as far as classes were concerned & in the matter of viewing demonstrations we were all on equal footing, we were seldom given privileges as regards getting a good view, & we preferred taking our luck with the rest, it was nevertheless very pleasing to have a door held open for us & to receive similar small attentions, also in hospital I never expected the men to do my work for me, tho' occasionally they did without consulting me, & yet in many ways they treated me well, they never swore at me though they did to a marked degree at each other. I never felt any lack of consideration & neither do I think they considered me a nuisance.[70]

Nevertheless, there were times when Alice and her friends felt they would rather have been treated as medical students than as women. When, during their fourth year, the class was arranged into teams for ward work, the four women, without consultation, were placed as a group within one 'clinic'. They would have preferred to have been placed in pairs in two clinics, to obtain a wider sample of cases that they could then discuss with one another. But their request was denied.[71] A further incident was rather more personal to Alice. At the end of 1934 she had passed her first professional examination with distinction. She had done particularly well in anatomy, with a mark of 85 per cent, and was the only woman to have passed the primary examination for fellowship of the Royal College of Surgeons, when it had been held for the first time in New Zealand in December 1934. In recognition of her achievement, Alice received the Scott Medal, traditionally awarded 'to the student who is judged by the Professor to have the best knowledge of Human Anatomy ... [taking] into consideration the records of the students in class examinations, practical work, and in the First Professional Examination'.[72] Nan Berry believed that, because of her success, Alice should also have been offered an appointment as a graduate demonstrator in anatomy on completion of her degree, but that she was taken aside by Professor W.P. Gowland, head of the Anatomy Department and a man with great personal respect for her, and told that the appointment would go to a man. Whether this was policy is impossible to establish since no records exist from Professor Gowland's time.[73] Women students had an edge over their male peers in only one training area: they were permitted to attend births at Red Roofs, the Salvation Army hospital for unmarried mothers, while the men were not. Women students were thus saved the necessity of having to come to some arrangement with hospitals in their home regions for at least part of their vacation between the fifth and sixth years in order to obtain their required 20 cases. This was considered quite an advantage, even though attendance at Red Roofs necessitated transportation by taxi, an expensive business.[74]

In November 1936, Alice passed the first section of her third professional examination. For the sixth year of their medical education the class would be distributed among the four main centre hospitals. Although they would return in November 1937 to sit the second section of their finals, the Dunedin student days were over. An impressive academic record, the recollections of fellow students and her later attitudes suggest that Alice felt happy and confident in the medical school environment. The combination of a committed intelligence, good health, an equable temperament, a firmly established work ethic and a secure and supportive family background had left her well placed to respond to the demands of the student experience. Any setbacks she may have suffered had been comparatively minor and were mostly shared with her female contemporaries. Their experience may have been that of a minority, but it was never one of individual isolation. At the end of their student days they exchanged photographs taken particularly for the purpose.[75] Now, on the brink of returning home and actively practising medicine, Alice's outlook seemed bright, but she was soon to discover that for a woman to enter medical practice on an equal footing with men posed more problems than getting a professional education.[76]

CHAPTER 2

Work and War

> *I'm beginning to get the hang of things and I think perhaps I might manage.*[1]

Alice's sixth student year at Auckland Hospital included ward work, operating theatre sessions, short courses of instruction and individual assessment by senior staff. When the medical superintendent, Dr J.W. Craven, referred to her in November 1937 as 'probably the most brilliant student the hospital had this year',[2] he was confirming that she fitted comfortably, and very competently, into the professional world. Yet it was only when a meeting of the Auckland Hospital Board virtually ordered him to employ her,[3] that Alice was taken on the staff as a junior resident medical officer (JRMO) or house surgeon the following year. Nor was she alone in this predicament. None of the women in her class had obtained a conditional appointment by the time they returned to Dunedin to sit their finals, although all performed well academically. Margaret Jackson and Nan Berry were placed in the top half of their class, and Alice was in the top tenth.[4] Because, in 1937, resident experience was not essential for full registration, they could have moved directly into an area of medical practice for which there was little competition. For women this usually meant employment with the Health Department, since they found it difficult to raise the capital to finance even a struggling private practice. But such positions offered only low pay and status and carried few prospects of advancement. Like their male colleagues, the women graduates of 1937 regarded resident appointments as being of considerable professional value and consequence. For this reason, competition for the posts was keen, especially in main centre hospitals.[5] Frustrated, the women complained to the dean of the Medical School, who was 'sympathetic in a mild sort of way', suggesting that when all the men had been fitted in there would 'probably' be some jobs left for them. Finally, Margaret Jackson went to Dunedin, Beatrice to Palmerston North and Nan to Greymouth, while Alice 'got into Auckland after a struggle'.[6] That struggle centred not on professional competence but on accommodation.

Despite the customary provision of a residence especially for house surgeons, accommodation for women doctors was a perennial problem because contemporary opinion could not countenance the idea of unmarried men and women living under the same roof. The issue did not arise until after graduation. Sixth year students were automatically placed in the main centre hospital nearest their own home, where they lived unless, as sometimes happened, they covered for a house surgeon for a short time. Since Nan Berry was the only resident at Greymouth the problem did not arise for her. In Dunedin Margaret Jackson was provided with a small flat near the hospital. Beatrice Nelson's living arrangements in Palmerston North are unknown, but women doctors were often accommodated in nurses' homes and this may have provided a solution for her. In Alice's case, both the doctors' residence and the nurses' home were full,[7] so she 'lived out' at Denestone, fortunately close to the hospital, during her resident year. This was so unusual and against the clear intention of 'residency' that, 50 years later, male contemporaries found it hard to believe.[8] They could shed no light on the episode, which seems to have been a non-event for them.[9] Nor is there any official evidence to explain this obvious compromise. A request from the Auckland branch of the Medical Women's Association that the hospital board should provide accommodation for women residents in any future rebuilding scheme can hardly provide the key.[10] Alice has left no personal record of these events and younger family members can recall only that there was a 'problem'. The most likely explanation is that, yet again, Alice received crucial parental support. Joseph Stanton certainly had sufficient influence and connections within local government circles and he took great pride in Alice's achievements;

he would have found it galling for her career to be checked in this way.

The underlying reasons for the 'problem' are easier to identify. While Alice's champions on the board, Dr E.B. Gunson and Mrs Mary Dreaver, argued that women doctors should have the same right of access to public hospital training as did men,[11] and while the board bickered with the hospital's medical superintendent about who had the authority to appoint staff,[12] this wrangle was really about the way the social role of men and women affected their career opportunities. The women of this year found it difficult to get resident positions because they were part of a large class and men were given priority, firstly because staff facilities were designed around the expectation that medical personnel would be male, and secondly, because of wider cultural assumptions that men were potential breadwinners and therefore were more in need of career advantages. Men had been given priority for resident medical officer (RMO) appointments at Auckland Hospital since the early 1900s and shortage of accommodation was still being used as a reason as late as 1947.[13] 'Living out' had also been permitted for two women residents in 1934, although their circumstances seem to have been slightly different since they, unlike Alice, did not request a boarding allowance of 30 shillings a week.[14] The situation was ultimately remedied, not because of women doctors' complaints but because the 1950 Medical Practitioners' Act made a year's resident experience mandatory before full registration was granted.[15] Hospital boards were then obliged to provide accommodation for women doctors. This was not the case in 1937, when Auckland Hospital was left with two medical men, whom it had no apparent problem in accommodating but some difficulty in finding a situation,[16] and Alice, whom it could not accommodate but whom it felt obliged, after some pressure, to situate. It was a sobering introduction to medical practice.

Despite the difficulties over her appointment, Alice clearly valued her experiences as a resident since, in 1939, she successfully applied for a senior RMO post at New Plymouth Hospital. The year proved a happy one. There was no problem with accommodation – she was given a modest flat in the nurses' home – and the hospital had a good reputation within the profession.[17] Now 25, Alice had blossomed professionally and personally and enjoyed life in its widest sense, expending vast amounts of energy on both work, which could stretch into 12- and 14-hour days, and recreation. Although she retained strong emotional links to her family, she was, for the first time, living as a self-reliant adult. Her description of a November weekend in 1939 demonstrates the love of simple pleasures, companionship and the driving need to be active that were to remain important facets of her mature personality. After work until midday Saturday she relaxed in the sun, knitting, before going swimming at Oakura with friends. After enjoying sandwiches, a glass of beer and a smoke, she chopped firewood before returning to New Plymouth. The party then went to the Alpine Club dance, leaving at midnight for Mount Egmont (now Taranaki), which they climbed until 3 a.m. After spending the rest of the night in a hut, they set out for the summit the following morning. On returning to New Plymouth, they added a final flourish by climbing to the top of a local landmark, Paritutu, to see the sunset. This was what Alice called 'a thoroughly good time'.[18] Nineteen thirty-nine was also the year when external influences would begin to provide unusual opportunities for her to expand her professional horizons.

At New Plymouth Alice took her meals in the residence where, as the year went by, the dining room wall was being used to display a map on which small flags marked the progress of approaching war.[19] For medical men the call of duty was clear. From 1940 to 1945 the medical students' magazine, *Digest*, recorded 430 graduates serving overseas, with 20 confirmed deaths.[20] Every aspect of Alice's personality inclined her towards active participation in the war effort. She not only shared most New Zealanders' emotional ties to Britain but believed strongly in the moral legitimacy of the struggle against Fascism. Towards the end of the year she wrote,

> ... this I do feel definitely, Britain is now pledged to this war, if she withdraws now she must lose any spiritual values which she may possess. If she is defeated, which seems an impossibility, but really isn't, then you and I must take the consequences ... That is why I think that the responsibility lies with each of us to do our bit.[21]

In the ordinary course of events, this was the time when an ambitious young doctor would be thinking of obtaining overseas experience. Margaret Jackson had already left for Australia in 1938, and Nan Berry did the same at the end of 1939. Alice remained in New Zealand. Although she did not make this decision with the idea of furthering her medical career, it placed her in a very advantageous position professionally. Trained medical personnel were at a premium to replace the large numbers of medical men joining up. Refugee doctors from Europe were unacceptable to the local profession:[22] their academic standards, cultural mores and politics were all suspect.[23] New Zealand's women doctors suddenly found themselves in demand. Towards the end of 1939 Alice began negotiations with Dr Edward Sayers, a popular general physician in Auckland, to act as his locum for the duration of the war.

Just who initiated this arrangement is unknown. Sayers later recalled, a little hazily by his own admission, that Alice had approached him, offering to try running his practice 'as a war service, seeing she could not go herself'.[24] Their only previous contact appears to have been during Alice's sixth year of study at Auckland Hospital in 1937 and her residency the following year. She apparently made a favourable impression, though, as a married man with a growing family, Sayers must have been under some pressure to maintain his practice during his absence overseas. They reached a definite arrangement early in 1940 and Alice left New Plymouth Hospital on 4 February.[25] She took a short holiday, which included a visit to the Centennial Exhibition in Wellington, and arrived back in Auckland eight days later. Over the following fortnight Edward Sayers familiarised her with the practice and they drew up an agreement by which Alice would take the first £400 of the profits after all expenses had been paid. Any income over that amount would be divided: one-third would go to Alice and two-thirds to Sayers. If profits reached £1,600, the proportions would be altered to half each. Alice was bound 'for the duration of the war, or rather until he [Sayers] comes back'. In the event of Sayers not returning Alice would have the option of buying his equipment and carrying on under the same arrangement for two years, when the practice would become hers entirely.[26] Only under these peculiar wartime circumstances could a virtually untried woman doctor have entered a successful private practice under such advantageous terms.

In this venture Alice once again received valuable family support. Her father acted as her legal representative and accompanied her to meetings where details of the locum were discussed.[27] She continued to live at home and so was relieved of the primary responsibility of running a household, though this domestic advantage would be undermined by her mother's increasingly frequent bouts of ill health. Nevertheless it was a period of great personal tension for Alice, a time when she was unsure 'how much of life is real and how much my own imagining'. In typical fashion she reached back to the yardstick of the old Protestant values to measure her new situation. It was not reassuring. 'It doesn't seem right that a golden opportunity like the present should really be real,' she confessed. 'I have done nothing to merit it'.[28] On the eve of taking over the practice, however, she addressed her situation straightforwardly:

> ... next week I shall have to stand on my own feet. I have very mixed feelings, but oh! I'm going to try hard ... you've got to look after your patients first and if there's any time left, then it should be devoted to keeping you fit to deal with your patients. That is the philosophy which I am adopting ...[29]

Private practice opened the doors to a new, risky, medical world but war made it easier to face the reality that this was not a sacrificial public service, although doctors liked to present their work in this light, but a business venture which needed to make a profit so that its owner might live, preferably at a higher than usual standard.[30] Even women doctors, who were supposed to be further above the venal considerations of commercial life than their male peers, could virtuously exercise business talents when they were protecting the financial interests of serving soldiers. As Alice put it herself, 'I have been much happier earning my £1,000 a year because I know that I'm doing a good thing for Dr Sayers.'[31] Nevertheless it was still a struggle. Perhaps in reaction to the shock of finding a young woman rather than an older man behind the doctor's desk, patients were occasionally so thin on the ground during the early months of 1940 that Alice feared the collapse of what had been a thriving concern. She was more than relieved when, two weeks after she began work, a new patient arrived at the rooms, and thrilled when a woman she had treated in hospital came particularly to consult her.[32] She worried when patients did not progress or questioned her diagnosis and found the business side of running the practice tedious. To boost her income, she made herself available to do anaesthetics and, in her spare time, attempted to keep up with professional journals. These strains were tempered by the obvious shortage of medical manpower in the city, which brought the sense, important for Alice, that individual effort really counted. She found the 'personal element' of general practice satisfying and at this stage preferred it to the thought of specialising.[33] As needs dictated, however, and her confidence grew, she began to extend her horizons. The origins of all her later professional concerns and activities are to be found in the war years, and among the earliest was the treatment of allergies.

When Alice took over his practice, Sayers was treating asthmatic patients for allergies. This was a new field for her. The topic was not taught at medical school in relation to clinical medicine but only as an aspect of bacteriology.[34] Sayers had become interested because he had an asthmatic daughter.[35] Determined to conserve his practice to the best of her ability, Alice immediately began to read on the subject. She sought the advice of Douglas Whillans, a hospital laboratory technician who had assisted Sayers privately with the preparation of solutions, yeasts and moulds for diagnostic purposes, and discussed pollens with Lucy Cranwell, a botanist at the Auckland War Memorial Museum.[36] Patients' allergic symptoms were relieved with various drugs, sulphonamides used for bacterial infection and the topical application of tar and mercury for eczema. The allergies themselves were treated by diet and programmes of desensitising injections, using extracts that Alice prepared at the rooms. At dawn on the slopes of Mount Eden, she collected grass pollens to be used in this way, and patients brought her the contents of their vacuum cleaners for the preparation of house dust extracts.

Alice later recalled this programme as very effective.[37] Her patients and the local medical fraternity must have agreed because she began to be regarded as an expert in this field. By 1944 she was presenting papers on allergies to her medical peers and the Registered Nurses Association,[38] and attempting to relieve the pressure of work in her practice by employing an assistant to make the extracts and do laboratory testing.[39] When Sayers returned at the end of the year they agreed that she should charge the same specialist fee as he did for such consultations, though she continued to ask for the usual general practice fee from her other patients.[40] The acquisition of specialised knowledge was a bonus for Alice in both professional and financial terms. It arose partly out of her own drive for professional excellence and partly because she entered the right practice at a time when it was still possible to achieve specialist status in some areas through experience and skill, rather than formal qualification. But this era was rapidly coming to an end and a further inheritance from Sayers which provided the foundations of her major specialty, paediatrics, could not take her so far.

When Alice became Sayers's locum she also took up his appointment as a visiting physician to the Plunket Society's Karitane Hospital at Mount Albert, beginning an association that would last until her death.[41] In the early 1940s Karitane hospitals specialised in the care of 'premature' babies (weighing less than 5 pounds or 2.26 kilograms) and those with feeding problems. Mothers were occasionally also admitted to be schooled in the nurture of these struggling infants. The sustenance of prematures involved the most basic technology: hot-water bottles and light bulbs covered with wet muslin to maintain humidity. Still, babies over 3 pounds (1.36 kilograms) usually survived.[42] Alice attended the hospital at least once a week, examining new admissions and advising the nursing staff on their treatment. She also counselled mothers and lectured Karitane nurses training at the hospital.[43] It was a valuable opportunity for a new practitioner and a future paediatrician, giving Alice regular contact with worried mothers and trainee children's nurses and establishing her in their eyes as an authority on child health. It also brought her into regular touch with other visiting doctors, including Dr Basil Quin, who became a lifelong friend and eventually a mentor, nominating her in 1970 for a fellowship of the Royal College of Physicians.

Not all these doctors were men. At Karitane Alice met Dr Helen Deem, the Plunket Society's medical director. A forceful widow, Deem had been the first holder of the Lady King Scholarship and the person responsible, over the 1930s, for revising Sir Frederic Truby King's dietary dogmas into a form more acceptable to the medical profession.[44] Alice also mixed socially with women doctors, including Margaret Thompson, Elizabeth Nannestad, Phyllis Moir and Elizabeth Cole. Their professional involvement varied, usually as a response to their domestic commitments, and Alice remarked, without comment, that some were not practising at all.[45] One woman doctor in particular showed that this need not be the case. Almost as soon as she took over Sayers's practice, Alice lunched with Dr Elizabeth (sometimes known as 'Kate' or 'Katey') Hughes,[46] a woman in her early 40s, of wide professional experience and active in Auckland medical circles. Hughes was assistant to Dr S.L. (Sammy)

Ludbrook in the children's wards at Auckland Hospital and wartime locum for Dr J.E. Caughey, a consultant physician. She had been married since 1925, the year after her graduation, and had two sons.

Although Elizabeth Hughes provides the most obvious professional model for Alice from the perspective of combining marriage, motherhood and a medical career, their personalities were dissimilar. She was described on her death as a 'shy retiring person, whose true worth was hardly recognised by more than a handful of people until towards the end of her life'. She found academic examinations difficult and never attempted formal postgraduate qualifications. None of this would apply to Alice, and there is no evidence that they formed an intimate and enduring friendship. Nevertheless, Elizabeth Hughes was one of the few women during Alice's lifetime to hold a senior hospital appointment.[47] She was also already involved in almost every new venture on which Alice would embark in the early 1940s. Both sought to enhance the role of women in the profession through the revival, in July 1943, of the Auckland branch of the New Zealand Medical Women's Association (NZMWA) which had lapsed over the early war years. During its previous, brief, existence in the 1930s, meetings had been occasional and informal. The new group decided on a more organised programme, with regular quarterly meetings at which members would present short papers, followed by discussion and supper. Topics ranged from heart disease, tuberculosis, anaesthesia and the immunisation of children, to menstrual disorders and the possible incidence of infections and discharges in women using internal sanitary protection. Alice took her turn as hostess, presented her first paper on the anaesthetic technique, 'Intravenous Pentothal',[48] and at the end of 1944, when Elizabeth Hughes became the group's president, acted as secretary.[49]

It is hardly surprising that Alice valued this contact with her fellow women doctors since, even within the context of war, she continued to experience professional frustrations that were purely gender based. At a meeting called to inform the local medical fraternity of their place in the Emergency Precautions Scheme, she was furious to discover that the proposed structure allowed her 'no niche at all'.[50] She became involved in 'active' service only with the development of an unofficial voluntary Women's National Service Corps (WNSC) in the city and this 'posting' came about through personal, rather than professional or official, contacts. The corps, which numbered among its officers Phyllis Boult, had been organised by Dorothy Hawkins, who had been an administrator in the women's division of the Royal Air Force in Britain during the First World War and, more recently, had become games mistress at Hill Top School. This was undoubtedly the channel whereby Alice became corps medical officer, giving recruits routine physicals. She also lectured members on aspects of health, including sex education. When she introduced the topic of venereal disease, many corps members were profoundly shocked.[51] It is tempting to see Alice as standing on contentious, even radical ground, but she was no Ettie Rout. Venereal disease had become a homefront problem that could not be ignored because, with the setting up of camps for United States forces involved in the Pacific campaign, New Zealand for the first time acted as a base for large numbers of troops on active service. As the rates of infection rose, official backing was given to various measures aimed to educate the public of its dangers.[52]

Alice's involvement was apparently unofficial. It seems to have been only her links with Dorothy Hawkins and the WNSC that led to the continuation of her lectures to Auckland servicewomen, both at Papakura Camp and at the Young Women's Christian Association (YWCA), after the corps had been formally integrated into the regular armed forces.[53] For her trouble she was to receive an unsought but valuable professional bonus. In 1943 Elsie Bennett, the YWCA's innovative and energetic wartime secretary, suggested that Alice should consider putting her talks into booklet form for wider distribution. Alice did not enter into this arrangement lightly. Although she favoured a more open approach to sexual matters,[54] it was one thing to address a private meeting but quite another to have your words circulated in print under your own name. She was only just gaining the confidence to begin challenging the conservative boundaries of her past, and had reservations about releasing a text that she considered 'pretty bold in many places'.[55] Her conflict is revealed in *Personal Relationships*, which was published in 1944 and directed specifically to young women in wartime. The sections describing biological reproduction, the physiology of human sexual organs and sexual intercourse, and the causes and symptoms of venereal diseases, are precise, clearly articulated, serious but not panicky, admirably constructed to fulfil Alice's aim 'to give straightforwardly the main facts of sex relationships, leaving to each reader the responsibility of making her own rules'. But, the foreword and a closing passage entitled 'Fundamentals' provided definite indications as to how such decisions ought to be made, and these were clearly in tune with established middle class sexual ideology.

Alice warned women of the dangers of promiscuity and left no doubt that she disapproved of allowing free range to the human 'sexual instinct'. For her, the proper place for sex was within marriage and she justified the postponement of immediate sexual gratification with the promise of richer future fulfilment. She stressed both women's particular responsibility in maintaining sexual decorum, particularly during the stress of war, and the importance to the nation of happy family life. She resorted to old Methodist principles by taking 'individual responsibility' as her theme and arguing that 'the future of our civilisation is bound up as much with the lives of individuals as with the movement of masses', making it possible to lose 'by decay from within all that our men are now fighting to protect from attack'. Even her suggestion that a woman had the right to demand medical proof of her husband's freedom from sexually transmitted diseases before marriage was an echo of the 19th-century feminist 'social purity' movement.[56]

Alice's great strength, however, even at this stage in her career, was that she was realist enough to recognise that her ideal sentiments did not have the same appeal for all women, that some did have sexual encounters before marriage and that this needed to be taken into account. She proposed that a woman, too, should submit to medical tests if she had had intercourse with a man who might possibly have venereal disease, 'for the sake of her children'. She also acknowledged that, even in the early 1940s, not all women shared the same aims, pointing out that 'reasoned and conscious control of the sex instinct is as necessary for the girl who would aim at a successful business career as for the girl who looks forward to the joys of bringing up a family'. She managed to balance conservatism and realism in just the right proportions to satisfy concerned officialdom. After consultation with the Health Department, 20,000 copies of the booklet were printed.[57] Excerpts were also featured in the *Mirror* magazine,[58] and probably provided the basis of a 1945 article, 'Sex and Instinct', which appeared under Alice's name in an untraced journal put out by the Auckland Young People's Club.[59] The whole exercise bolstered her confidence. In December 1944 she wrote, 'My book is off the press, – pamphlet really, but I like to call it a book. I'm quite proud of it. A forward [*sic*] by the Minister of Health, & Govt. have ordered 20,000 copies. I'm not sure what they're going to do with them.'[60]

Although sex education was a traditional role for women doctors, it is unlikely that Alice's work would have made the same impact in normal circumstances. Until the 1960s only social crises brought discussions of sexuality into the public domain. War conditions had placed her under the spotlight and they were also making her unusually visible within professional circles. Because there were fewer young men about, keen and competent medical women like Alice were more likely to be noticed by their seniors, and to receive essential personal patronage and opportunities to participate more fully in their profession. By 1944, she had become involved in the debate surrounding 'socialised medicine'.

Until the 1930s doctors had largely avoided political confrontations with the government because state involvement in health services had been limited and based on participatory criteria of which middle class professionals approved. This apolitical stance had become increasingly difficult to maintain since the Labour Party had come to power in 1935 with a flourish of socialist rhetoric and a garnishing of parliamentary representatives with origins in the early, and ideologically extreme, 'Red' Federation of Labour. Concerned that cost raised a barrier to health care and eager to avoid the taint of 'charity', the new government had set about constructing a Social Security Act that contained provisions for a universal 'free' health service to be funded by income-related taxes. In this new scheme, general practice would be organised on a panel system in which doctors would undertake to care for registered patients at a set annual fee paid by the state. The doctors' professional body, the New Zealand Branch of the British Medical Association (NZBMA), argued that this would turn independent professionals into salaried civil servants and interfere with freedom of choice for both doctor and patient. It preferred a subsidy system based on individual consultations and graduated according to the patient's income. A prolonged and bitter debate ensued.

Within the profession, the only open challenge to the NZBMA attitude came from a few specialists based in Auckland. Calling themselves the Medical Study Group, they were led by Douglas Robb, a general surgeon in private practice. His differences with the medical establishment had their origins during the late 1930s when he had attempted, as a recently qualified specialist, to institute reforms at Auckland Hospital. His actions had alienated senior staff and resulted in his exclusion from professionally important hospital appointments. Robb was regarded as a medical radical but his inclinations were essentially meritocratic and liberal. He did not support a system where an impersonal state dictated terms.[61] As he wrote at the time:

> the people have in recent years lost their authority, and become cogs in the great machine of the State. Signs are not wanting in Britain and other parts of the Empire that our ancient robustness, independence, and sense of personal responsibility in life may be weakening. The freedom of personal initiative that is theoretically enjoyed at present is, in actual fact, becoming more and more frustrated in our health services by the contradictions that have grown up with them.[62]

Robb proposed taking advantage of the social and economic disruption caused by the Depression and the outbreak of war to reorganise medical services. He saw salaried medical officers not as state servants but as professionals freed from the need to concern themselves with bread and butter issues and given the time and opportunity to devote themselves wholly to the pursuit and practice of medical knowledge. Suggestions of this kind, along with his open criticisms of the existing situation, brought him into sharp conflict with the conservative medical lobby.

Elizabeth Hughes was also a member of the Medical Study Group, and it was probably at her invitation that in July 1940 Alice, the youngest and by far the least professionally experienced member, became involved. So recently almost thwarted in her own career path, Alice was attracted by Robb's liberal ideas based on progressive individualism and status earned by merit. By 1943, when the group published a small book, *A National Health Service*, she was its secretary. In 1986 the only surviving contributor, Howard Gaudin, recalled that the book's central ideas were '90 per cent Robb's' but it was democratically presented as a group effort, with members listed alphabetically as co-authors. By a stroke of fate Alice's name topped the list, and the book commonly appears in bibliographies under the authorship of 'Bush, Alice, et al.'.

A National Health Service argued for the restructuring of both professional and bureaucratic areas of health care. New Zealand would be divided into regions, each with a Health Board that would co-ordinate all health care in the area and be responsible to a National Health Council. Boards and the council would consist of a combination of elected and appointed members, lay and medical.[63] General practitioners would no longer practise individually but in groups from local medical centres. Each district would have a large base hospital, confined to inpatient care, and departmentalised in recognition of developing medical specialties. All outpatient procedures, including consultations, examinations and investigations, would be carried out in an adjacent building called a polyclinic, which would also provide reading rooms and other educational facilities. Patients would benefit from efficient, accessible health care, while doctors would work shorter hours with regular incomes and more opportunities for study. The existing power of the administrator would be reduced in relation to senior medical staff. Both public and private medical practice would be encouraged, to avoid 'putting all our eggs in one basket'.[64] The whole scheme could be funded within the resources already being raised by social security taxes. Alice fully supported Robb's crusade, and her active participation in his campaign offered a valuable apprenticeship in the tactics of placing issues before professional and public forums. Robb was certainly a model of confidence. 'Douglas is full of ideas of our group sending down a representative to instruct the new Govt. whatever it may be,' Alice wrote.[65] She shared the platform with him at a meeting of the Progressive Book Club, publishers of the book,[66] and, on her own, spoke to women's groups around the city on 'social medicine'.[67]

Through one such engagement, a talk in June 1942 on 'The Clinical Method of Medicine', a proposal that some hoped might include birth control clinics,[68] Alice was drawn into early membership of the New Zealand Family Planning Association (NZFPA). This organisation, committed to improving family life through sex education and increased access to contraceptive advice for women, was already supported by Elizabeth Hughes and Dr Elizabeth Cole. Alice was a willing convert and in August the Auckland branch secretary of the NZFPA informed the national executive in Wellington that she was a recent addition, 'who we think will be excellent', to the branch's referral list.[69] The list, sent to women who wrote complaining that they could find no doctor willing to give them contraceptive advice or to fit the necessary devices, contained 21 doctors nationwide.[70] Since instruction in birth control was not included in undergraduate medical training Alice was no better, but certainly no less, informed on such techniques than any general practitioner in the country. In 1943 her links with the NZFPA were formalised when the organisation's headquarters was transferred to Auckland and she became a member of the national executive.

Association with the Medical Study Group also encouraged Alice's interest in mental health, a field regarded with suspicion by most of the medical fraternity. *A National Health Service* contained an appendix, aptly entitled 'Forgotten Men', dealing with deficiencies in this area. Psychology was not regarded as necessary to undergraduate medical study and psychiatry was a postgraduate qualification, with training available only outside New Zealand. When a Psychiatric Society was formed in Auckland in December 1943 by private practitioners, representatives of mental hospital staff and neuropsychiatrists attached to United States military and naval hospitals in Auckland, Elizabeth Hughes, who had previously held a fulltime appointment with the Mental Hospital Division of the Health Department and currently ran a children's psychological clinic, invited Alice to attend.[71] Further encouragement was provided by Eva Fischmann, a German refugee and Freudian psychoanalyst who had arrived in Auckland in 1939 and established a private psychotherapy practice.[72] In September 1944, after hearing Alice speak, Fischmann sent her a note that demonstrates the appeal of Alice's personality and approach to those, particularly women, standing outside the strictly defined boundaries of the medical world: 'Everytime I hear you talking I am fascinated by your warmhearted & clearsighted appraisal of things – you prove, I think, how important it is that women take an active part in every way of life.'[73]

At this time Alice was so taken with the importance of mental health that she seriously considered becoming a psychiatrist.[74] In future years this would become an increasingly common career choice for medical women, partly because of personal inclination but also because of structural changes introduced to overcome severe understaffing in a medical area that suffered from lack of professional status, even persistent stigma.[75] Although there were no inducements such as flexible working arrangements and incentives to postgraduate training in the 1940s, Alice was acutely aware of the lack of expert personnel at any level. In 1945, when the NZFPA established a

Family Guidance Centre in the city to offer 'help and advice with the wide variety of problems that crop up in personal relationships and in the rearing of a family',[76] she energetically supported the enterprise but despaired of the dearth of trained people to staff it.

> They are hoping to establish a bureau where psychological advice could be dispensed to folks in difficulties over their marriage or their families. A v. sound idea ... but fraught with difficulties, not the least of which is the staffing problem. Mrs Eva Fischmann is the only person available at the moment, I think she'd be v. good, but the amt. of time she can give is limited, & as she herself says there are disadvantages in having the thing run entirely by a foreigner. She really is a v. nice person.[77]

The establishment of the Psychiatric Society was only one aspect of a wider movement in Auckland – the expansion of postgraduate education in the form of two- to three-day seminars centred on particular areas of medical interest. These had been stimulated by the arrival in the city of United States armed forces' medical bases staffed by highly trained personnel familiar with the latest professional developments. Their presence exerted an intellectual attraction that Douglas Robb could not resist. He was instrumental in setting up the Auckland Postgraduate Committee as an organising body while other members of the Medical Study Group were active participants in their own fields. Alice, as a recently qualified doctor, made the most of these new opportunities to extend her knowledge, but she was also expected to contribute. At the first paediatric course in February 1944 she presented a paper on 'Common Allergic Disorders'.[78] The same year she was elected to the executive of the older Auckland Clinical Society, where cases of special interest were presented at evening meetings. During the second half of 1945 she offered two papers, which appeared in the *New Zealand Medical Journal (NZMJ)* the following year, her debut as a contributor to her profession's national publication.[79]

These interests would influence Alice's later life but perhaps the most important aspect of her involvement with the Medical Study Group was its politicising effect: for the first time, she was actively pursuing change within her profession. By 1944 the government had compromised over the medical provisions of its social security scheme to the extent that it had agreed to a fee for service for medical benefits, guaranteeing a payment of 7s 6d for each consultation and allowing doctors to make an additional charge if they wished. Only the mechanics of payment (whether the patient or the doctor should obtain a refund from the government) remained to be settled. When, that same year, the NZBMA produced an interim report on the future of medical services, the members of the Medical Study Group were miffed to find that their book did not appear in the bibliography. Alice complained, 'We are doing our very best to make the [NZ]BMA meetings less of a farce & to encourage the expression of enlightened opinions, instead of resigned acceptance of the plausible arguments of the aged.'[80] Moreover, she was prepared to express her opposition at the NZBMA Auckland branch meeting called to discuss the Planning Committee Report. When the method of payment dominated the debate on general practice, sidelining 'Utopian ideas such as clinic practice', even though a group of Taranaki practitioners was keen to try the idea, Alice was incensed.

> I remarked that it was no more practical to bring the majority of doctors back to collecting fees from the patient instead of from the doctor [sic] than it was to survey a new field & consider a new form of practice which would be a definite advance. There was a bit of desultory discussion & finally Dr Cronin came forward with a motion that certain groups in the proffession [sic] who had a mind to do so, e.g. the N.[ew] P[lymouth]. doctors, should be allowed to give clinic practice a trial. I seconded it. You should have heard the impassioned speeches protesting against this selling of the medical profession to the Govt. . . . & when it went to the meeting our motion was sadly lost. Perhaps I aim too high, or perhaps I'm just incompetent, but I cannot feel that under present conditions I give the best possible service to my patients.[81]

Despite her ardour, Alice still lacked the confidence of experience. She agonised over the consequences of nailing her colours to the mast. Could she continue to speak publicly in favour of clinic practice and remain a member of an association that had 'straight out' condemned it? Should she offer to resign before she was asked to do so? Although she believed such a step would place few practical disadvantages in her way, she had to confess that she was 'ill-suited . . . to be a rebel'. The comparative equanimity of her older and more experienced colleagues emerged when Alice sought the opinion of the NZBMA branch president and fellow study group member, James McMurray Cole, who suggested she let the matter lie and see what happened.[82] Alice's morale must have been considerably bolstered when, shortly after, he asked her to consider nomination for the Auckland branch executive of the NZBMA. Even so, her feelings were mixed.[83] After some thought, she decided not to put her name forward because she thought she would 'make a better fist of it in a few years time'.[84] In fact Alice never took up such an office, but she had learnt a significant lesson: it was possible to challenge the establishment and survive.

The experience was edifying in another sense. In 1940 Alice had decried Labour's medical proposals under the social security scheme as 'a few political leaders ... [dictating] to a whole people just how long they shall work for how much'.[85] Now, in 1944, she was criticising her own professional organisation along much the same lines. For the first time she had seen that a conservative interest group could inhibit the individual freedom she valued so highly. This was to be the foundation of all her later political differences with her profession. By war's end she was already critical of several developments, complaining that doctors had 'for too long shut their eyes to the need for cooperation between medical & other social services', that they did not 'really face up to the responsibility of their privileged position', and that, with recent advances in medical science, 'the good dr. is inclined to become arrogant c. the knowledge that he truly can deal out life or death'.[86] These were all issues that Alice would take up in the future, but in the immediate postwar years she had more pressing concerns. She had become a married woman and a mother.

CHAPTER 3

Marriage

> *I realise that if I gave you up now I would be giving up forever my long cherished hope for my own home & my own family.*[1]

Nothing more clearly defined the difference between men and women doctors than the effect of marriage. The right wife could give a young doctor a great deal of support. She freed him from the day-to-day concerns of the domestic scene, could fill in as receptionist or nurse, represented him in the community and supported him emotionally.[2] For Alice, as for most medical women, marriage was to prove more of a challenge than a career support structure. She seems first to have seriously considered marrying in 1938, but the relationship, which had developed over her student years, broke up. The failure of this first strong emotional bond to someone outside her family was painful for her. She later recalled her feelings at the time.

> At 'Varsity I ... was smothered by a senseless loyalty to a very mediocre person which derived largely from a puritanical feeling that because I'd let him kiss me I must love him forever, & partly from pity. Then he let me down, when he no longer needed me to assuage his own loneliness & homesickness. I swore after that I'd not take into consideration the hurting of a man's feelings, they could damn well look after themselves,

& I turned my back on Puritanism & started out to have a good time. That was when I went to N.P. [New Plymouth] & there I had a taste of what good fun life can be. For the first time in my life I saw myself as an attractive woman and it warmed my heart . . . Maybe I was nearer the truth in my original puritanical outlook on life, but I only know that it stunted my life for over 6 yrs.[3]

Alice's idea of turning her back on Puritanism might be more accurately described as living the life of a mature, 'respectable' single woman in the late 1930s. She smoked quite heavily but drank moderately. When she described herself as a 'pretty chaste woman',[4] she meant that she was romantically unattached. That is until the end of August 1939 when she was introduced to Faulkner Bush, sole-charge teacher at an isolated country school in Moawhango, just north of Taihape.

Alice and Faulkner met at the New Plymouth Hunt Club Ball on a blind date arranged by a local journalist and friend of Faulkner's, who must have had a fair degree of optimism in his make-up for they were not an obvious match. Alice was quiet, controlled, a professional woman from a family whose social standing was impeccable. Faulkner was loud, brash, employed in a job that could only just be considered a profession and came from a family which had seen better days. His father, George Arthur Bush, was one of five sons and two daughters born to Robert Smelt Bush, a resident magistrate, and his wife Eliza, daughter of John Lees Faulkner, an early Tauranga trader.[5] George earned his living at various times as a miner, an assayer and an accountant and served overseas during the Boer and First World Wars.[6] His first marriage ended in divorce and in 1910 he had married Faulkner's mother, Adeline Muriel Dempsey. Their son was born the same year.[7] By the time Faulkner met Alice the family had experienced several reverses. In September 1930, when George was secretary of the Te Aroha Jockey Club, the local Trotting Club, the Agricultural and Pastoral Association and the Terminating Building Society, he committed suicide in a car parked outside a private hospital in the town, leaving a compromising letter that involved one of the nursing staff. The coroner brought in a verdict of suicide while temporarily insane, referring to evidence of 'nerve trouble' since Bush's return from the war.

The tabloid newspaper *Truth* had a field day. Faulkner, who was 20 years old at the time and a student at the Auckland Teachers'

Training College, was deeply affected by his father's death, and the subsequent publicity and legal proceedings. Even after his mother had made a second, happier, marriage to Alfred Hamilton, whom Faulkner affectionately referred to as 'the Step',[8] times remained hard for several years.[9] Unlike Alice, Faulkner had personally experienced the effects of the Depression. For the first two years after qualifying as a teacher he could not get fulltime work. By 1938, when he became sole teacher at Moawhango, he had wrought himself a persona that was an effective carapace against further pain. He was a big man, very fit and fond of sport. In both dress and manner he could affect a carelessness verging on boorishness. He was inclined to direct this sort of behaviour particularly toward those in authority or those whom he felt were socially pretentious. During weekends Faulkner enjoyed the company of other teachers in the district. They converged on Taihape, spending their time at the tennis club, the pub and a local teacher's residence, where they discussed and debated the alternative political and economic ideologies that surfaced during the Depression years. These included the rejection of imperialism, laissez-faire economics, war, the establishment, charity and the banks. They were for anti-colonialism, a reformed monetary system, pacifism and an egalitarian society where the state would provide education, health and welfare services accessible to all. They were not natural allies of trade unions nor did they seek wholesale structural revolution. They believed the problems of production had been largely overcome; only a fairer system of distribution was needed. Although they looked favourably on developments in the Soviet Union and often made use of Marxist language and analysis, very few became Communists, but to traditionalists in 1930s New Zealand they looked very 'Left' indeed.

In a small provincial town like Taihape, this rowdy, argumentative, intellectualising group gained some notoriety, particularly when they supported the pacifism of the new Methodist minister, Les Clements. Faulkner became very close to, almost protective of, Clements who, in turn, discerned a sensitivity in Faulkner that was revealed to very few.[10] It was a friendship that would last a lifetime, though Faulkner was not easy to know. His persona at this time was deliberately elusive. He introduced himself to strangers as 'Warren' Bush, and it was probably an indication of the serious nature of his interest that he told Alice his real name shortly after they first met.[11] Most people seem to have found him something of an enigma. His temperament was mercurial: 'Not for me the placid content of the cud-chewing cow,' he wrote.[12] Conversely, many of his basic values were rigid, including his concepts of behaviour appropriate to women. How could Alice, a product of the establishment and someone who honoured its values, become involved with this man who constantly challenged both? To her he must have seemed a creature apart. Nevertheless they were strongly attracted to one another. Faulkner travelled to New Plymouth on odd occasions when he could get a lift and Alice could arrange some time off, but they kept in touch mainly by telephone and mail. Within this correspondence lies Alice's response to the first real challenge to her established world view and some valuable insights into their relationship.

Alice was immediately attracted to Faulkner because his provocative intelligence, or what she would later describe as 'an appreciation of your brain', appealed to her natural curiosity.[13] She envied his evenings with his teacher friends in Taihape, referring to them as time spent in 'mutual education'. 'I need evenings like that too,' she explained, 'I need someone who can talk about something other than hospital ... your solace has been books ... my comfort has always been people.'[14] Only a few weeks after their first meeting she wrote,

> much as I like an argument just for its own sake, much better do I like to be able to put down just what I think I think & test it against what someone else thinks, & now I have found you it is a golden opportunity ... I find it almost impossible to think coherently to myself, for a long time I have thought practically nothing at all for that very reason, but now I find myself holding long conversations with you, about all sorts of things, great & small, so you see you are clarifying my mind.[15]

It was indicative of the place of women in New Zealand society during the mid 20th century that men seldom entered into intellectual conversations with them.[16] Alice had long enjoyed what she called 'yarns' or 'chats' with older men of an intellectual bent within her own circle, but these were people with family and professional responsibilities whose views were very much in tune with, indeed had nurtured, her own. Faulkner had the time, the emotional inclination and the intellectual curiosity to share in a stimulating discourse that focused on Alice alone. Over the 12 months of their courtship he spent hours writing letters of up to 15 pages and insisting Alice reciprocate, forging lines of communication that were to form the keystone of their relationship. 'I have had 32 letters since Labour Day, 7 weeks,' he wrote proudly on 13 December, 'but I'll wager you have had more.'[17]

If Alice hungered for debate, a banquet of exotic dishes was now laid before her. Faulkner introduced all his current hobbyhorses, redirecting her recreational reading from the lightweight popular novels she usually favoured to works published by the Left Book Club. It seems fair to assume that she had never heard Britain's struggle against Germany articulated in quite the way Faulkner proposed when he wrote to her a little over a month after their first meeting.

> We are fighting, if at all for the protection, perpetuation and prostitution of a lousy system of materialistic Imperialism wh. is altruistically (?) alluded to as "civilisation" or "the path of progress" . . . we are battling to bulwark British bank balances. The side issues of freedom, democracy, etc. are just padding . . . might I suggest you consider our present system as being based on profit & surplus value, all production being for profit.[18]

Alice was conservative but she was also game and certainly did not want to terminate the new-found acquaintance. She started off tentatively,

> Your letters made me feel ashamed and thoroughly ignorant . . . Please bring the Left book . . . I will do my best to read it. I like to study them, though I don't always agree with them. . . . Communism, I fear, I have never studied in any detail . . . but I can't imagine it being practicable, nor is it possible even to experiment in it without establishing a dictatorship, & that seems to me to be a major evil. The two things above all to be striven for are freedom of thought & equality of opportunity, & the first at least must immediately be abandoned with the creation of a dictatorship.
>   . . . if you will prepare for me a short homily on the elements of socialism and the evils of capitalism . . . you will find me a willing, if not a very bright pupil. I didn't realise until I started to think about the subject, just how vague my ideas were.[19]

It was not long before deference was dropped. Alice was too honest to be able to maintain this stance for long. Exchanges sometimes became stormy, as these two strong-minded individuals each drew on their own, very different, experiences to validate their views. Their approaches, too, were different. Alice's viewpoint was never limited to the black and white that tended to constitute Faulkner's spectrum. She was prepared to adopt the role of examiner to his preferred role of propounder and to test her theories so as to proceed to a coherent whole in a way that Faulkner often did not. Under this unflinching spotlight, she began to take a wider range of ideas into account and found that many of the views she had held unquestioningly were open to argument. She confessed, for instance, that while she did not support the redistribution of wealth through income tax, which was to underwrite the benefits provided by the welfare state, this stance conflicted with her views on the limits of free will.

> One question which I can never decide for myself is this, is it right that the workers in a community should support the drones & maintain for them a standard of living as high as their own? To most of the people I know such a question would allow of no argument, but holding as I do the belief that free will, if indeed existing, is extremely limited, then I rather think the answer is yes, at least that should be the logical conclusion, & yet a great part of my makeup is entirely against such things & my natural inclination is to the belief that many things – luxuries and material goods should be always the reward of industry.[20]

Despite Faulkner's assiduous tutoring, Alice's political outlook remained comparatively intact. Her entire cultural background militated against her conversion to 'socialism'. In tune with her class, Alice believed that Labour politicians were at best well-meaning but incapable of practical government. In 1945 after Bill Parry, Minister of Internal Affairs, had met the Medical Study Group she wrote,

> An interesting study of a type of politician, an idealist, for which one must give him credit, especially when one considers that his ideals have survived through a pretty tough time when material things must have been of importance because of the struggle necessary to get them, they were not nurtured by culture & education. . . . If only one could couple his idealism with an intellect capable of longer vision one would have someone worthy to carry the responsibilities of Govt, as it is one feels that his efforts are doomed to failure because he is incapable of initiating

an organisation which is likely to be permanent.... I've always felt that at least some of the labour people had fine ideals, what they lack is the ability to put them into practice & so they have failed the people.[21]

Neither could she conceive of class in its Marxist sense. Her one passion in life, she said, was 'people as individuals'.[22] It was not a group's relationship to sources of economic power, or the conflict of class interests, but class culture that defined the term for her.

I still can't agree that a classless society is a possibility, you must have leaders for the people, and there straight away you have a division into classes, those who lead, and those who follow. Even if you gave everyone the same amount of money ... people would divide themselves into classes by the way they spent it.[23]

To Alice, challenging existing structures seemed unnecessary and she continued to express notions of the mode of political change in a style that would have gladdened the heart of any early 20th-century Protestant prohibitionist. For her 'the fundamental problem [was] not in the method of administration but in the evil of human nature'.[24] 'Would not a change of heart in the people make it possible for an ideal world to materialise under the present system?' she asked Faulkner.[25] The solution she favoured was education in its widest sense. 'There's still only one antidote,' she explained, 'and that is education, in general and in particular, in schools and out of them.'[26] Nevertheless, individuals, especially those who had done well, had a duty to contribute to the greater social good. When she wrote in April 1940, 'I believe that every privilege carries its responsibilities and my responsibilities must be considerable for I count myself as among those who have great privileges. Life has been too good to me not to feel a big debt to be paid back',[27] she was expressing a belief that would underwrite her actions for the rest of her life.

Alice's religious beliefs, too, were tested by Faulkner. Doctrinal discussions revealed areas of uncertainty. Alice already doubted the existence of life after death, though she believed that something 'beyond our comprehension' might live on. She found the doctrine of original sin unsatisfactory because she could not reconcile herself to any known method of bringing about its essential complement, 'the Great Solution'. She confessed she often went to church and did not take Communion because 'I think one should not accept it unless one feels more or less in harmony with the teachings that it symbolises'.[28] Alice seems to have felt that she had missed a revelation.

> I can't quite get my beliefs straightened out. Intellectually I believe that Christ was and is the Son of God, and I am always hoping that some day I will experience a real conviction of the importance of the fact. I've had glimpses of something at times, but I fear that I have never given the requisite amount of time to my search for truth.[29]

It was the application of Christian principles to the organisation of everyday life that really appealed to her. When Faulkner struck a worldly pose, describing Christmas celebrations as 'This barbarous custom of gourmandising just because a baby was born 2000 years ago,'[30] Alice was quick to react.

> Can you really honestly say to yourself that to you there is no significance in the event.... Mankind truly has failed to meet the standard set for him, but to millions of people that event provides the inspiration for all that is good in them & preserves them from the utter despair which must otherwise be the inevitable result of this failure ... looked at in the right way it can be a great inspiration.[31]

New Testament Christianity provided Alice with moral authority for her worldly activities. All her life she had the disconcerting habit, for those who might oppose her, of backing an argument with a biblical quotation. Her supporters spoke of her 'mission' in life,[32] her critics of her 'crusading zeal'.[33] Nor could she ever quite shed the puritanical element within her nature: she was not inclined to austerity but there was always an underlying compulsion that the good things of life must be 'paid' for.

Animated debate over particular points would continue but Alice and Faulkner came to an agreement on one matter. They were discussing marriage. Although they had spent comparatively little time together, the intensity of their correspondence had deepened their emotional and physical need for one another. But there were problems. Alice nurtured a deep desire to marry and have children but she also had to consider her family, to whom she remained close, and Sayers, whose practice she had undertaken to keep running during the war. The situation was compounded by the fact that Faulkner fell short of generally accepted notions of what constituted a 'good' prospective husband. The ideal personified by Marjorie and Joseph still reigned supreme. Husbands were breadwinners, wives stayed at home and had children. Faulkner wished to marry a woman who not only came from a 'better' family, but whose job carried greater rewards and status, and who apparently intended working after she was married. This struck deeply at a man's self-image in the 1940s. Men who, for reasons of lesser financial contribution or status, were perceived not to be 'the head of the house' were ridiculed. Although the demands of war forced some modification of women's roles, these were regarded as temporary aberrations under abnormal conditions. In 1943, *Better Business*, a magazine with predominantly male readership, ran an article on working women which illustrated how bizarrely any permanent change to accepted norms would be regarded: 'In years to come we may glimpse inside the happy home Mother, feet resting on the mantel, pipe between her teeth, engrossed in the daily paper, while father, apron round his waist, takes his turn at cooking the dinner and getting the children to bed.'[34]

It took a very confident man to overcome this kind of raillery and Faulkner was not a confident man. When Alice sent him details of the agreement she had reached with Sayers, Faulkner complained that, by contracting to stay in the practice until Sayers's return, Alice had not considered him. He grumbled that they had agreed that she would work no longer than two years and that 'the work, your dough [money], wh. seems to be going to be fairly substantial, plus your other interests, will take you from me'.[35] Finally he challenged her directly,

> Tell me too how much you are enjoying the work, for it may help to assess my status. Tell me, lady, on your honour, if you had to choose me or the job, wh. would you take? No conditions, just that plain choice. Perhaps you will be angry at this, well, I promise to be patient.[36]

Alice's reply left no room for doubt, revealing not only her deeply ingrained sense of honesty and fair play but also the central place Faulkner now occupied in her emotional life.

> you or the job . . . I can't see the point in making such theoretical decisions, but since you've asked I've tried to be honest. I'd stick to the job, my darling. That's just a plain answer. I have put in no conditions

whatsoever, but am I allowed now to expand a little? In considering this I assume conditions to be just as they are at the moment viz. me entrusted with the practice & being relied on by Dr. Sayers, & you a free agent, needing me only as a luxury. Don't misunderstand me, but you probably will. What I'm trying to explain is this, if you forced such a choice on me now I would consider you were behaving like a spoilt child. If I chose you I would lose both, for I'd be forever regretting my breaking of faith & I know that in the end I would blame you for that. I'd lose the feeling that I value so much, that you bring out the best of me, & I fear my love would die. I realise that if I gave you up now I would be giving up forever my long cherished hope for my own home and my own family. There would never be anyone else but you. I'd spend the rest of my life justifying the choice.[37]

Alice was a woman of her times, and a conservative one at that. She did not see her insistence on continuing with her work as a radical challenge to women's accepted social role. Rather, she argued, she was fulfilling obligations she had incurred both in her personal life and as an advantaged individual in society. Her further attempts to overcome Faulkner's reservations emphasised the mutual benefits to which her income would be directed, the need for her to repay the money she had been lent for her education, the altruistic nature of her calling and her belief that her medical career would not last forever.[38] She had already directly linked the need to succeed in her career to her personal commitment to Faulkner. 'I daren't fail,' she had written to him in mid-February, 'for that would be letting you down as well as myself.'[39] As late as July 1941 she was still suggesting,

When this war is over, as perhaps it may be quite soon, I think perhaps I'll give up the job, or a good deal of it & just be a good wife. Would you mind? It would mean living very quietly without any frills, but one would be able to devote all one's energies to doing one thing well.[40]

But central issues, such as women's customary economic dependence on men, continued to surface even during the war. In June 1940 Alice urged Faulkner not to accept a married man's allowance if he entered the services because 'that allowance is made so that you may support your wife, it's not in recognition of any increased efficiency or value on your part ... well I don't need that support'.[41]

Alice had to contend not only with Faulkner's misgivings about her job but also about her family. He felt overwhelmed by the Stantons' social advantages and their strong and supportive family ties seemed to constitute a clannishness he could not breach. Alice made no secret of her intense family loyalties and the great affection in which she held her parents. Faulkner, gnawed by insecurity, could not accept her assurances that this would not threaten his own position in her life. Alice was more of a stoic than Faulkner. She believed he was the man for her and was prepared to take things as they came. Faulkner did not have the same equable temperament and insecurity brought out the worst in him. At the end of January 1940, when Alice took him to Deep Creek to meet the family for the first time, Faulkner, by his own admission, 'performed dreadfully'. When he spoke to Alice's father about his intentions, he found Joseph 'as always, very courteous and kind, but to put it euphemistically it was clear I would not have been his favourite pick for a son-in-law'. This unnerved Alice considerably and it was a few days before she re-established her equilibrium, intensifying Faulkner's trepidation.[42] For Alice, part of Faulkner's attraction had been his difference and his persistence. Both were now problems. While she struggled to establish herself in Sayers's practice and placate her family, Faulkner pressured her to marry him sooner rather than later.

In February, when Alice travelled by train from Wellington to begin work in Auckland, she broke her journey at Taihape to spend the weekend with Faulkner. Her mother was not happy about this. She would have been even less happy had she known that, during the weekend, Alice and Faulkner took it into their heads to marry immediately. They woke Les Clements in the middle of the night and asked him to perform a ceremony the next day. Clements had to explain that this was not legally possible.[43] Alice returned home a single woman but as the war worsened Faulkner increased the pressure. Towards the end of May, when he was urging her to set a date for their marriage, Alice made it clear that this rush was not to her liking, though she avoided challenging him directly by placing her ideas in the context of advice to a theoretical son.

> It creates a bad impression when a man makes demands on his fiancée, she may accede willingly to them but at the same time she would appreciate recognition that there is no justification for them. After all a

woman gives up very much more of her freedom when she gets married, than a man does, & when she finds it going while she should still be a free agent she certainly can't be blamed for having grave doubts as to what life will be like when she has formally promised to honour and obey.[44]

One area that must have concerned Alice's parents about her relationship with Faulkner was her new-found interest in radical social and political theories. They would have been unaware, as was Alice and even, one suspects, Faulkner himself, of the ephemeral nature of their future son-in-law's leftist leanings. Now and then hints of déclassé origins in his political radicalism emerged. 'My sympathies are all against the Tories – not by birth but by what I am pleased to call reasoning,' he wrote to Alice in late 1939.[45] When he compared his opinions with those held by Alice's father, he did not speak as a member of the lower classes; in fact, his attitudes towards that sector of society were often somewhat patronising.

> Now as to whether it is your father or I who is wrong. I take it he has lived all his life in the really narrow confines of Akd. I, by chance of fate, have lived more with the common man, and it is possible that I may understand more of his problems than the city dweller... On the whole they are as decent people as any other sector of society, less polished and conventional maybe, but fundamentally as good.[46]

It is perhaps helpful to remember at this point that when Alfred Stanton was working as a storeman in Auckland, Robert Smelt Bush was sitting on the magistrate's bench in the same city. If only Faulkner's father had not let the side down. His family's slide down the social scale left Faulkner with a resentment that he never successfully overcame. For this reason Alice could always be assured of her husband's steady support when she took on the establishment. When she was less ready to challenge its values, his attitudes could make life very uncomfortable for her.

The impasse over the implementation of the medical provisions of the Social Security Act became the focus of their opposing political viewpoints. It also provided Faulkner with a neat challenge to Alice's protestations that hers was a socially concerned profession. Their debate makes it quite clear that initially Alice had shared the distaste of most of her fellow professionals for the government's proposed capitation scheme. In April 1940 she echoed the NZBMA's principal arguments when she maintained to Faulkner that three essentials had to be considered in any reorganisation of medical services: maintenance of the competitive aspect, some form of payment by the patient and a 'good standard' of remuneration to the doctor.[47] Although she claimed to be 'a lot more in favour (or should I say tolerant to?) socialism than I used to be,'[48] she saw the proposed system as basically impersonal and levelling. Alice also believed that Sayers's practice, for which she had made herself personally responsible, would be at risk as a hybrid of specialist and general consultation, neither of them large enough to sustain itself as a separate entity. Given her lack of specialist expertise, her only practical recourse would be to nominate herself as a general practitioner under the conditions of the act, thus abandoning the specialist part of the practice and effectively rejecting many of Edward Sayers's patients.[49]

Such opinions summoned up all Faulkner's anti-élitist passions. He reminded Alice of a homily she had recently written for his edification on 'striving', which ran:

> ... don't you honestly think that you feel happier for a little striving? ... the whole tendency of nature is to go forward, that is obvious on any study of botany or biology & to keep in rythm [sic] with nature we must go forward too ... I believe that man finds truest happiness when he has best developed all his possibilities. When I say that happiness comes from striving I don't mean striving to appear better than the next man, I mean striving to be better than one was before, & using real values, not necessarily the superficial values of the world.[50]

With these expressed principles, asked Faulkner, how could she maintain that the competitive element would necessarily be absent from a state medical service 'because you have told me that real striving comes from one's desire to better oneself, irrespective of beating the other fellow'?[51] When he compared her earnings favourably to those of a 'wharfie', Alice was stung. A wharfie's wages were 'all pure profit', she informed Faulkner. 'Besides I reckon that I work a good deal harder than the watersiders that I have seen at work ... I don't think it's possible to make everyone equal. It simply can't be done.' Doctors, she maintained, 'only do like everyone else, they put a price on their services and the public can take it or leave it, there is no compulsion, and there's always good sound medical attention available in the hospitals'. Although she confessed that living on a flat income all her life would not appeal to her, she believed she could,

> But I know a lot of people who are not like that . . . if the complete socialisation of Medical service comes in N.Z. the standard of general practice will fall. . . . Ambition is the greatest stimulus in the world today . . . if you take away ambition you must have something very powerful to put in its place or the world will just go backwards.

Perhaps unnecessarily she added, 'I'm not feeling at all communistic just now.'[52]

But she was feeling liberal and Alice's entry into the activities of the Medical Study Group at this point brought a merciful end to the debate, prompting her to write only three days later, 'I think it's time we stopped squabbling & prepared to back up the Govt. even if we [the medical profession] don't approve of them in peace time. I'll go into a socialised medical service without a murmur if the[y] introduce it . . . I'll keep the practice together, somehow.'[53] Faulkner was pleased and proud of Alice's participation in the Medical Study Group and in the production and publicising of *A National Health Service*. He wrote a long letter (unfortunately lost) giving his 'views on your book', but he assured her he was '100% in agreement c. its general principles my criticisms being concerned c. the administrative side',[54] and was gratified to see an advertisement in the *Standard* presenting it as the work of '8 eminent practitioners'.[55] Despite her involvement, Alice was not unconditionally sold on the idea of a salaried state service. There were times, she confessed, when some of the more onerous jobs required in medical practice were sweetened by the 'contemplation of the extra guineas'. But she allowed that a properly organised and funded service could lighten such tasks with 'improved facilities', as well as mitigating the 'hopelessness' of 'trying to bring health to homes where all the conditions are against it, & trying to struggle on without proper technical aid because the patient can't pay or because the services are not available'.[56] She also began to tire of Robb's habit of introducing his 'hobby horse' at what she considered were inappropriate times, 'ruffling the surface of a beautiful clinical discussion'. 'I must watch for myself,' she added. 'I'd hate to think people would have to blush for me as I blush for

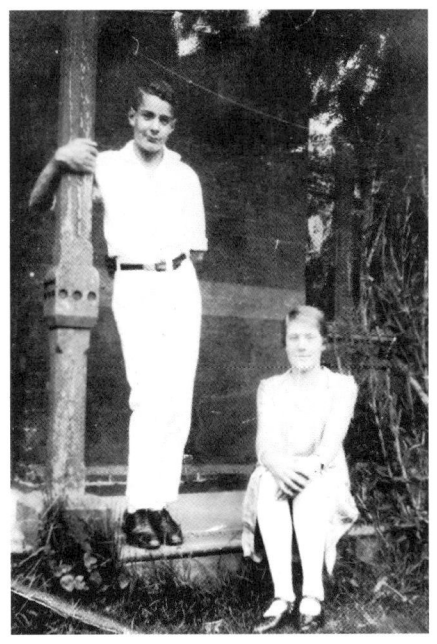 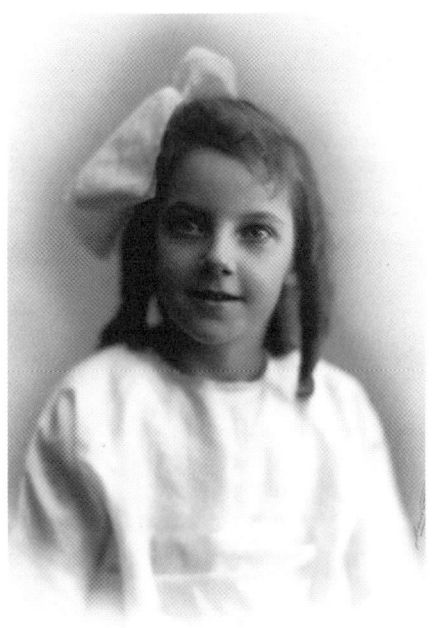

ABOVE LEFT: Alice's parents, Joseph Stanton and Marjorie McMaster, before their marriage. *Patricia Rogers (MC)*

ABOVE RIGHT: Alice, aged five years. *Christine Moorhouse*

BELOW: Marjorie and Joseph in the 1920s. *Patricia Rogers (MC)*

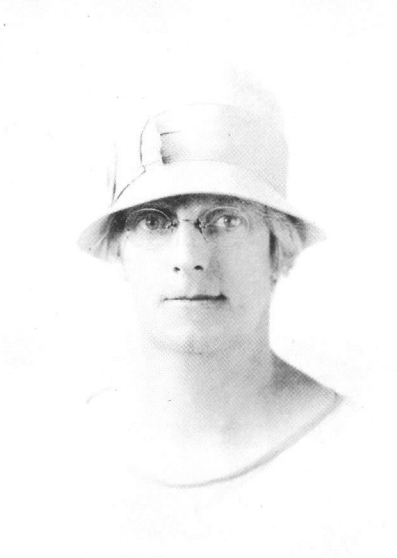 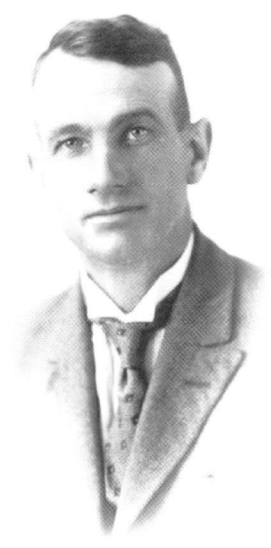

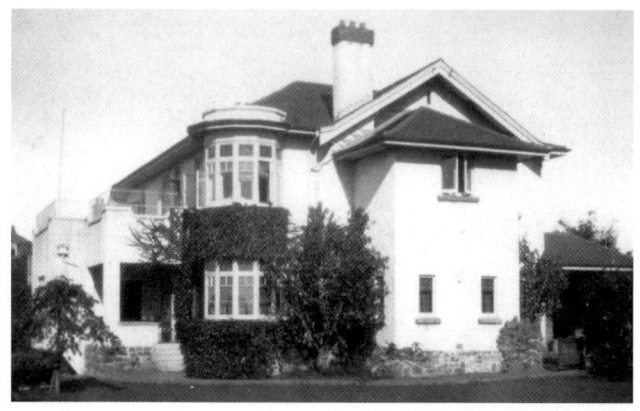

LEFT: Denestone, Alice's home for most of her life. *Patricia Rogers*

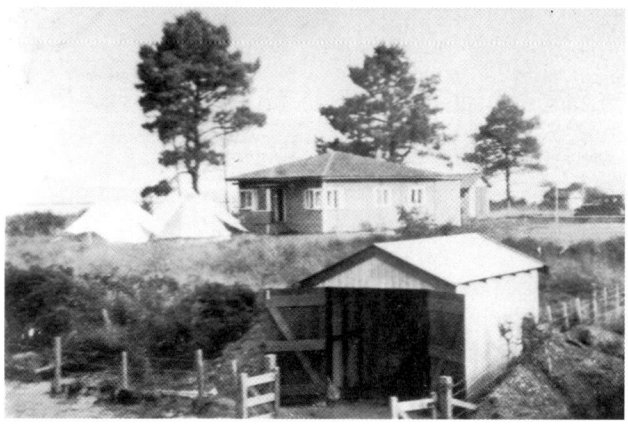

ABOVE: Deep Creek. The land on which the house and hard clay tennis court were situated now forms part of the Waiake Beach Reserve, Torbay. *Patricia Rogers*

LEFT: Alice at Deep Creek, 1920s. *Patricia Rogers*

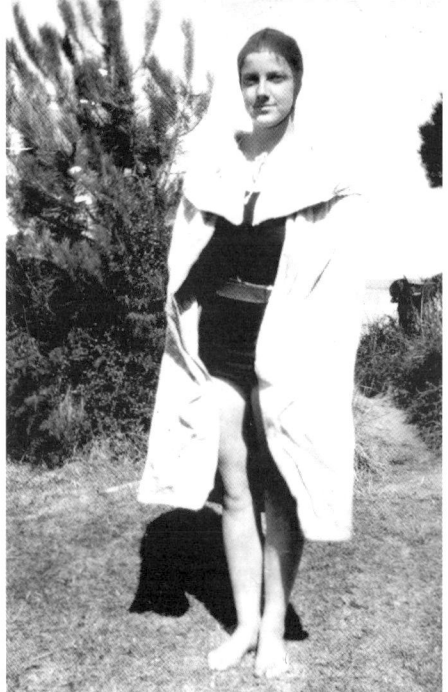

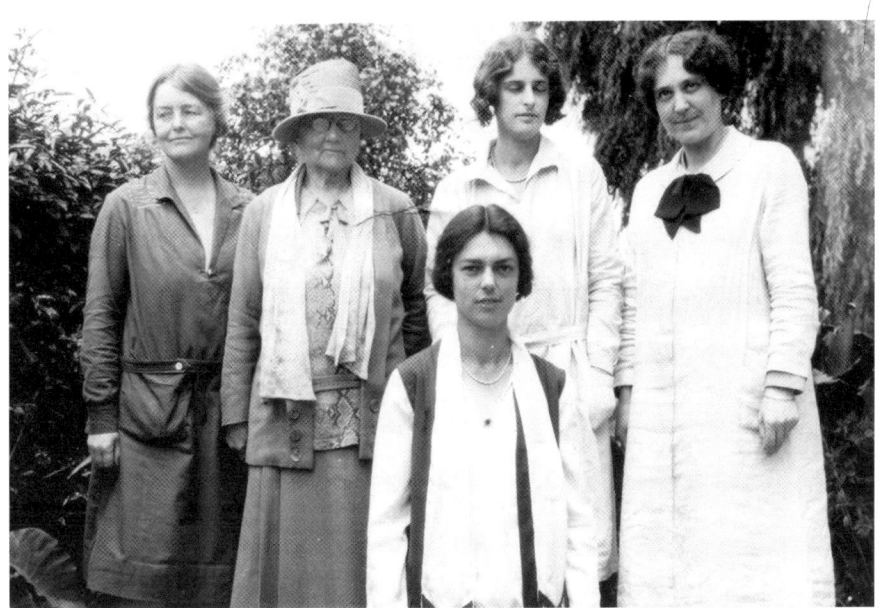

ABOVE: The staff at Hill Top School, 1920s. From left: Miss Boult, her mother, Mrs Boult, Miss Howard, Miss Stitchbury, Miss Leighton. *Hill Top School*

BELOW: Diocesan School for Girls, 1920s. *Diocesan School*

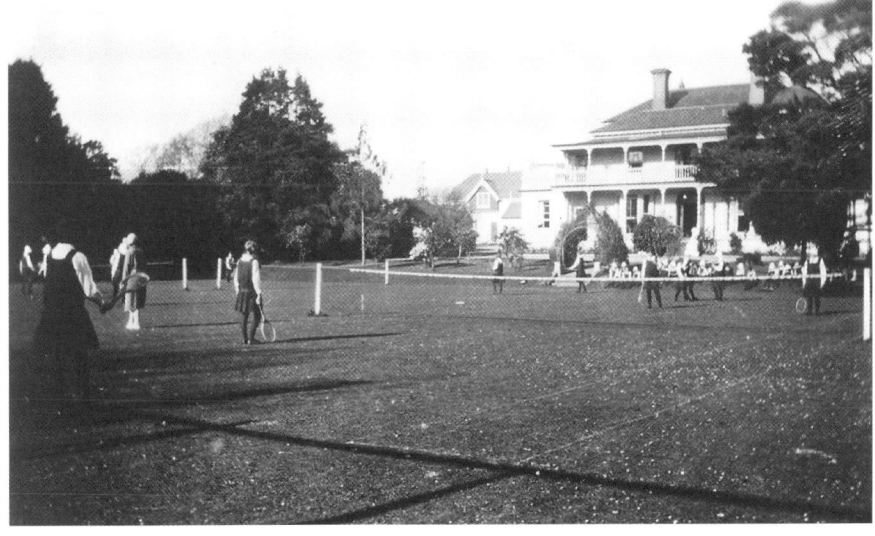

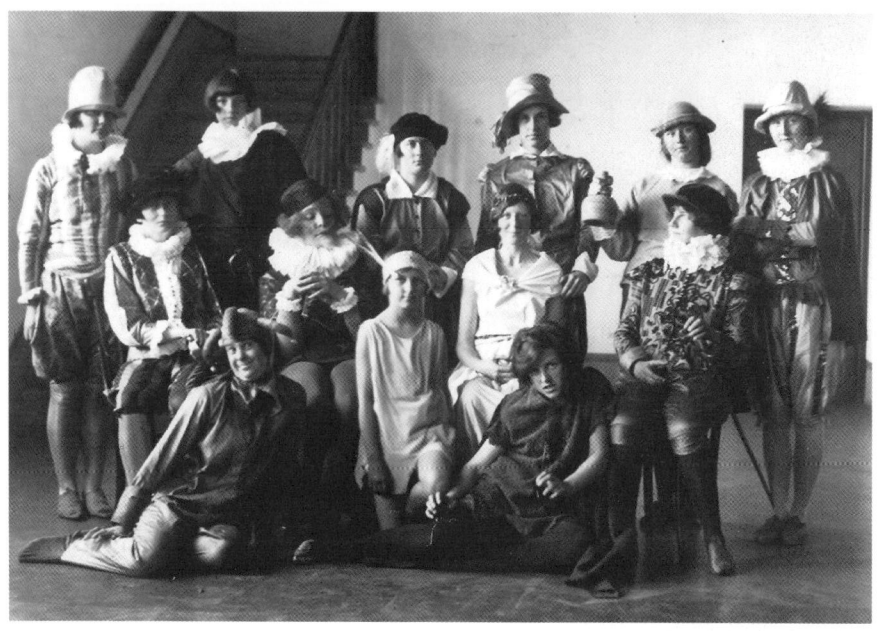

ABOVE: Alice (seated, far right) as Antonio in *The Tempest*, Diocesan School.
Babette Pilcher (MC)

BELOW: Alice, standing second from right, in Diocesan School Hockey Team, 1931.
Diocesan School

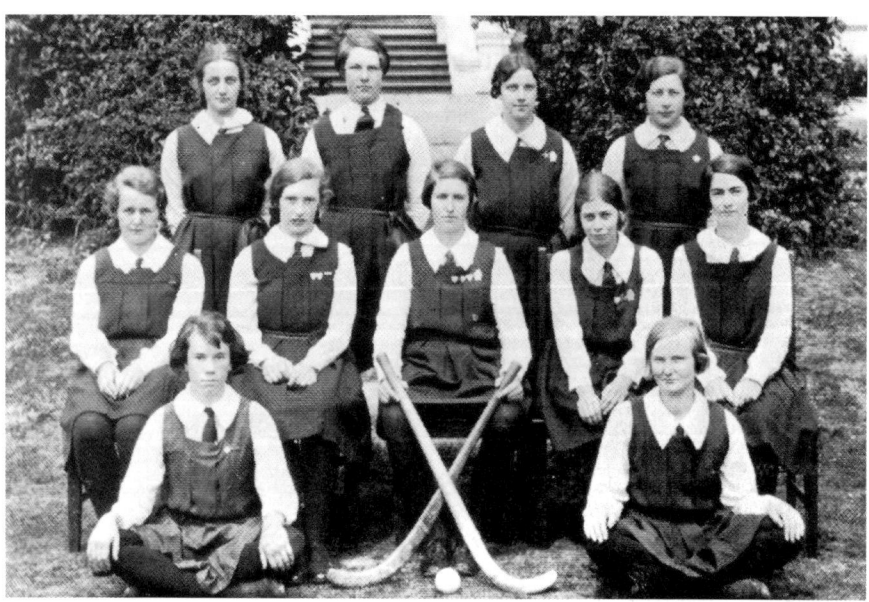

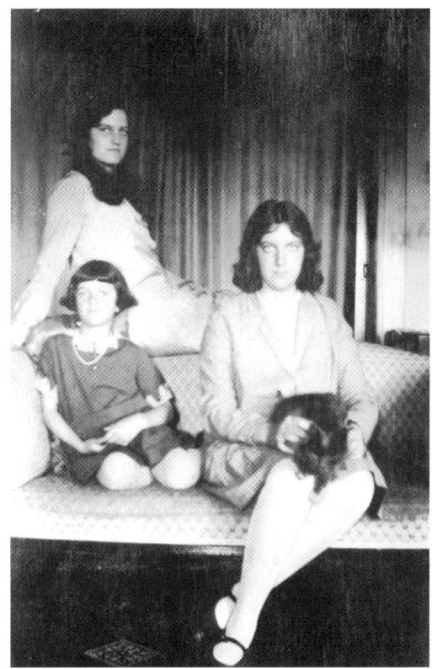

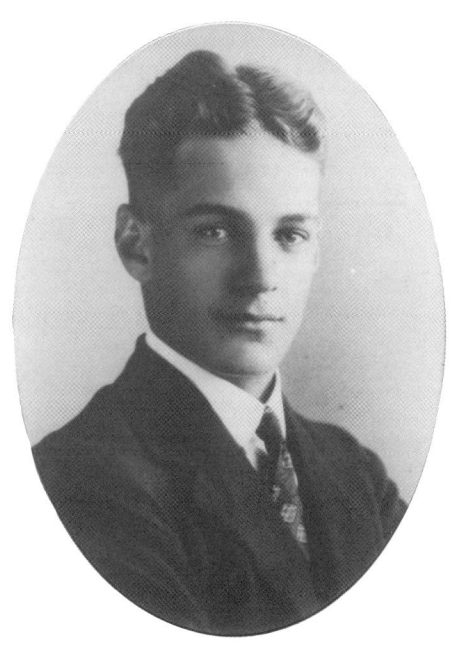

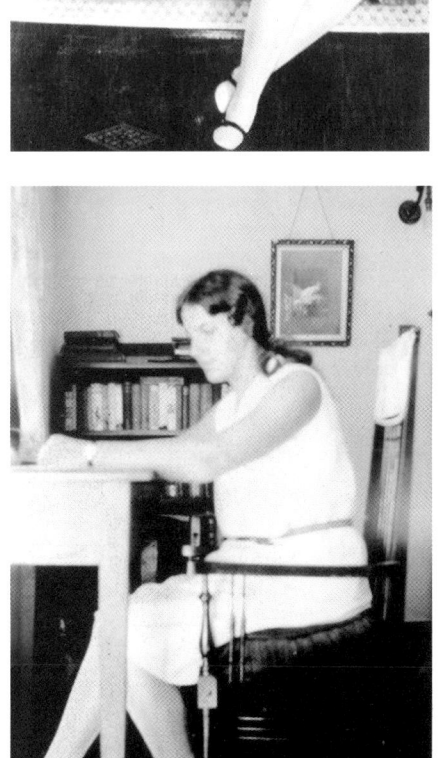

ABOVE LEFT: Patricia (at rear), Aileen and Alice (holding Christopher Robin, the cat) at Denestone, early 1920s. *Patricia Rogers*

ABOVE RIGHT: Warwick Stanton, early 1930s. *H. G. C. Merritt*

LEFT: Alice at her desk, Denestone. *Patricia Rogers*

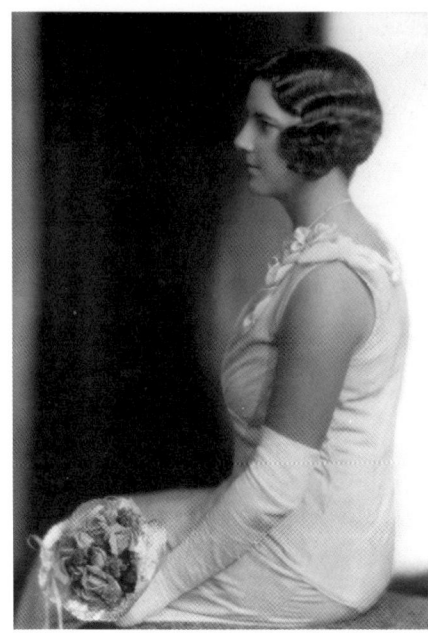

TOP: Alice 'comes out' at Government House, Auckland, June 1932. *Andrew Studios. Courtesy Christine Moorhouse*

CENTRE: Alice and Ida, flanked by fellow students, Dunedin, mid-1930s. *Christine Moorhouse*

BOTTOM: Class photo, 1934. Alice, looking every inch the dedicated student, is on the left of the front row. Margaret Jackson (later Chieffi) and Nan Berry are seated, far right. *Dr A. H. Berry (MC)*

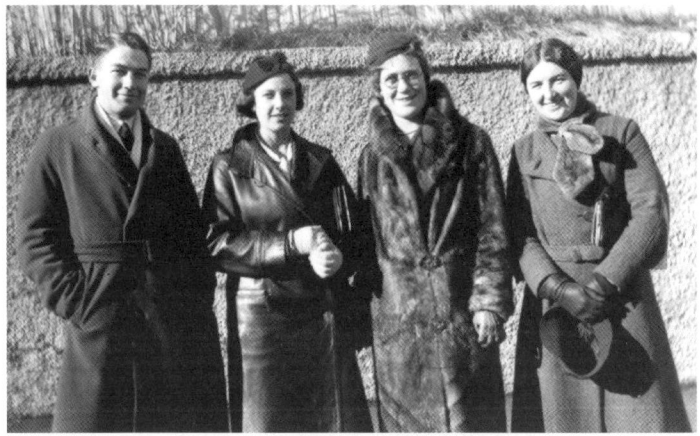

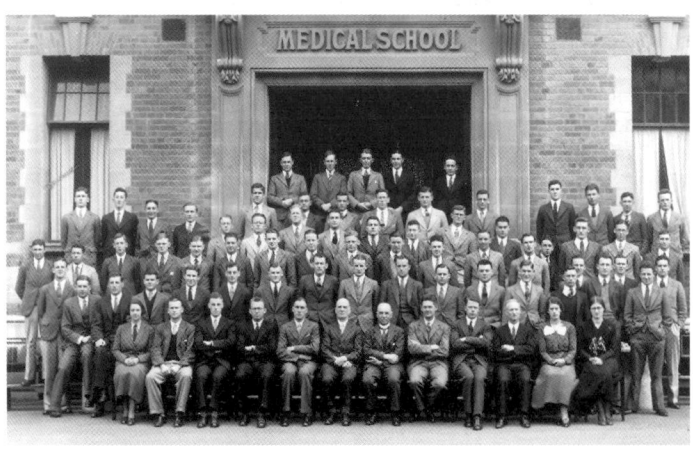

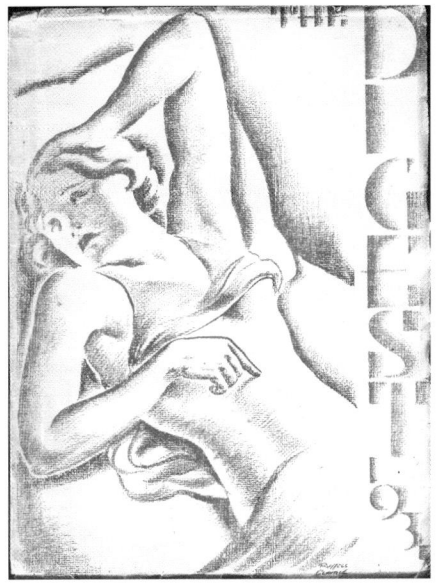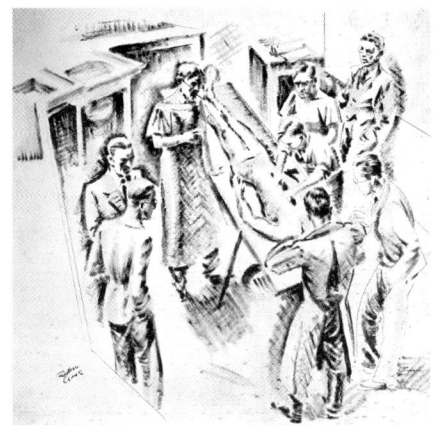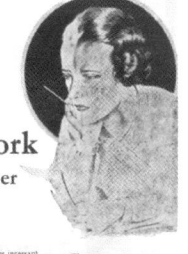

ABOVE AND RIGHT: The medical students' magazine, *The Digest*, 1935. Women appear as patients, or the victims of frazzled nerves. The serious demands of medicine are faced solely by men.

BELOW: Alice (second from left, front row), Lady Vice-President, Otago University Student Executive, 1936. MC

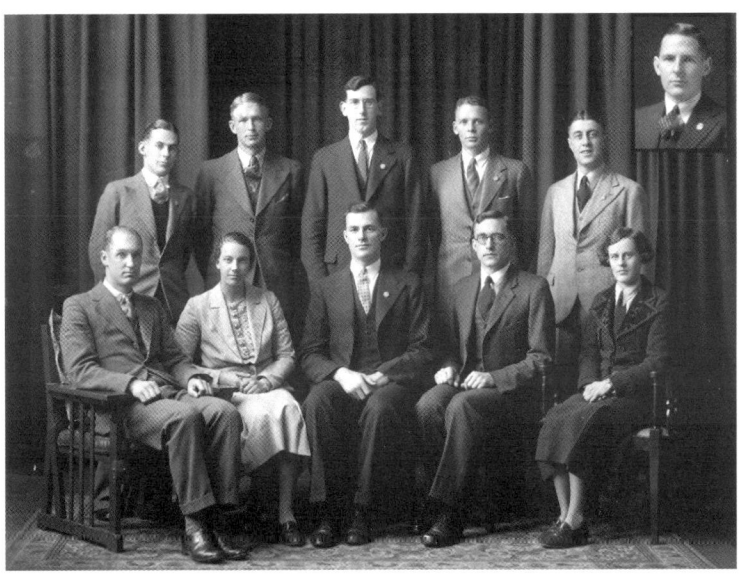

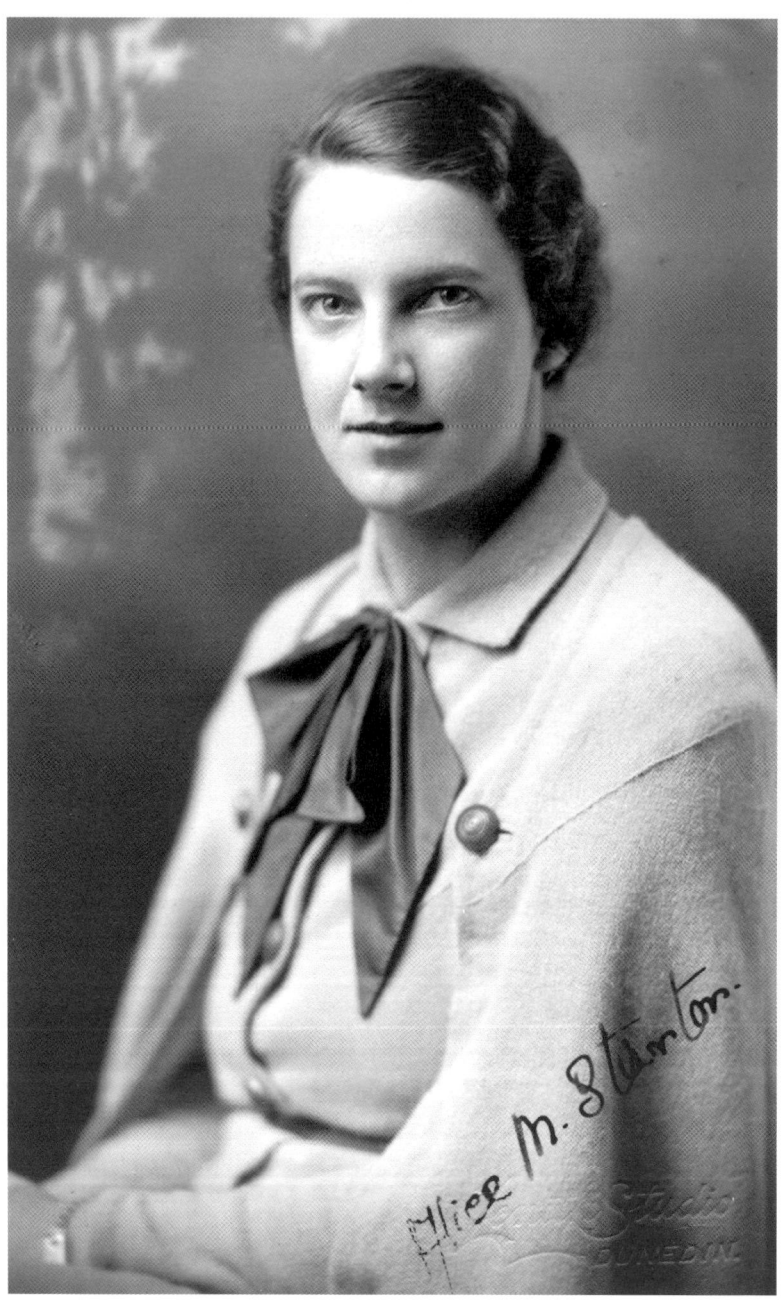

The signed photograph Alice gave to Nan Berry on the completion of their time at the Otago Medical School. *A. H. Berry (MC)*

Douglas sometimes.'⁵⁷ Those who were associated with Alice in later life might be permitted a smile.

By this time Faulkner had become almost completely disillusioned with the Labour Party, particularly the cabinet, which he described as 'Tory as the Nationals'.⁵⁸ He had begun toying with the idea of supporting ex-Labour dissident John A. Lee, a man whose personal qualities were remarkably similar to his own.⁵⁹ He was also inclining towards a career change. During a stay at Denestone over Easter 1940, which went more smoothly than his first visit, he had declared an interest in taking up law. This disclosure brought to the surface all the tensions which Alice's decision to marry Faulkner had invoked. In a family discussion following his departure, her mother approved of this new direction on the grounds that it was not good for the couple's future happiness if Alice's accomplishments were 'greater' than her husband's, not only for financial reasons but because of 'his standing in regard to other men'. Joseph, however, felt a legal career was not 'very feasible' for Faulkner. There was general talk of the necessity of 'city life' and developing 'more or less to the common pattern'. Alice, who duly reported these discussions to Faulkner, admitted she was in a quandary herself. She could not admire 'the servant who buried his talent' and had to agree with her father when he suggested that, in the past, Faulkner had sometimes 'taken the path of least resistance'. On the other hand, while she wanted him to 'make the effort', she did not want him 'spoiled and veneered over with convention'. Reading her letter the following day, Alice clearly recognised that she could not have it both ways. She added a final paragraph, 'On second thoughts, dearest, I don't think this is a very good letter.... I think that you are marvellous & just the one & only person who can save me from being a useless encumbrance of the earth.'⁶⁰ Despite further suggestions from Alice of a career in writing, or a move from primary to secondary school teaching, Faulkner enrolled with a coaching college and proceeded, over the remainder of 1940, to study Latin to matriculation level; the subject had not been available to him at Te Aroha High School. He gained a pass of 70 per cent at the end of the year and began law studies at Auckland University College in 1941.

By this time he was a married man. At the beginning of July Alice had told her parents that she and Faulkner had decided to marry on 17 August. Although it was to be a quiet wartime ceremony in the Diocesan School Chapel, attended only by members of their immediate families, Faulkner was a bundle of nerves. When he picked up his suit, made to measure for the occasion, the jacket was too big. This put him completely off his stride. The bride, who was already demonstrating a casualness in her choice of clothing that was to become something of a hallmark, wore a suit of blue novelty weave (selected with the help of her mother and sister, who had not been impressed by Alice's own earlier choice), with navy hat and accessories. A shoulder spray of pink hyacinths and fox furs, a wedding present from her parents, completed the ensemble. Accounts of the wedding appeared in the local press, describing Alice as a doctor who would 'continue her practice in Auckland for the duration of the war'.[61] But Alice signed a marriage register which left blank the space provided for her 'Rank or Profession'. During the ceremony she promised to 'obey', something she had discussed with Faulkner before the wedding. 'Yes, I shall say "obey",' she wrote on 12 July. 'I suspect I shall have to carry it out anyway.' After her death in 1974 an older and wiser Faulkner added, 'That wd. have been the day!'[62]

After a fortnight's honeymoon at Deep Creek Alice returned to work. Because of the war, the generosity of Joseph and Marjorie and financial factors that related directly to Alice's professional activities, the couple began their married life at Denestone. Alice had to impress the reasons for this on Faulkner, who was understandably uneasy about the wisdom of such a move: 'It would of course be ideal to have a flat of our own but we can't do that cheaply because we'd have to have reliable help to answer the telephone, we couldn't do it under £5-6 a week.'[63] Even so, Alice's marriage, and the failing health of her mother, who died on Christmas Day, 1942,[64] increased her domestic responsibilities. Paid household help was scarce. The number of women working as private domestic servants dropped by two-thirds between 1936 and 1945.[65] The war years saw a succession of cooks and domestics at Denestone, most of whom Alice engaged and supervised. Rationing and the reduction of home deliveries added to household concerns, but the war brought one compensation. For a time Alice's sister Patricia, now married to Dacre Fox Rogers and the mother of two small daughters, returned home while her husband served overseas. During this period she assumed much of the responsibility for the running of the household. It was obviously a large one. Denestone was still home for Allenby, whose legal career had been delayed by military service, and for Aileen, a science undergraduate at Auckland University College. Relations were always welcome to stay, so that even after February 1945, when Patricia and her family left to take up farming in Hawke's Bay, seven adults and two children were still living in the house.[66] Alice did her share of the practical work, including the bottling of fruit and tomatoes, the making of jam and sometimes the cooking and laundry.[67] She found it a frustrating and exhausting experience, complaining to Faulkner,

> This housekeeping business is more tiring than the practice of medicine. ...You men just don't realise how lucky you are. Taking all in all, even admitting that in wartime men have some pretty tough luck, I still think it's a man's world, & that we get the rough end of the stick. If it weren't for the nice superior feeling that one can enjoy as a woman, knowing that one endures the greater hardship, I would almost wish I'd been born a man. Smug? yes I am about that. If you had to deal with my domestic problems for a month you'd be ready and willing to go back to the army.[68]

Marriage also created a problem, both personal and professional, regarding Alice's change of name. She discussed this with her family and with Faulkner. In letters written at the time he seemed non-committal and insisted on leaving the matter to her, but his later recollections admit to some serious conflict.[69] At first Alice decided to 'be Mrs Faulkner Bush, or Dr Alice Bush as circumstances dictate. ... It will be easier to change now than later, and I always have condemned women who wouldn't take their husband's names.'[70] In this Alice appears to have been more conservative than Joseph, who expressed the view that it was 'quite common for girls to get married and continue in their business under their maiden-name'.[71] Paternal pride was probably not entirely absent from this consideration. Dr Alice Stanton eventually became Dr Alice Bush by evolution. In the 1941 Auckland telephone directory she was listed as Dr A. Stanton Bush, by 1943 as Dr A.M. Bush.[72] Possible patient confusion was avoided, and both family pride and husband's self-esteem preserved.

Alice's marriage eased much of the tension in her personal life but one irritant remained: Faulkner was still opposed to personal involvement in the war effort. He continued to sympathise with the ideals of pacifism and argued that the Labour government had no public mandate for conscription. He asserted the mobilisation of Japan would make home defence a greater priority than the dispatching of New Zealand troops to war theatres in Europe and the Middle East. These were not original arguments but there was another, more particular, aspect to Faulkner's dislike of the idea of military service: the connection that had been made between his father's army experience and his later, troubled, years.[73] There was also Faulkner's aversion to authoritarian structures, and a resistance to submersion within a group, which became manifest when he did take part in service life. Since Alice believed that militant pacifists should be interned for the duration, that conscription would have a 'tonic effect' on the country and that New Zealand's first duty was to sustain the British in their struggle, their discussion of the issues involved was typically lively.

Although Alice argued that it was necessary to fight 'for the ideals of freedom and equality',[74] she found the human cost of war repugnant. When the men of the *Achilles* marched through Auckland in February 1940 her feelings were mixed.

> I felt that it was only right and proper that we should do these men homage, for they did a great job of work, but . . . it's heartbreaking to think that courage and skill should be so degraded, that we should commit murder and rejoice over it . . . I can see no antidote, the war must be fought, and it is the nature of war that man shall kill his brother, and yet how I loathe it.[75]

Nevertheless she entered wholeheartedly into the war effort, delaying the purchase of her household linen until sales tax came into operation as 'a small contribution' and investing in war bonds. In comparison, Faulkner dragged his feet. By the end of 1939 he had faced the fact that his commitment to pacifism was insufficient to sustain him through possible internment, though he retained some admiration for those prepared to travel that road.[76] By February 1940 he had applied for entry into the air force, which was vastly more popular than the army and had a substantial backlog of applicants awaiting interviews. Consequently no real progress was made and after his marriage Faulkner filled temporary teaching posts in Remuera and Papatoetoe. On 4 December 1940 his number came up. He formally entered the army on 26 March 1941 and went into camp on 28 May the same year as a member of the 9th Heavy Regiment, New Zealand Artillery.[77]

The combination of service life and law studies, which Faulkner could continue under the special arrangements for serving soldiers, diverted him to a certain extent. At the same time, the war imposed its own demands on relationships. It had already provided the rationale for an early marriage; now it was to do the same for parenthood. When Faulkner was graded for overseas service he and Alice decided that the time had come to start a family. On 23 September 1943, Alice gave birth to a daughter, Lesley Elizabeth.[78]

CHAPTER 4

Circles are Broken

> *I have considered various possibilities . . . it's a sort of vicious circle, one needs to be doing hospital work to get the higher exams before one can get started on the hospital work.*[1]

Alice took three months' maternity leave but after less than three weeks at home she was complaining to Faulkner of the dullness of a life where 'the stimulus of work' was missing.[2] During her absence, Dr Adah Platts-Mills, who had rooms in the same building, looked after her patients. Although Alice felt 'very queer . . . a bit shaky writing the prescription'[3] when she first returned to work, within 10 days she was fitting eight home visits, two anaesthetics, her own meals and the breastfeeding of her child around a full session at the rooms.[4] Faulkner, who had been transferred to the Medical Corps in September 1943 and was awaiting embarkation for the Middle East at Trentham military camp, had assured her that he wanted her to continue working, arguing that she owed it to the community and adding, 'Would hate you to relapse into soulless domesticity'.[5] But Alice clearly did not want her professional commitments to detract from her performance as a mother, vowing on her first day back in the practice, 'I promise you the child won't be neglected'.[6]

The engagement of competent care for her baby was the least of Alice's domestic problems. The Plunket Society's Karitane infant nurses were available for short-term work in private homes and Alice employed four of them over the first year of her daughter's life. A middle class mother's use of this kind of proxy was unlikely to open her to criticism but it was not cheap. Alice was paying a total of £5 15s a week in board and domestic expenses, leaving her only £1 5s from her salary after the deduction of social security tax.[7] On top of this the practice profits for 1943-4 were down by around £250 on the previous year. 'I reckon that the infant cost the firm close on £300,' Alice wrote to Faulkner. 'But I reckon she's worth a lot more than that, & I don't think that E.G. [Sayers] will grudge it.'[8] Fortunately Faulkner had confidence in Alice's arrangements and gave her his full support when, after the departure of the last of the Karitane nurses and a rather unsettled period at Denestone, she needed to compromise a little. During 1945 a widow, previously employed by the family as a cook, brought her own young son to live in the house and looked after the two children during the week as well as doing the 'upstairs' housework. Both children had the run of the place and they would often go with Alice in the car while she visited patients.[9] On Lesley's second birthday they had a joint party,[10] and Alice assumed responsibility for them over at least part of the weekend. Indeed, she was scrupulous in avoiding any differentiation between the two children and was furious when 'someone, I don't know who', suggested to her helper that such equal treatment was inappropriate, provoking a period of tension that took some time to resolve.[11]

Despite Alice's positive approach to the care of her daughter, there was an emotional cost. Employment of a Karitane distanced her from sole autonomy over Lesley's care, and it took discipline not to interfere during the week when the nurse was in charge.[12] When the baby cried before her four-hourly feed was due, Alice had to steel herself not to respond. 'I've been trying to be strong & not go in to nurse and suggest feeding her before time,' she wrote to Faulkner. 'When she really cries I feel that I must comfort her, it's quite different from hearing any other baby cry, it takes all my strength of mind to tell myself that its [sic] right and proper that she should cry sometimes & that it really is good for her.'[13] By the beginning of Lesley's second year she became visibly upset when her mother left for work and Alice began to question 'whether it's really a fair thing to have a family and then leave it to other people to bring up . . . I wonder whether I'm letting the poor little soul down, & whether it's rather a miserable life for her having a doctor for a mother'.[14] Alice also discovered that her medical training did not exempt her from an overcautious concern about her child's health. She found these experiences professionally edifying. 'All these little trials', she wrote to Faulkner, 'are making quite a good doctor out of me. They do help one to understand the patient's point of view.'[15] They also helped to extend her professional interests. By the time Lesley was 13 months old, crying was no longer considered a beneficial exercise. 'I don't think it's good for a child over 6 mths. to be left to cry herself to sleep,' Alice informed Faulkner. 'I am confirmed in that opinion by the Psychiatrist at the Hospital for Sick Children.'[16]

Alice also soon realised that theory did not always fit easily with practice. 'Already,' she confessed to Faulkner, 'I find myself constantly falling below my own standards of what a mother should be.'[17] 'If you can't raise that child better than anyone else could I'll eat my hat,' Faulkner replied.[18] Nevertheless they began to modify their ideas about the suitable size of a family. Earlier estimates had ranged as high as six children,[19] but by mid-1945 both were agreed that two might be better, although Alice rationalised her own argument around the concept of the family breadwinner in a curiously convoluted way.

> I think 2 will be just a nice family for you. I don't think you can be expected to have yr. life curtailed & controlled for yrs. & yrs. because there's always a little one to be considered. I did used to think I'd like 1/2 doz ... but there's no question that they are rather constricting. Even c. 2 I can see all my leisure time pretty well occupied for the next 10 yrs. & if there were more I'd have to drastically limit my practice of medicine & that would mean yoking you hard into the business of bread winning.[20]

By then Faulkner knew that the last thing on Alice's mind was drastically limiting her practice of medicine.

Edward Sayers was released from army service at the end of 1944 but he had already discussed the future with Alice during earlier periods of leave. He proposed their remaining in partnership at a specialist level, forming the embryo of a group practice that might later expand to employ a fulltime laboratory technician and possibly a radiologist. Alice wrote to Faulkner, telling him of Sayers's suggestions and they discussed her future career at some length by way of the vagaries of the wartime postal service between New Zealand and Italy, where Faulkner was stationed at Bari with No. 3 New Zealand General Hospital. During this correspondence Alice put some concrete proposals to Faulkner. 'You must understand,' she wrote, 'that you & the family come first, tho' I admit that I'd be sorry to give up the job.' Did he approve of her continuing in her profession? Would he be prepared to live in Auckland for the next five or 10 years? Would he object to her going to the United States for three to six months before his return if the opportunity arose?[21] This was clearly crunch time. Alice had arrived at the crossroads and wanted to continue, not only with fulltime medical practice but at the highest level. Would Faulkner agree? It seemed he would.

> We agreed long ago that it wd. be a pity if you thought of giving up the work & you know that I neither expect nor want you to, until such time, if any, as *you* may feel disposed to toss it in. So all future plans are to be made on the basis that you go on indefinitely . . . I've already become reconciled to a city existence apart from any medical considerations . . . I'm 100% c your ideas on the form of practice you want to adopt – it's a gt. chance, to society as well as you.[22]

He emphasised his support by requesting a screed of information about their present financial situation, when she planned to go overseas, how much that would cost, whether it would be too much to combine this with a pregnancy, what plans she had made for Lesley's care while she was away and whether he should come home and do this. 'I'll be awaiting your answers c gt interest & suggest super thrift in the meantime,' he concluded.[23] Alice would need this kind of wholehearted backing to achieve the specialist status that Sayers had suggested as the basis of their future partnership, but she had already made her first moves in this direction. Eleven days after Faulkner wrote this accommodating letter she was appointed part-time assistant visiting physician to the children's wards at Auckland Hospital.

Hospital appointments were essential in advancing a postgraduate medical career beyond general practice but women had had even less success at this level at Auckland Hospital than they had obtaining residencies.[24] Positions were advertised biennially, although incumbents were usually reappointed. More than one application increased the chances of success and in January 1944 Alice had lodged two as an assistant physician: one at the new Green Lane Hospital, the other (her first preference) in the children's wards at Auckland Hospital. This was currently held, and reapplied for, by Elizabeth Hughes, but only as insurance against the failure of her bid for a senior post in the infectious diseases block. When the hospital board rejected all applicants for the senior vacancy, Elizabeth Hughes retained her old job while the Green Lane post went to another woman doctor with postgraduate qualifications and overseas experience superior to anything Alice could offer. Alice was offered work as an anaesthetist; there was a serious shortage of manpower in the area.[25] This placed her in a dilemma.

> I have heard from an unofficial source that they are adopting the policy that anyone wanting a job on the Hon. staff must first serve their turn as anaesthetist. . . . it would be quite sterile as far as valuable experience goes. On the other hand if that policy is to be adopted it seems that the sooner I become an anaesthetist, the sooner I can cease to be one.[26]

Alice had made no further moves when the hospital board, following some pressure from senior medical advisers, and after readvertising, decided to give Elizabeth Hughes the senior post. This gave Alice a second chance and she promptly forwarded a fresh application for Hughes's old job, supported by a testimonial from Sammy Ludbrook, the senior children's physician.[27] On 25 September 1944 the board accepted her and Alice was jubilant. Apart from undoubted professional advantages, she had gained a certain £300 a year.[28] She immediately cabled Faulkner: 'HAVE BEEN PROMOTED   GREETINGS TO THE BEST OF FATHERS . . . ALL MY LOVE . . . ALICE BUSH'. His reply was curiously muted.

> Well, I guess you will be very pleased c things & sitting on top of the world, albeit alone, wh. I think is a bad thing. I'm glad for your sake, but it seems to me a comparatively poor appointment for one so worthy. What do you think? At least the ice is broken now anyway . . . I do hope you will find the work interesting, & happy, & that it will lead to far, far greater things, & to spheres in wh. you can do even more excellent work. I fancy you are more professional than maternal deep down, & in any case why shouldn't you be? You do pretty well at both & I'm certainly

not criticising. That's honest. I just want to be home. I'll bet when I arrive you'll be in the States, or some bally thing will go wrong .... So many of the things I plan never seem to eventuate.[29]

This was rather different in tone from his letter of less than three weeks before, but Alice felt very positive about the whole situation and particularly happy working with Sammy Ludbrook,[30] a visiting physician at the hospital since the 1920s and a well-known specialist in child health in Auckland.[31] She was to attend the children's wards three mornings a week and on Sundays.[32] At the same time she contracted to a three-year partnership with Edward Sayers. He would retain a two-thirds interest in the practice and she, after payment of £200, a third. Sayers still had a significant reputation in Auckland. When he resumed work he was already booked for almost two weeks ahead and Alice had all the work she could handle.[33] By January 1945 they were employing a receptionist and two nurses. Sayers resumed his senior post at Auckland Hospital, but did not reclaim the Karitane appointment so Alice now held two hospital appointments. Only a lack of formal postgraduate qualifications stood between her becoming a 'complete specialist & perhaps [taking over] a full halfshare' of the practice.[34]

Probably because of the limitations of civilian travel during wartime, ideas of going to the United States were abandoned for something more immediately at hand. For many years the only postgraduate qualification available within New Zealand had been a doctorate in medicine (MD). It required a thesis based on original research with an examination dependent on the quality of the submission.[35] The establishment of the Royal Australasian College of Physicians in 1938 had provided an alternative, with membership (MRACP) attainable by examination alone and requiring travel only across the Tasman. Initially, the MD seems to have appealed to Alice more,[36] but over the middle months of 1945 she began to favour the MRACP because of the difficulty for a general practitioner of setting up a research project. She made one, unsuccessful, attempt to set up a clinical trial at the beginning of 1944 after an elderly woman patient reported that she had cured herself of diabetes by drinking an infusion of the green berries of the poro poro (*Aviculare solanum*). When Alice found her condition had improved, she set up a programme of blood sugar testing on a reliable and accessible non-diabetic – herself. For several weeks, she dutifully drank the bitter-tasting liquid and then took samples of her own blood, which were analysed by her sister Aileen's future husband, and later professor of chemistry at Auckland University, Alan Odell. By the end of the year the results were disappointing and she did not proceed further.[37]

From then on Alice concentrated on the MRACP, extending her hospital experience by relieving during Elizabeth Hughes's periods of leave from the infectious diseases wards and accompanying senior physicians on their rounds. Her directed approach attracted their patronage. Sayers, a foundation fellow of the Australasian College, was particularly supportive, discussing cases, lending her the latest textbooks, involving her in giving a joint paper on asthma at a postgraduate conference on chest diseases and setting up evening study sessions with her and Ronald Caughey, a younger medical man and future colleague.[38] 'Just now I'm enjoying a wonderful opportunity,' Alice enthused to Faulkner. 'I can discuss all my problems with Ted, & I've learnt more medicine in the last 4 mths. than in the previous 4 yrs. put together.' She gave up all except the clinical meetings announcing that 'the political side of medicine can go hang in the meantime'.[39] Things simply could not have been going better when, towards the end of 1945, the opportunity arose for her to sit the MRACP examination without leaving the country. The *NZMJ* announced it was to be held for the first time in New Zealand, in Wellington, in February 1946.[40] But before that date Alice's private world had been shattered.

When Faulkner had entered the army he had done so with little relish. His tension was revealed in the staccato tone of a letter hurriedly written to Alice around the time of his embarkation: 'Keep child unspoilt. No thrusting of her before family or public – nor of me. Read yr. journals. You have promised to live only for child & work in my absence. Well, here is the test right now.'[41] Alice had tried to transmit some of her own confidence to Faulkner. 'May you be allowed to keep your dear personality intact,' she began.

> I don't want you to change for I love you so dearly as you are, & yet I know that no change in you will alter the fact that you & I belong to each other, we may sometimes even strain against the bonds, strive to hurt each other but that is in reality only hurting ourselves. But against all logic and through all change, both within & without is that deep affinity, that oneness of which Lesley is the personification.[42]

Faulkner's experience of army life did not add to his self-esteem. He worked as a ward orderly in the hospital in Bari, a position that his seniors, and almost everyone was his senior, appeared to regard with little consideration.[43] Being ordered about by sisters of the Army Nursing Corps exposed his essentially conservative attitude to women.

> I make no comment on their professional performance but I don't find working c them v. exhilarating ... The general idea, no matter how good the dame may be, is just repugnant. They hold too high an office in the outfit, & too high an opinion of themselves.[44]

Faulkner voluntarily spent extra time on night duty simply because there were fewer sisters around and that shift, calling less on his time, gave him more chance to study. As a reluctant and lowly component of a medical hierarchy, Faulkner's experience as a serving soldier compounded rather than relieved the difficulties he faced in coming to terms with marriage to a woman doctor. He resorted to his old tactic of challenging Alice with the claims of her profession, taking a particular delight in medical progress that had its source in lay people,[45] and professional resistance to socialised medicine remained a useful bludgeoning tool. Loftily he pointed out that education had continued to function efficiently as a state enterprise though, he challenged, 'one would not expect the obscurantist B.M.A to agree with that ... The fear of becoming a civil servant ... is anathema to the genteel M.B.'s.'[46] Such arguments placed Alice in a defensive position.

To add to his unhappiness, Faulkner, like many men who served overseas, believed that his countrymen and women had no appreciation of the conditions, frustrations and hardships experienced by servicemen. Worse, he grew to believe that Alice did not and that she and the family were not keeping him fully informed of events at home.[47] He had been particularly upset when Alice had written telling him that she had attended a servicemen's hospitality centre at Government House on an evening when Diocesan School old girls were required to provide hostesses. Faulkner not only disapproved of 'social' war activity,[48] he held firm opinions on the behaviour appropriate to married men and women who, for any reason, might be temporarily separated. He seems to have found the idea of his wife going out dancing with anybody else particularly distasteful.[49] Alice's professional ambition became Faulkner's ally in maintaining their relationship along lines acceptable to his ideas of constancy and he would remind her that the achievement of formal postgraduate qualifications was a more appropriate pursuit for her while he was away.[50] Over the two years of his absence Alice was regularly exhorted to spend all her 'spare' time on concentrated study. At the same time, Faulkner saw Alice's increasing involvement in her profession as a potential threat to their future family life and he began to suggest the possibility of various assignments, either in New Zealand or overseas, to which one or both of them would somehow travel in order to conceive another child.[51] So Alice found herself simultaneously urged to work to the limit and to give priority to motherhood.

During his overseas service, Faulkner's unhappiness occasionally assumed the proportions of true depression. In mid-1945 he reached the nadir.[52] Although the war in Europe was over, there was no official indication of future troop movements and he feared that his division would be diverted to the Pacific.[53] Mail, always unreliable and slow, was held up. In mid-May he complained that he had received no letters or parcels for three weeks, only a cablegram that he could not understand.[54] On 9 July he wrote to Alice offering her her freedom and pouring out a catalogue of woe. It was not that he no longer loved her, he was quick to point out, but it seemed obvious to him that they were increasingly at odds in their opinions and attitudes, and that his views, not hers, were changing. Part of the letter was devoted to a particular aspect of their relationship.

> Rightly or wrongly, it seems to me that your career is slowly but surely claiming more & more of you, & leaving less & less for other things & for me. I can't blame you, for I walked into the position with my eyes wide open, & with the advice of older & probably wiser people before me, but you will agree that, if I'm right in assuming this to be the case, it won't make post-war life any easier. I'm not blaming you one little bit, just trying to show you what an impossible set-up it would be for me. Moreover, I wouldn't ask you to give it up. I think you would, if the choice came to such a position, be far more useful to society in your present role than as the talented but idle spouse of a misfit & most probably failure. Please don't consider yourself under any obligation to chuck in the job, whatever happens. All I ask is that you don't overdo things to such an extent that the child suffers . . .

> Incidentally, I'm also a little weary of being the spouse of a prominent person – I know it's not your fault & that I saw such possibilities, but it doesn't help any. I love you & only you, & I love that child, but I still can't see that that is enough in itself on wh. to base future stable union. What am I to do? I wish I knew. I get no further ahead with these problems after 3 months of puzzling.[55]

This letter must have hit Alice hard. Her own high standard of personal loyalty had never faltered and she had supported Faulkner in time-consuming ways that must have added to any personal stress she was already suffering. She had plied him with letters and parcels of comforts, purchased and posted textbooks and consulted university staff and regulations on his behalf. At his request she had saved every copy of the *New Zealand Herald* for the whole of his absence, now and again discarding, from long lists of dates he sent to her, those that he had been able to read in Italy.[56] She kept him supplied with photographs of their child, bought a movie camera and film (both hard to get at the time) and had people in to take home movies of Lesley. Despite her increasing workload, she had tried to study but, as she attempted to point out, a practice spread physically all over Auckland which included a significant amount of home visiting, exhausted her physical and intellectual energies. She feared she might have lost the ability to study.[57] These factors, and the other medical responsibilities that were as necessary to her eventual success in postgraduate work as formal study, made it difficult for her to make progress. Her domestic responsibilities, not a gay social life, took up every spare moment. She had tried to convey to Faulkner the stress of her lifestyle, even before she had a hospital appointment.

> Life has been hectic. Take last wk. Sun. night 2 calls after dinner. Mon. night op[eration] till 7.30 then went on to Dinner with Douglas R[obb]. for whom I'd been giving the anaes[thetic]... & on my way home had to stop and spend 1/2 hr. fixing up an intravenous drip for the subject of the op[eration]. Tues. night finished my calls at 10 p.m. Wed night 4 visits before B.M.A. meeting that finished at 10 p.m. Thurs. night at home, studied a textbook on the thyroid gland, Fri. night the Reids to dinner & I had to rush off at 7.30 & another call at 9.30. Sat. night just got settled by the fire with my journals when the child awoke & took considerable time to get her settled again. Sun. night worn out, & read magazines until an early bed. What a life! How can I swot under the circs?[58]

Less than a month after writing this letter, Alice was suffering from extreme physical and nervous exhaustion. The demands of her patients and the broken nights with Lesley stretched her nerves to breaking point.[59] Not without a degree of guilt, she arranged to take a week's holiday, leaving Lesley in the care of her nurse and the practice in the care of Adah Platts-Mills. She spent a few days at Ngawha Springs in Northland, in the company of her friend and patient Phoebe Meikle. She had to confess to Faulkner that motherhood had taken a greater toll on her energies than she had anticipated, but this was not the least of her unreal expectations of herself and, in the best self-mortifying manner, she coupled these with a sense of false pride.

> I would have liked to have done without holidays while you were away, to have devoted my life unfailingly to my work, with the child for restfulness. But it just didn't work . . .
>
> I despise myself for not being able to keep going indefinitely but I could not see the sense in courting a complete breakdown just for my pride's sake, so I solace myself with the thought that having a baby is probably a strain on the nervous system and that mine hadn't fully recovered. I hope in the future to be a little more strong minded – to stand up to things even if they are pretty strenuous.[60]

Fortunately Alice had arranged to take another holiday in July 1945 and she found the reserves of strength to face Faulkner's despair and to respond to this crisis as she had to earlier ones, with a measured understanding of her husband. She began carefully. 'Thank you for the offer of my freedom, but truly I don't want it. That is my well considered opinion.' She then went on to agree that they did have differences, that at times he did make her angry, indeed he did have faults, but 'underneath there is something that I admire & respect & love, all the more perhaps because sometimes I have a suspicion that I haven't got it'.[61] But in further correspondence she did not duck the issue of her career and its place in their relationship. Perhaps, Alice suggested, the very qualities that he had once found attractive in her had proved more difficult to live with than he had expected; her intelligence a menace 'because it pits itself against your own', her success a source of irritation rather than a source of pride. This was something he must come to terms with. 'I have nothing to offer you for compensation,' she continued, apart from the fact that

'I know myself too well to be able to pretend to myself that I really count in real values'.[62]

Alice was no longer the young woman who had written to Faulkner in May 1940.

> I once wrote a very fine essay on women's right[s] and privileges. I am essentially an anti-feminist & I maintain that women lose far more than they gain by attempting & even accomplishing a man's work ... take women surgeons for instance. They are doing great work in the world today, & some original work too, but I am of the opinion these things are done equally well by men, & there is nobody to do the work of mothering that the women surgeons have left undone. Of course its possible that it would be better for all children to be brought up in the mass by scientifically trained nurses, male or female, & in that case, women will have to occupy themselves with something else.
>
> ... my chief ambition is to make my husband happy & bring up his family, that is of course appallingly old fashioned, but then I know that I was born about 50 yrs too late.[63]

Now, in 1945, he received letters like this,

> You say you can be happy only in a set up wherein you & I meet on an equal basis. I agree ... The crucial point is what is this equality. Would you consider it exists in the average home where the man follows his vocation & provides the money & the woman, whatever her talents or aspirations might be is tied to the washtub, the sink, or the children, or if there should be enough money, she may have the choice of a life of frivolity or voluntary social service ...
>
> My idea of equality in marriage demands that each partner should be free to develop thier [sic] own talents to the fullest extent that is possible, admitting their joint responsibility to provide a home & companionship & supervision for the family.[64]

What had happened? For a start their relationship had developed. In May 1940 Alice had written to Faulkner, 'Would you like a real big argument when you come up? or shall I be nice and feminine & agree with everything you say?'[65] Things had obviously moved on from that level. In those five years Alice had experienced a full professional life and she had enjoyed it. It had been hard, exhausting work but she was now well placed to establish herself firmly within professional structures. She had the commitment and the ability, she was in partnership with a leading physician, had two hospital appointments and had attracted the patronage of leading professionals. Moreover, she was possibly now, for the first time, supported in her ambitions by feminist theory. In July 1944, she met Dr Edith Summerskill, British feminist and parliamentarian, who was visiting Auckland and spoke at a public meeting in the town hall. Alice was attracted by Summerskill's personality, describing her to Faulkner as 'a fighter, loves a bit of opposition I should think, plenty of self confidence and a v. nice easy manner'. She was rather more reticent about the 'subject matter' of Summerskill's public address, which she reported as containing nothing 'terrific just an appeal to women to take their part in the planning of the world, and a reminder of the hardships our predecessors suffered to get votes for women'.[66] Alice may well have taken more from Summerskill than this nonchalant assessment implies. Edith Summerskill championed the rights of women not only as mothers and homemakers but also to a life outside the home. She held that participation in one sphere actually enhanced activity in the other, so that professional women gained a greater understanding of people's lives if they were also mothers; she wished that it would be possible for some men 'to go through this humanising process'.[67]

The insistence that motherhood augmented a woman's professional capacity was an extension of the late 19th-century version of middle class feminism that had underwritten women's entry into the medical profession and allowed for either a domestic or social mothering role, but not both. Summerskill's was undoubtedly an empowering message for many women with sympathies similar to Alice's. In September 1943 the wish that 'our best equipped women should have marriage and children as well as career' had been cited in correspondence as part of the 'creed of the Auckland Association [of the NZFPA]'.[68] The personal encounter with Summerskill may provide the final key to Alice's unflinching determination from 1944 to further her career. Her attitude to marriage and motherhood had not changed. She wanted a family of her own and a good relationship with her husband and children. Her new agreement with Sayers included a maternity leave clause.[69] The demands of general practice had proved difficult to reconcile with her desire for family life, but specialisation seemed to offer a means by which she might fulfil all her aspirations. 'My chief aim at present,' she wrote to Faulkner, 'is that I should qualify to practice [sic] as a specialist & so be able to carry on without neglecting either you or her [Lesley].'[70] All she needed to secure her new ambition was a postgraduate qualification, but she needed it quickly. It was most unusual to hold a visiting hospital appointment without one and competition was increasing as a host of medical ex-servicemen returned seeking to re-establish themselves. The decision to hold the MRACP examination in New Zealand had put this essential qualification within Alice's grasp. Fortuitously, Faulkner was already pulling himself out of the trough, ready once again to take up familiar themes. 'Forgive me if I appear to nag,' he had written at the end of July, 'but just how soon can you get that M.D.? ... Would you consider seriously the question of Part 2 of the family, if and when you would like it. .... It is for you to make any decisions and I'll abide by them.'[71]

Although his moods continued to fluctuate, Faulkner had surmounted the last major crisis connected with his army service. During 1945 he had been appointed admitting clerk and found 'what was for me, the most congenial and satisfying job in the whole hospital'.[72] After four years in the army he gained two promotions in rapid succession, ending his war service with the rank of temporary sergeant. For the rest of the year he directed his energies into more positive efforts to improve his lot: a campaign to get home as quickly as possible and plans, which ultimately came to nothing, to stand for Parliament as a soldiers' representative, in the mould of John A. Lee. Alice was far from convinced of the viability of these proposals, but she offered Faulkner her support though, typically, she held out no false hopes to him. Both felt that they had weathered the storm. Their prospects seemed bright and they were content to see out the final months of their separation equably. But the bitterest blow of all was yet to fall.

From her earliest days Lesley was an extremely active child, very restless at night. To keep her covered, Alice used a sleeping bag, which she sometimes pinned to an ordinary bed in the absence of a cot. When Lesley was suffering from a cold one Saturday night in early November, Alice humoured her by allowing her to sleep in the sleeping bag in her bed. Early in the evening she went to look at her daughter, who was lying quietly, obviously settled for the night though not yet asleep. Alice went downstairs, wrote to Faulkner and did some reading. When she retired to bed herself about 10 o'clock she found 'a hump at the side & no head on the pillow, I ran around & lifted the blanket & there she was hanging by the sleeping bag cold & limp'.[73] She immediately swung into action, calling for her sister Aileen, starting artifical respiration, injecting coramine into the child's heart, then adrenalin. Aileen telephoned Edward Sayers and F.P. Furkert, a surgeon and near neighbour, who massaged the heart and continued with artificial respiration while Alice administered oxygen. The child did not respond. Edward Sayers arrived and he and Furkert dealt with the police. Then, as her father was away, Sayers took Alice home to his wife, Jean.[74]

Lesley's death was perhaps the greatest crisis in Alice's personal and professional life. She was faced with the trauma common to any parent who experienced the loss of a child, but her grief was compounded by the intensity with which she had planned and carried out her parenting role, the tender age of her daughter, the tragic circumstances of the death and, above all, any implications Alice may have drawn from her dual role as professional woman and mother. On top of all this, she was separated from her husband and communication delays kept her ignorant of his response for some time. She had no word at all from Faulkner until a cablegram arrived on 12 November, nearly 10 days after their daughter had died. During the same period she had sent three cables and written three letters. Until 7 December, those letters that did reach her were written before he had received the news and continued to refer to Lesley as a living child. Over this period Alice experienced an intense sense of isolation. Although friends and relations flocked to support her, they could not, she wrote to Faulkner, 'speak the language that I speak, I feel that only you & I can talk about Lesley & understand each other'.[75] Only after she had received his cable did she feel 'so much better, we have established contact once more and we live again in the same world'.[76] In the first crucial days of her bereavement, Alice was forced to find within herself some way to overcome her terrible grief. Her self-questioning letters to Faulkner chart her internal struggle. Had she been a 'good', a 'true' mother? Had she loved her child too much? Had something she had done, or not done, contributed to the accident?[77]

One source of comfort might have been a strong religious belief. Lesley had been baptised an Anglican, a decision that had stimulated Alice's interest in attempting once again to define her own faith. She and Faulkner had discussed the matter keenly over the early months of 1944 but had reached no more than agreement that formal commitment to a church was a responsibility they owed their child. Alice was not convinced that the good life could be lived only by Christians;[78] indeed, she feared 'that by all the canons of the established church I'm a heretic'.[79] The Christian promise of life hereafter had not comforted her at the time of Warwick's death and nothing had happened since to make it any more effective when she lost her daughter.[80] But her recent interest in mental health had the potential to provide a counterbalance to her diminished religious faith. Alice had come to believe that mankind's 'craving for a personal God' lay not in the expectation of divine intervention but in the desire for individual understanding.[81] In the past this, and the absolving of guilt, had been part of the culture of religion. In the future these tasks would be taken up by the guardians of the psyche and their handmaidens, social workers and counsellors. Similarly, just as religion had been a motivating and authorising force for women's involvement in life beyond the home, the caring, scientifically marginal mental health professions would offer them particular opportunities. As the 20th century advanced, increasing numbers of medical and lay women would be attracted by the holistic, inter-personal, anti-mechanistic nature of its therapies, which explored the emotions and could both recognise and inform their own life experiences.[82] Alice seems already to have undergone this conversion by the time of Lesley's death.

The importance of overcoming guilt had already modified her inherited values to a surprising degree. Earlier the same year, she had proposed that couples separated by war should agree to

> have as good a time as possible ... continue to love one another, but let the enjoyment of friends of either sex be considered no disloyalty ... if they could only have their fun without feeling that giving in to temptation once or twice has spoilt forever their love and loyalty there'd be fewer men coming home to empty lives. A revolutionary doctrine I admit, but I reckon it's sound psychology.[83]

This was not only counter to Alice's own wifely constancy but also diametrically opposed to Faulkner's views (and the argument was addressed to him), so it represents a fundamental shift in her attitudes. Alice would continue to refer to New Testament morality to justify many of her social crusades but it was her commitment to mental health and the need to avoid the destructive personal effects of guilt that would provide an ongoing, although not always obvious, authority for her more radical views, those with which conservative Christians could not agree. Later debates surrounding sexuality would make this clearer but, at the end of 1945, the immediate value of Alice's interest may well have lain in giving her a philosophical lifeline to revive her innate vitality. Four days after Lesley's death, she wrote to Faulkner, 'you know I am not one to indulge in foolish morbid self accusation,'[84] but it was not until the end of November that she decided they must have more children, though they should not let this unhappy experience make them overprotective parents.[85] Alice also found great comfort in her career; she had never related its demands to Lesley's death and returned to work the day after the funeral. She had arranged to attend a postgraduate conference on nervous diseases for the rest of that week and she found it helpful to keep her mind off the searing experience. 'Back at work,' she wrote after a visit to Lesley's grave, 'I felt that I could breathe.'[86] It now seemed to her more necessary than ever to sit the membership examination for the Australasian College. The preparations would provide a rehabilitating self-discipline; success in the examination would restore her confidence in herself and leave her with something to offer her husband on his return.[87]

Although stunned by the death of his daughter, of whom he had seen so little, Faulkner drew on all his reserves to support and comfort his wife. Perhaps the magnitude of the loss and Alice's real vulnerability inspired in him an unusual confidence and he was stalwart and sensitive in his response. His cablegram to Alice was addressed to her rooms. Whether or not it was his intention, she felt this to be a symbol of his continued support for her career, and he did not once suggest that she should not continue with it. He refused to apportion blame and tried to place their personal grief within a universal context.

> You must not reproach yourself for anything – I can't see why you should. . . . No child ever had a more loving mother, no worthless male so wonderful a wife. I know you will carry on with the work & find comfort in helping others – we are not alone in grief & because of our own sorrow we become more sensitive to others.[88]

Alice, her father, professional associates and friends tried to get Faulkner back to New Zealand as soon as possible. Even so he did not embark from Egypt until mid-December. On New Year's Day, 1946, he wrote to Alice, 'Saw the S[outhern] Cross a couple of nights ago lowdown [*sic*] on the horizon & the bow pointed straight to it – sentimental perhaps, but it was good to see, as it meant just Home.'[89] His ship berthed at Lyttelton on 13 January 1946 and two days later he arrived by train in Auckland. On 1 February he and Alice left for a holiday in the South Island. On the way they spent three days in Wellington, where Alice sat the examinations that were to make her the first New Zealand woman member of the Royal Australasian College of Physicians. They returned to Denestone at the end of the month to face, for the first time, life together in a world that was not at war.

CHAPTER 5

Full Use of Her Talents

> *Every girl should be trained to make full use of her talents, and to develop to the full her personality.*[1]

The war years had unsettled Alice's life on many levels but one thing that emerged intact was her faith in the power of the individual to influence social change. She was not sanguine when she looked about her, but she had already determined that the world could be put to rights and that she and Faulkner had a part to play. In late 1944 she wrote to him,

> I agree with you that the moral and ethical state of society is punk, but doesn't that fill you with a desire to correct it, to weild [sic] every little bit of power and influence that you possess to improve it? One can't be human and not recognise that one has a stake in humanity, one can't pass by on the other side where the world is concerned . . . you & I have to fight with all our brains and all our strength so that our children and other people's shall have a chance.[2]

This was just the sort of talk Faulkner liked to hear. He found it easier to accept the demands of Alice's career when she played the traditional medical woman's role of social benefactor. During the war he had visited a contemporary of hers who was living and practising in Italy and found her 'attitude to medicine' to be 'just too purely pathological ... a career rather than a calling'. The 'elements of true greatness', he had assured Alice, 'were with you & not c her'.[3] But even this potential for social good would not overcome his initial difficulties in facing daily life with a woman doctor working full time and heading towards specialisation. Before taking on the problems of society Alice had to divert a considerable amount of energy to sorting out the 'little world' into which she had hoped she and Faulkner could 'retreat ... somewhere where we can get a respite from strife'.[4]

Partly because of the acute postwar housing shortage they continued to live at Denestone. Although there were often quite large numbers of people living there, the household ran reasonably smoothly. Help was still employed but Alice's greatest domestic asset was Aunty Betty, a retired nurse and Joseph's oldest sister, who had come to live with her brother. Energetic and helpful, she was regarded by Alice as 'a jewel' and,[5] until her health failed in the mid-1950s was a capable resident supervisory presence who fitted happily into the family. Reintegrating Faulkner into domestic and civilian life was more of a problem. Recognising that this was not an easy time for him, Alice tried to smooth his way but, as a fulltime working professional woman, she faced particular difficulties. Although he would grow into the role of supportive husband, Faulkner did not start out any better, or worse, than most men of his time. The demands of Alice's career had their place while he was overseas but he did not find them as agreeable on his return home. The immediate postwar years would almost destroy their marriage.

Not only was there now potential for face-to-face conflict on a daily basis, but differences had to be ironed out in a house where several other family members lived. Moreover, despite the fact that he had diplomatically vacated the spacious main bedroom for Alice and Faulkner, Joseph was still the head of the house and Alice continued to act as his confidante and, when necessary, as his hostess. 'We all adhered to Joe who was the true father figure,' Faulkner wrote in later years, 'and a wonderful father too.'[6] But at the time he did not find the situation easy and he was not a man to hide his feelings: 'you can be very difficult sometimes,' Alice wrote to him while he was visiting his mother in 1946, '& to know that underneath you really appreciate things can be cold comfort.' Alice turned to her new professional interest, suggesting to Faulkner that he should undergo psychoanalysis to help manage his obvious stress. Since Faulkner had described this technique in 1940 as 'largely bunk, a whim created for the luxury of the expensive hypos' [presumably wealthy hypochondriacs],[8] it says much for her powers of persuasion, or Faulkner's unhappiness, that, at the end of March 1946, he began regular analysis which he eventually found beneficial.[9]

At the same time Alice made it quite clear that she would be continuing with her professional ambitions. Over 1946 she steadily advanced her plans to travel to London as a candidate for membership of the Royal College of Physicians (MRCP), the acme of postgraduate qualification by examination. Many of her male peers who had served in the armed forces were already going directly to Britain from their service postings, funded by rehabilitation schemes that included both study bursaries and travel costs.[10] Alice would have to pay her own way. She planned to leave at the end of 1947 when her contract with Sayers terminated but, since passages on ships were at a premium, preliminary bookings were made at the end of 1946.[11] A few months later, Alice discovered she was pregnant. She and Faulkner were overjoyed; they had been trying to conceive from the time of his return, but an infant was going to significantly increase the cost of the trip. A Karitane nurse, Lola McKellar, was engaged to care for the baby while they were away, but this added a return adult fare, her fee and keep to their total expenditure. The question of finance was a constant worry to Faulkner, particularly when the Education Board refused him leave without pay, making his future teaching career unsettled.[12] Alice seems to have shouldered much of the expense, since Faulkner believed that the venture cost her all she had saved since entering private practice.[13] It is likely, however, that he was expected, and would have wished, to make some contribution and this may well have emphasised in his eyes just how much smaller his earning capacity was than his wife's.

Alice knew exactly what she wanted, but Faulkner seemed unable to come to a decision. He completed his law degree in February 1946 and began fulltime study for a master's, using Education Board leave and rehabilitation finance. At the end of May he entered a returned soldiers' course on full pay at the Auckland Teachers' Training College and, though he completed his second degree, he returned permanently to teaching in November 1946. Faulkner later put this unexpected change of direction down to the lack of encouragement he felt he received from those with whom he and Alice had raised the idea of his entering the law. To him, this seemed to be a rebuff for the energies he had put into his studies, which he had seen as an answer to criticism for 'not having made better efforts at "self-improvement"'.

> I think that [the lack of encouragement] fixed it and Alice said "OK if you're in the law and you do any good I'll have to eat into my thing to be more social with you than I would if you were a teacher". So that was just about that. The term back at Training College on pay settled it early.... She was with me all the way.[14]

But, given Faulkner's already fragile self-esteem, could it really have been as simple as that, and was he with Alice all the way?

It seems not. While Alice continued with her preparations, he continued to agonise. Alice worked until the day before she gave birth to a son, Peter Joseph, on 17 September. By now she was 33 and Faulkner 37 years old.[15] In November she took the baby with her when she travelled to Wellington to attend a postgraduate course on paediatrics and then on to Dunedin to make some last-minute arrangements concerning her overseas trip. Before she left she had written to the Auckland Hospital Board requesting that the 11 weeks special maternity leave she had been granted be extended until the end of her present term of appointment 'as I am hoping to travel to England early in the New Year'. Since she expected to be away for over 12 months, she added, she would not be reapplying for her position in the 1948 biennial staff elections.[16] Even at this late stage, Faulkner did not seem to have decided whether he wished to be involved in the enterprise, or even in a future married life with Alice. On 22 November she wrote to him from Dunedin,

> when I get back we will have to get underway with preparations & I shall be requiring your assistance. You will be able to tell me whether you would rather have your freedom. This is the first time I have been away for any length of time since you came back. I feel it is a good thing, you can take stock of things & make up your mind whether I am worth putting up with the obligations that my presence involves. I feel that your analysis must now be sufficiently advanced for you to put it to some practical use, you should be able to bring an unclouded judgement to

bear on your problems & make up your mind whether you want a wife & family or not, & if I am the right one. You can't have it both ways, a bachelor existence with a wife in the background – not with me anyway, though I promise not to make unnecessary demands upon you. Your son will make demands too, you know, & it's only by meeting them you'll enjoy the full glory of being his father.[17]

Obviously they had reached a crisis point in their relationship. Alice was determined to continue with both her career and her marriage; Faulkner would have to decide if he wished to be her husband on these terms. Faulkner finally made up his mind to go with Alice. They sailed from Lyttelton for Britain on 20 December 1947.[18]

Despite Faulkner's doubts, the trip to Britain proved as important to their personal lives as to Alice's professional life. For the first time they functioned as a nuclear family unit. Their tiny flat in Wimbledon was their first 'home' in that sense, free from extended family and inherited customs and routines. This period set the pattern for many of the small practices of their future married life. Faulkner relieved Alice of the day-to-day management of their financial affairs. He also helped in small ways on the domestic front and took Peter for walks on the common and to the shops, enjoying with his son the experiences war had denied him with his daughter. Alice's courses usually involved weekday attendances and Faulkner did some teaching in London so that the Karitane nurse often took time off during weekends, leaving Alice, Faulkner and Peter to enjoy family life. At other times Alice and Faulkner would go on walking tours, leaving Peter with Lola. In many ways, however, this was an unreal phase. Faulkner would still have to return to everyday life as the husband of a practising doctor and his time away may have dealt the death blow to his own career. When they returned to New Zealand he was nearly 40 years old and had spent much of the previous decade out of teaching.

For Alice the experience was undoubtedly a professional success. She was in her mid-30s, could expect to work for at least another 20 years and was at a similar career stage to her male peers who had lost time through war service. But she was also the mother of an infant son who had broken nights and would be settled by no one else. The stress of gaining her membership hung over her head for the whole of 1948 and in June she forgot to sit her preliminary paper. While doing a course in Cambridge, she had tea with Margaret Gatman, a New Zealand woman doctor visiting England. When the latter confessed to Alice that she felt guilty because she was neither working nor studying, Alice answered, 'Don't'.[19] By the time she and Faulkner had packed and embarked for the voyage home, on 6 May 1949, Alice was 'tired and ready to rest' and in the early stages of another pregnancy.[20] Although she took up her medical interests on her arrival in New Zealand, she did not return to work until the new year. Life at Denestone was also quieter. During their absence Joseph had been appointed to the Supreme Court bench so spent more of his time out of town, and the rest of the family were living in homes of their own. On Christmas Day, with the birth of her second daughter, Christine Mary, Alice felt she could truly make a new beginning. She wrote to a family friend, 'when I see my children together I know I shall be able to feel that the bitterness has gone from old memories, and only the sweetness remains.'[21]

Nevertheless Alice still badly needed Faulkner's support to continue with her career in postwar New Zealand. Although increasing numbers of married women were entering the paid workforce, these were generally difficult years to balance the demands of a family and a job. On the one hand, a booming export economy, a protected manufacturing industry and a shortage of labour created both a demand for women workers and a host of desirable products on which extra household income could be spent. On the other hand, family-focused government policies and the security promised by the welfare state encouraged a much wider section of the community to aspire to the previously middle class ideal of family life based on a single, male, breadwinner. These developments resulted in considerable practical problems for employed married women, especially those who were mothers. They usually worked in jobs that lacked social status, were poorly paid, not particularly interesting, offered few opportunities for advancement and had no childcare facilities. The usual solution was to work part time; the justification, their economic contribution to the household income to buy 'extras'. Women's work was therefore subsumed into their family identity.[22]

Even so, ideological tensions remained. During the late 1940s, popular magazines that had encouraged women to participate in the war effort now carried authoritative articles urging them to focus their energies on husband, family and home.[23] By the early 1950s proponents of these theories claimed the added authority of science when Dr John Bowlby issued a report for the World Health Organisation (WHO) entitled *Maternal Care and Mental Health* (later published as a book, *Child Care and the Growth of Love*). Bowlby, a child psychiatrist, had become deputy director of the Tavistock Clinic in London after the war.[24] In 1950 he was temporarily appointed to the WHO to study the mental health of children living in institutions – not refugees but those 'homeless in their native country'.[25] Central to Bowlby's findings was the notion of 'maternal deprivation', that the early experience of 'a warm, intimate, and continuous relationship with his mother (or permanent mother-substitute) in which both find satisfaction and enjoyment' was essential for a child's development and future mental health.[26] 'Maternal deprivation', with its intensification of the mother's role and its preference for almost any kind of home care over institutionalisation, signalled a major shift in childcare ideology and was taken up by various groups to different ends. Among the causes Bowlby listed as contributing to the failure of the 'natural home group' to care for the child was 'Full-time employment of mother'.[27] Alice, with her well-paid, interesting and socially acceptable career could avoid many of the practical problems of other working mothers, but her particular interest in early childhood and the psyche should have made her especially vulnerable to Bowlby's arguments. How could Alice both support his thesis (and she did) and work long hours when her two children, particularly her infant daughter, were within the age group that was at maximum risk?

We know that Bowlby's theories appealed to Alice because her papers contain a review of *Maternal Care and Mental Health*, undated but fairly certainly written soon after the report's release, which offers no criticism of its research, argument or conclusions. To see Alice as a Bowlby convert, however, would be inaccurate. Rather, they were fellow travellers. His interest in mental health, the first five years of a child's life, the provision of marriage and child guidance services and the training of physicians, nurses, social workers and others in psychology, were already shared by many of those preoccupied with family and child welfare. They were based on psychosexual theories and new approaches to education and child development that derived from several sources, including Havelock Ellis and Sigmund Freud. Elements of this new philosophy had been introduced to New Zealand as early as the 1930s by visitors such as the educationalist Susan Isaacs, returning New Zealanders such as Dr Maurice Bevan Brown, and immigrants such as Dr Enid Cook. Relevant literature had been transmitted throughout the country by educational networks, particularly the New Education Fellowship, and the emerging social sciences. Central to this ideology was the concept that

> It is the conditions of life in the earliest years which most determine the future – whether a child becomes mentally ill or delinquent, or develops into a useful and satisfactory parent and citizen.[28]

Parents therefore needed to be educated

> ... in the mental and emotional development of the child as a person and the importance to its future life in the community of establishing in the home the habits of right relationships – parent and child – child with child, etc.[29]

By the time Bowlby's writings appeared, groups were already established which championed these new ideas and regarded the early Plunket Society and kindergarten focus on nutrition and authoritarian socialisation as limited and outmoded. Instead, they concentrated on nurturing the mental and emotional health of parents and children through education, psychological understanding and enriched personal relationships. Here was the inspiration for the concern of Parents' Centres with natural childbirth and early bonding, and Play Centres with parentally involved preschool education. The Family Guidance Centre, Marriage Guidance and the New Zealand Family Planning Association looked to the relationship between parents themselves and its influence on their children. To achieve their aims they needed to overcome traditional ideas of sexuality as a 'closet' subject and challenge existing associations between birth control and immoral or extramarital sexual activity, or, in the case of condoms, venereal disease. Contraception was now to be seen as essential for more acceptable ends, spacing births and allowing parents time for a more intense relationship with their existing offspring while they continued to enjoy a sexual life free of the fear of pregnancy and of the frustration and tension so damaging to their own mental health and bonds within marriage. They would pass these benefits on to their children by their happy example and free discussion of sexual matters, avoiding inhibitions and ensuring good marital relations for the next generation.

Since the early 1940s, Alice had been mixing in circles where such ideas were freely discussed, and involved in activities and groups that were fostering them. Her familiarity with them meant she read Bowlby's writings more accurately than many. Although he occasionally extended his argument to extremes, at one point talking of a mother-child relationship in terms of the 'provision of constant attention day and night, seven days a week and 365 in the year',[30] Alice recognised that the institutionalised children Bowlby had studied had suffered 'serious interference' in familial relations.[31] For this reason she did not believe his book was one for the average parent, a category which, under these criteria, would have included herself. Rather, it was 'for those whose privilege and responsibility it is to guide and instruct parents of today and tomorrow and help them with their problems',[32] and here she clearly did include herself because she was referring to

> ... doctors, who must sometimes send children into hospital ... nurses who care for them there ... members of the Child Welfare Department ... Orphanage Boards ... the Matrons and staffs who care for the homeless child. Schoolteachers would find here the reasons why some children present almost insoluble problems at school, and Magistrates and Probation Officers would gain greater insight into some aspects of their work from a study of these pages.[33]

Alice's later writings reflect the concerns she shared with Bowlby about the need for quality parenting, measured principally in terms of emotional nurturing in the child's earliest years, but she had absorbed this message long before. It was the problems arising from institutionalisation that made this work important to her. These contributed to her and Bowlby's approval of early adoption when a single mother could not immediately support herself and her baby.[34] Such ideas were also influential in Alice's approach to hospital paediatrics and the care of the mentally ill, but, unlike some fervent supporters, they did not lead her to interpret Bowlby's writings as an argument against any mother working or spending time outside the home. She fully agreed with Bowlby's argument that mothers of very young children should not be forced to work purely for financial reasons, a contingency he argued could be overcome by realistic, graded, family allowances with the largest benefits for mothers of children under three years of age. Then, children should be able to cope with attendance at a day nursery.[35] The idea of family benefits that could help to keep mothers out of the paid workforce was widely supported in a post-Depression, postwar world. For many women, sub-standard housing, lack of basic amenities and often poor health meant that they could do without the extra burden of going out to an unrewarding job. Alice herself found it 'deplorable that any mother should have to park her babies in a day nursery and go out to work just because the family finances cannot be met otherwise.'[36]

Any suggestion that she was promoting a broader argument – that mothers should not work outside the home at all – is removed by her already established support for equal pay,[37] and the context in which this statement was set. It appeared in an essay entitled 'Is Motherhood Enough?', published under Alice's own name in a booklet called *Men and Women*, produced by the National Council of Churches in New Zealand in 1953. It was therefore written almost concurrently with her Bowlby review and argued that for women to restrict their role to the purely domestic was good neither for them nor for their families, though the alternative would depend on 'circumstances, financial considerations, individual aptitudes and ambitions'. Some women might choose to re-enter the paid workforce, some to follow other pursuits, but all, Alice proposed, should be trained for a career which

> should be considered not just as a means of keeping herself and filling in time until she gets married, but in its relationship to her whole life, something that is worthwhile putting an effort into in the first place, and which will enrich her marriage by giving her experience and understanding of the realities of life, and something to which she can come back when her domestic duties become less onerous and allow her more freedom.

Since this essay, with its implications of self-fulfilment and possible economic independence for women after marriage and motherhood, was written at a time generally regarded as a feminist wasteland in New Zealand, it is worth looking at in some depth. 'Is Motherhood Enough?' illustrates the way in which, lacking a contemporary coherent feminist ideology, Alice co-opted and extended old and new authorities to sustain her position. Even Edith Summerskill's arguments, so cogent during the war, were not central here. Alice paid more attention to the advantages for individual women than to any benefit their special qualities would bring to their job or the community at large. Where Alice did address community good, in an introductory paragraph headed 'The Principle', she relied on the Nonconformist belief that individual advancement would ultimately result in communal advantage, underpinning this argument with an allusion to the parable of the talents.

> ... to live the full life includes the development of all those talents with which we may be endowed. It is not selfish to desire to enrich our own lives to the fullest extent to which we may be capable, it is our bounden duty, for though individuals we are also "members one of another" and the good of the whole community is the result of good things accomplished by its separate constituents.

There were also direct and indirect references to the various interests of the groups she was supporting and their potential role in enriching the lives of women and their families. She presented birth control as a practical necessity. Parenting was still seen as an important part of women's experience, but 'Is Motherhood Enough?' urged that it should not predominate, arguing that 'human life is broader and deeper than the mere continuance of the race' and several times citing the necessity for small families if women were not to be confined to the domestic scene for too long. At the same time, Alice did not downgrade the value of work in the domestic area. She pointed out that many women enjoyed such activities and she saw no reason why paid domestic service should not become 'quite a popular profession' as long as the attitudes of employers were 'more humane' than they had been in the past: there must be proper working conditions, reasonable hours of duty and 'a status in the community commensurate with the responsibilities they [domestic workers] undertake'.

Alice's interest in emotional and mental health was discernible in the priority she accorded to personal family relationships over household tasks such as cleaning and cooking, and in her suggestions that every woman needed 'to develop to the full her personality', 'to find herself completely satisfied'. She urged women not to accept relationships which demanded that their needs be made subservient to those of other family members. She described a husband who was unable to accept his wife 'as an equal' as insufficiently mature, 'demanding that his ego be built up by having a woman to wait upon him'. Neither should a mother's ambitions be overridden by those of her children, since an 'intelligent and capable woman' would 'seldom find herself completely satisfied to remain just the housekeeper while her growing children forge steadily towards their own independence'. Nor did Alice accuse the working mother of maintaining a lifestyle that would lead to symptoms of maternal deprivation in her children. It was the more mundane problem of lack of household help and child minding services, not the dangers of separation, which Alice cited as barriers for mothers taking paid work until the youngest child was at least school age. Too intense a relationship between mother and child was actively discouraged as

> too heavy a burden to ask any child to bear. A mother is a better mother for having a full and satisfying life of her own, she will love her children the more happily for not feeling sacrificed for them and as she loosens them from dependence on her she may become their loved and much valued friend and advisor.

Perhaps the most striking feature of 'Is Motherhood Enough?' is its combination of theoretical argument with practical advice to sustain mothers in their new, challenging role. Despite Alice's relatively advantaged career and domestic situation her suggestions were based on shared experience, down-to-earth and within the reach of most. Although she diplomatically described a husband's 'willing cooperation' as 'the first essential' in lightening the working mother's domestic load, Alice urged her readers to make sure that their first earnings were directed towards purchasing

> an electric dishwasher, to be followed by any other gadget that will make the housework easier. Only when the mechanical labour of housework is reduced to the absolute minimum will she find life anything but hectic unless reliable help is available.

Even with mechanical aids and smaller families, working mothers needed to develop 'a proper sense of perspective'. They must accept that they could no longer do everything and confine themselves to those things that no one else could do. Housework and cooking did not rate highly when there were children to consider. But mothers were also assured that limited time with one's children was not, of itself, limiting, since

> the reality of family life lies not in the number of hours that the members spend in the home, but in the personal relationship that exists between them. The woman who devotes to her children one hour each day, may be closer to them, and have more influence over their development than a woman who considers she spends her whole waking time at the service of her family, but who is so occupied with the material aspects of that family's comfort that she fails to maintain the one essential of accessibility to the small child, without which she must always remain a somewhat shadowy figure.

It was at this point, where theory met practice, that Alice was uniquely qualified to address the problems of working mothers and in this sense her essay can be seen as a vindication of her own struggle, a demonstration that she believed it had been worthwhile. No 1950s woman was more aware that maintaining a relationship acceptable to one's husband and children within an unusual lifestyle was extremely difficult. Alice had argued that specialisation within her profession would allow her to control her commitments to accommodate her family's needs. In theory this was true. She had 'office hours' in her private practice, and regular 'sessions' at Auckland Hospital and at Karitane. She kept one afternoon a week free, intending to spend that time with her children. But it was not long before theory broke down. There were unexpected calls, meetings, speaking engagements and medical conferences, all of which meant nights out and sometimes several days away from home. Phoebe Meikle, in her autobiography, *Accidental Life*, recalls a story Alice told her.

> She and her daughter Christine, then about four years old, were playing a ball game when Alice saw it was time for her to leave for the hospital. Christine cried and begged her not to go. "But, darling," Alice said, "Mummy must go and look after the little sick children." "Why don't you dead the little sick children", said Christine.[38]

Phoebe Meikle points out, quite rightly, that 'because upper-middle-class working mothers were rare, their children found more difficulty than they would today, in sharing their mother with a profession'. Given adult hindsight and in a different social climate, Christine would not voice the same criticism,[39] but Alice was dealing with a problematic present. There must have been many occasions when she linked the complaints common to all children directly to the demands of her working life, producing the same niggling doubts she experienced when Lesley cried as she left for work. The fact that Alice took as much delight and satisfaction from motherhood as she did from her career can only have intensified her dilemma. In later life she vacillated untypically when expressing herself on the experience of working while her children were young. She told journalist Valerie Davies that she regretted returning to work so soon after their birth.[40] On the other hand, speaking to a group of fellow doctors, she was sanguine in addressing the conflict between the demands of family and profession: 'I've no doubt their [women doctors'] children have felt ill used at times, but then how few children find their parents without fault'.[41] But in a letter to Peter, a belated attempt to mark his 21st birthday over two weeks before, she ruefully admitted to feeling 'very guilty' because she had not written 'in time for the very day'. 'Perhaps that is typical of my attempts at motherhood, important things have sometimes been put off,' she added.[42] The letter, which was never posted, was found by Faulkner after her death.

Alice's problems in adjusting her personal and professional lives obviously continued long after she had written 'Is Motherhood Enough?'. Although she and Faulkner eventually reached a comfortable accommodation, their marriage was always unusual in that the demands of Alice's career dominated the couple's choices. Underpinning Faulkner's gradual acceptance of this situation was the fact that he was less driven than his wife. He enjoyed teaching and was good at it, but he could take or leave work. For Alice, it seems often to have been the reason for life. Faulkner's postwar career path was therefore considerably less demanding on their domestic arrangements. It was not until 1964 that he was appointed headmaster of Avondale Primary School after 14 years as '3rd man' on the staff of Manukau Intermediate School.[43] At the same time, Alice's belief in the value of education meant that she respected Faulkner's work. She also supported him in practical ways, transporting him to and from meetings (he did not drive), turning up at special functions, speaking at a headmasters' meeting and 'judging' the babies at a school fair.

There were also emotional factors to be taken into account. Faulkner learned to identify with and take pride in Alice's professional achievements, but his anti-élitism still tended to surface when she mixed with her medical colleagues outside working hours. He could be morose and grumpy and was sometimes seen to 'put Alice down' in social situations.[44] In May 1955, when Alice was elected first New Zealand woman fellow of the Royal Australasian College and travelled to Sydney to have her fellowship conferred, he stayed home with the children while she was accompanied by her father. Faulkner did not record why Joseph, and not he, escorted Alice and his story gives no indication that this was a matter for contention, though he does say that, during her absence, he was 'sad' on one occasion and 'depressed at night' on another.[45] A letter from Alice, written while she was in Sydney, suggests that he had refused to go.

> I couldn't help wondering all along the line whether you would have enjoyed it. I think you would have you know, or would you have been like Margaret Dods? who was just cross with her husband because she didn't get a chance to tell Mr Menzies how bad she thought his speech was. I would rather like to know her better, I think she is interesting, but perhaps a bit uncomfortable at times.[46]

The fact that Alice did not opt to have her fellowship conferred *in absentia*, shows that she was prepared to accommodate Faulkner only to a certain point. The Sydney trip provided the kinds of professional and social opportunities that delighted her. She visited the Institute of Child Health, the Mosman Spastic Centre and Dr Clare Ibister 'with whom I had a most delightful hour – she has 4 children and a very good reputation here as a Paediatrician & has written good articles in journals'. When she and Joseph dined at the home of a Sydney judge Alice revealed the artless side to her character, which allowed her to take particular pleasure in special events. She wrote of the 'delicious food', and 'all the trappings, Finger bowls & wines', and of a fellow guest 'who wore real pearls, & I'm pretty sure her earrings were real diamonds'. The ultimate, the 'thrilling occasion', though, was her installation. After dinner with Professor Lorimer Dods and Dr Howard Williams ('the best man in Australia where the really sick child is concerned'), the party proceeded to the Great Hall at the university.

It was a gay scene with many kinds of academic robes, & a good deal of gold lace around .... the other Fellows were presented to the President & had to bow to the G[overnor]. G[eneral]. I went up 2nd. I think I must have had just the right amount to drink, for I felt that it was a triumphal march, & walked with firm step & made my curtsies with such confidence that I was afterwards complimented on all sides, & even by the G.G. himself.

Menzies oration was, I think, a masterpiece.... Then to supper ... the President introduced us to the G.G. who chatted most charmingly for a few moments ... & then to top it all Ted [Sayers] took us off to someone who introduced us to the P.M. & he & father got quite deeply into some legal shop & I just stood by happily. Daddy was in fine form, genial, & not too hearty, & I was proud of him & pleased to be able to help a little in giving him what was I think, quite a thrill.[47]

Alice's account of this event also indicates her ongoing commitment to being a good daughter, which would continue until Joseph's death in October, 1963.[48] It must have been very frustrating for a rumbustious character like Faulkner having to share his wife's attentions with a father-in-law who was composed, courteous, generous, a successful public figure through his own effort and the recipient of a knighthood in 1957. What was worse, Faulkner recognised that the qualities he admired in Alice, a mixture of modesty and determination, humility and pride, were ones she shared with her father.[49] In later life, when Faulkner reflected on relations between them, he rationalised any tension

> For her part, she was always an excellent daughter, and knew him as a Father Image all right [sic]. She always felt that what he wanted done should be done. There were times when I thought I suffered as a result. Looking back it's so easy to see how false that was.... Perhaps it was me and I didn't like having to share her.[50]

Unlike Joseph, Faulkner was never the model middle class spouse. Placing himself in Alice's life after her death, he looked to this very difference. 'Thinking this a[.]m[.] of my unsuitability as a husband for Alice,' he wrote in December 1974. 'No other woman Dr in NZ has attained her eminence however acceptable their spouses. Sh[oul]d have thought of this before Joe died.'[51] In this he may well have been right. Alice, as a mature married woman, was prepared to challenge the system if she thought the ends justified the means. Joseph, the lawyer, was not. Alice herself reflected on that difference in terms of professional perspectives in a speech to the Medico-Legal Society delivered a few years after Joseph's death.

> ... doctors and lawyers are just about as different from each other as women are from men ... for we do look at things almost from completely opposite points of view. ... To the lawyer, sin is almost a concrete thing, he can define it, indeed with his laws he says what is sin and what is not. ... But from the point of view of the doctor sin is a very different matter ... we are not too certain that we know what it is, and we are even more uncertain whether we know who was responsible for it and indeed whom we should punish. And I am afraid we lack the simple faith that punishment will keep sin under control.[52]

As much as Alice loved her father, and kindly and generous though he might have been, life at Denestone became more relaxed after Joseph's death as the little formalities that had been maintained in deference to him began to slip away. Visitors who might have expected pomp and ceremony behind the still imposing facade were met by an almost shabby interior, but first impressions were soon overcome by the vitality of occasions when conversation buzzed and ideas flew. Alice was generous with her home for meetings, receptions for overseas visitors, accommodation for family, friends and sometimes even strangers. She loved a party and people and had a loyal band of supporters who would help on such occasions.[53] It was not a lifestyle that would have found favour with the fastidious or the pretentious but it certainly suited Faulkner. It was a rejection of the ostentation and display of wealth which he had always found so unnerving. Alice was 'always so right in her priorities,' he wrote, '& forget the unessentials – this suited me & was another reason we did so well together'.[54]

Time, and a considerable commitment from Alice to their 'little world', resolved almost all their difficulties. Faulkner found a comfortable niche for himself in the classic New Zealand male retreats of sport and beer. Here he could create his own persona, raising the roles of sideline commentator and pub debater to an art form.[55] Alice was happy for him to have these outlets. Coming as she did from a family where many of her father's contemporaries had been and remained 'temperance folk', she had found Faulkner's drinking difficult to accept, but this issue was resolved between them as early as 1945,[56] and there is no evidence to suggest that it was ever a major bone of contention. Faulkner claimed that Alice only once suggested he should cut down and she never became teetotal herself. Given her professional interests, Alice was probably better prepared than most women to handle any personal relationship problems that came her way. It may well have been no revelation to her to have read a comment Faulkner made after her death: 'I feel equality with men while drinking'.[57]

Alice and Faulkner's relationship was both unusual for its time and yet painfully of it. Jock Phillips has examined the stresses that arose from the mixture of assertiveness and the 'psychological need for a wife who would succour and support him', a 'new "Mum"', which New Zealand men brought to marriage from the 1920s to the 1950s.[58] Alice's correspondence articulates this delicate, and ultimately unsatisfactory, balancing act. During the first years of her marriage she frequently addressed Faulkner as 'Precious Child' or 'P.C.' but soon after Lesley's birth she began dropping the term and in August 1944, when Lesley was almost a year old and Alice's career was burgeoning, she wrote,

> You may know now, once & for all, that I didn't marry you because you were helpless. I married you as an equal because I believed that you too had a soul, & that real things meant more than superficial ones to you, as I like to think they do to me. Forgive me darling, but sometimes I feared I might have made a mistake, & that I would have to mother you all our life together. That gave me a lot of pleasure, the mothering, but I've just wondered what would happen when I wanted to do the leaning. I've lived on with that hope deep within me that my original feeling was right, & since you went away [in the army] the conviction has been growing, & with it my love for you, it isn't just a mother's love, my own, or just the passion of youth, both these come into it, but as well there is a dependence, a feeling that only you can make all things right. Do you understand? Don't ever be deceived by my show of independence ... I need you just as much as any shrinking violet needs her man.[59]

Even in later life, when social roles were beginning to change, Faulkner's personality remained the same uneasy combination of brashness and sensitivity. That Alice was painfully aware of his feelings is evident in her letters to him. Whatever their content they always ended with assurances of her complete devotion – although this stopped short of imposing his restrictions on herself. In 1965 she wrote,

> I think of you often. It would not be truthful to say that I miss you, for life is so packed full there is not time for more, but repeatedly I bless you for the maturity and tolerance which have allowed me to follow a way of life, which has led to this most stimulating experience.[60]

It was not until the early 1980s, as his own life neared its end, that Faulkner could himself reflect:

> As time went on I became more & more proud of her, & more & more co-operative & helpful in her activities. I think Alice was tough enough mentally to reach the top whatever I did. Like her father she was tremendously determined ... I must say that, in real terms, any "sacrifice" I made was minimal, & immeasurably recompensed by the life I was able to lead with this supreme woman.[61]

It was really a matter of accepting the inevitable. By the 1950s it must have been clear that determination and aiming high were both essential and continuing elements of Alice's personality.

CHAPTER 6

The Specialist

> *All fields of medicine are open to women. In the practice of paediatrics however, they probably have a real advantage and perhaps that is why in this country those women who have specialised in medicine have tended to concentrate on the younger age group and women specialising in adult medicine are rare.*[1]

Alice's approach to her mature medical career was characterised by the same urge to push boundaries that she applied to her personal life. During her lifetime, the career paths of women doctors tended to reflect their accepted social roles, concentrating them in what were generally regarded as low-status areas of the profession: public health, preventive medicine, sex education and the care of women and children. They did not usually advance to postgraduate qualifications and seldom competed with men for higher positions.[2] Although Alice concerned herself with preventive medicine, sex education and the care of children, she challenged the view that these were less important than the ground-breaking advances in medical technology which made popular medical heroes. She also competed with men on equal terms for higher qualifications and positions.

Nor does she fit neatly into the more general suggestion made in a 1972 survey of practitioners, that ultimate specialist status in medicine was more often the result of 'fortuitous circumstances' than the culmination of long-term strategies.³ 'Fortuitous circumstances' did undoubtedly play a part in Alice's career path, but so did commitment and strength of purpose, and long-term strategies were not absent or unfruitful. The unique professional opportunities of wartime New Zealand, the fact that Edward Sayers's practice attracted a considerable number of child patients,⁴ and that she inherited a Karitane Hospital post from him, could be described as fortuitous. Her preference for the Auckland Hospital children's wards in 1944 (if she were given the Green Lane appointment, she had written at the time, it would be 'better than nothing'⁵) was strategic. So, too, was her 1946 decision to work unpaid as a visiting paediatrician at the obstetric unit set up by the Auckland Hospital Board in vacated American service hospital buildings in Cornwall Park.⁶ Although the opportunity to sit the MRACP examination in Wellington in 1946 might be seen as fortuitous, commitment and strategy were also necessary. No concessions were made for those who wished to specialise in children's medicine which was, at the time, seen as adult medicine writ small and subject to exactly the same examination requirements as those undertaken by general physicians.

This was even more the case with the MRCP, with its demands of travel to Britain and submission to the most rigorous professional assessment. The examination was divided into three parts. The first consisted of two three-hour written papers and a shorter clinical section. After successfully completing this step, candidates proceeded to a viva. This was conducted by two pairs of examiners who posed a series of questions that could relate to almost any area of internal medicine, usually with some kind of pathological evidence as the starting point. Failure meant starting over again, but a good pass at this stage ensured that a final viva before the president and censors (examiners) of the college was almost a foregone conclusion.⁷ These events took place in an atmosphere that combined extraordinary tension with exquisite formality. To candidates the vivas seemed 'like an eternity'⁸ and the final one, when they faced the assembled hierarchy of the college dressed in their regalia, was a costumed theatre of power as daunting as a high court. One New Zealander who became a member during the late 1930s recalled being barely able to write the cheque to pay his membership fees after this ordeal because of the continued shaking of his hands.⁹ The failure rate was high and it was common to sit more than once. Alice first sat in April

1948, then again in July 1948, but did not succeed until January 1949. She followed Alice Campbell Rose (later Tallerman) (1927), Theodora Halls (1932) and Rosalind Latter (1935), to become the fourth New Zealand-trained woman doctor to achieve membership of the college.[10]

Because the London college did not run preparatory programmes for candidates,[11] there are no official records of the courses that Alice attended in Britain. In this she was, like her male peers, entirely on her own, and some of her choices reflected her particular interests. Before her departure she sought introductions to 'all the people who matter in the psychiatric world',[12] so it is very likely that she visited the Tavistock Clinic, which was not only a centre for the study of the psyche but also had a Department for Children and Parents and ran an Institute of Human Relations.[13] While in London she went to meetings of the Association of Allergy and visited the Fleming Institute, an allergy clinic.[14] She spent some time in Newcastle, Cambridge and Oxford.[15] Because an MRCP qualified doctors to practise as general physicians, she also sat for a Diploma in Child Health, generally regarded as a lightweight exercise in comparison with an MRCP but then the only formal qualification in paediatrics. As part of her preparation, she attended a course at the Children's Hospital in Great Ormond Street and visited Child Welfare Centres.[16] Towards the end of her stay she took part in a BBC Pacific radio programme as one of three women speakers comparing maternal and child health services in England, Australia and New Zealand.[17] Speaking to a meeting of the AKMWA after her return to New Zealand in mid-1949 she recalled her British experience in terms of widespread slum areas, an extensive school medical service, subsidised milk powder and free cod liver oil for children, a masseuse working with the congenitally spastic and the interest taken in the 'natural' childbirth theories of Grantley Dick Read.[18]

Alice's return at just this time may have been in itself a 'fortuitous circumstance'. New Zealand now had full employment, a booming economy and a newly elected National government cautious about interfering in popular social policies introduced by Labour. The family benefit, state housing at reasonable rentals, a minimum wage based on the premise that a male worker supported a family, free education and subsidised medical care gave the population the confidence to revert to a long-term trend that had been disrupted by Depression and war: more of them were marrying, and at a younger age. The result was a rapid rise in the birth rate, which continued until 1961.[19] These developments provided not only an expanding patient pool over the rest of Alice's working life but also governments and parents in a much better position to foster the health and welfare of children. And the Auckland Hospital Board was expanding and restructuring its services in the immediate postwar period, taking over United States' military hospitals in suburban Cornwall Park and Middlemore. Moreover, the idea that child health constituted a medical speciality was beginning to take root. In 1949, the Director-General of Health initiated a survey into the medical staffing of public hospitals in New Zealand. When the superintendent-in-chief of the Auckland Hospital Board saw the results he commented,

> It is surprising that Wellington and North Canterbury have neither a full-time nor a part-time pediatrician; but what is more surprising is that the Director-General of Health – (or the official who wrote on his behalf) – should infer that on grounds of economy this is a desirable state of affairs. In my opinion it is high time that the necessary appointments in this important speciality were made at all large hospitals.[20]

The same year, accommodation for children at Auckland Hospital, which had been the subject of criticism for some time, was transferred from the 30-year-old Princess Mary Hospital, a grandly named but outmoded two-storeyed brick structure, and an adjacent wooden building, to three wards in a recently vacated servicemen's block bordering the Domain. It was a spartan, 'temporary' affair but optimists continued to call the new premises the 'Princess Mary Hospital'. Those with their feet more firmly on the ground referred to the 'Princess Mary Block', or simply 'Princess Mary'.

Although children would continue to be admitted to specialist surgical wards in Auckland, Green Lane and Middlemore hospitals, and the new National Women's Hospital would deal exclusively with neonates, during Alice's lifetime Princess Mary remained the principal paediatric unit within Auckland Hospital Board structures. In 1949 it contained 120 beds, more than half of which were occupied by medical cases under the care of Sammy Ludbrook and his assistant.[21] This, along with the rising pressure to treat paediatrics as a speciality, provided the opening for an additional senior appointment at the beginning of 1950. Alice was tailor-made for the job. Since it was a new position, there was no sitting candidate and other applicants were either not as well qualified or could be accommodated in alternative positions for which they had also applied.[22] Had she delayed her re-entry into hospital medicine, her future career might have been very different. In February 1953 the president of the NZBMA referred to a survey in the Auckland province which had revealed that nearly half the doctors practising were now 'specialists'. As a result there were 'men with very high qualifications who cannot see any hope of securing the hospital appointments without which there can be no fulfilment of their careers'.[23]

Alice clearly felt that she held no sinecure, setting about consolidating her situation with a will. Within the hospital system it was customary for visiting doctors to supplement their primary appointment with at least one secondary post. In April 1952 Alice successfully applied for the position of physician-in-charge of an Allergy Clinic established at Auckland Hospital for inpatients and referrals from outpatient clinics.[24] The appointment was made when the payment of visiting staff was to be changed from a set stipend to a sessional rate, based on the number of 'tenths' of a week worked, so in June 1952 Alice's salary jumped from £650 to £865. This compared very favourably with the £470 then earned by assistant paediatricians with the same qualifications, if a little less practical experience and no secondary appointments.[25] During the same year she earned £25 for her teaching efforts on behalf of the Branch Faculty of the Otago Medical School, an obligation that was picked up to various degrees by senior medical staff.[26] Alice also took on unpaid responsibilities as a result of her hospital work and entered into the wider activities of the visiting staff, including membership of various hospital committees. These ranged from an advisory committee on the setting up a day school for children suffering from cerebral palsy,[27] to acting as a staff representative on the hospital board's Investigations Committee.[28] Alice was also a member of the Combined Medical Staff committee, which dated from the 1930s. She had taken a modest part in its deliberations before she went overseas.[29] On her return she re-entered its ranks with some authority when she correctly diagnosed a case of lymphatic leukaemia in a clinico-pathological exercise organised by a senior surgeon.[30] Membership of this influential body reflected the male dominance of visiting hospital appointments. There were a few women members, but there is no record of their holding office until 1970, when subcommittees of surgeons, physicians and paediatricians were established. Alice, the only woman included in any of these, became chairman of the Central Committee of Children's Specialists.[31]

Even in the mid-1950s, Alice was well-placed within hospital structures. When Ludbrook retired in 1954, she became the longest-serving senior paediatrician at Princess Mary. By that time hospital appointments in paediatrics had virtually dried up and paediatricians who would work with her for the rest of her life were already employed by the board. The care of children might be a woman's natural sphere, but at this level her peers were all men. Grahame Fox had replaced Ludbrook as a senior at Princess Mary and Ronald Caughey acted as assistant, while J.D. (Jack) Matthews and Leo Phillips held the paediatric appointments at National Women's Hospital. The barriers to entering hospital employment at this level persisted for some time, despite the pressure of increasing patient numbers, because the paediatricians themselves argued that there was insufficient private practice available in Auckland to sustain another part-time hospital appointment. Instead, the sessions of existing appointees were extended. It was particularly difficult to establish a private paediatric practice in the 1950s. General practitioners were more accustomed to referring children to various kinds of surgeons, neurologists or other medical specialists who took adults too. Those who were acutely ill or suffered from long-term problems that needed reassessment were usually sent to hospital. Alice's established reputation as an allergist would provide a valuable augmenting clientele for her own private practice.

Just before her appointment to Auckland Hospital she had taken a flat in a residential block, Cintra, in Whitaker Place, off Symonds Street. It was set up as both professional rooms and living accommodation for a nurse receptionist, whose wages were adjusted to pay her rent. This job went to Lola McKellar, the Karitane nurse who had accompanied Alice and Faulkner to England. She remembers that the practice was soon ticking over.[32] From the beginning Alice saw mostly children, but there was also a smaller but steady stream of adults. They came not only for the treatment of allergies and asthma but also for more general problems, including counselling or contraceptive advice. Since paediatricians were not usually to be found in provincial centres in the early 1950s, child patients came from the middle of the North Island and all areas to the north. For most of Alice's professional life, allergists remained a rare breed. Allergies were comparatively common, killed few, but made life a misery for many. Sufferers could exhibit seasonal hay fever, chronic rhinitis, asthma, eczema (and to these Alice added a variety of gastro-intestinal disorders and 'many systemic symptoms commonly considered to be psychogenic in origin'), in response to inhaling pollens, dusts, animal danders and the spores of moulds in the air, eating particular foods, or coming into skin contact with certain substances or some bacteria.[33] Identifying allergens was a process of trial and error which began with establishing the patient's history, paying special attention to their domestic and working environment and early feeding problems. Suspicions aroused here were further examined by skin testing and diet trials.[34] Multiple allergens and the effects of emotional tension or physical disability provided complicating factors.[35] Some families had a tendency to allergy.

Management of this problem could be a long and wearisome business, severely taxing the patience of both doctor and sufferer. Those with mild symptoms sometimes preferred to put up with them rather than embark on special diets, extended courses of desensitising injections, or the tedious maintenance of a dust-free home environment; the passage of time often brought about a cure sooner or later.[36] Within the medical profession, this field held little attraction for those fascinated by high technology, dramatic turnarounds and clear guidelines. It required a willingness to experiment in areas that were not always open to scientific demonstration and the confidence to take any resulting criticism. Because of her openness to new ideas, there were few things Alice would not try to seek relief for her patients. These included the contribution of disorganised binocular vision as a trigger in cases of asthma,[37] and the use of comfrey and hypnotism for the relief of respiratory obstruction.[38] In later life, she referred two cases of advanced cancer in children to a controversial and ultimately discredited therapist, Milan Brych.[39] Such a broadly based attitude was more unusual then than it might be considered today, but Alice's belief in cow's milk allergy (as opposed to intolerance) seems to have drawn most criticism from her peers. She placed its incidence in New Zealand at around 2–3 per cent,[40] and she was not mealy-mouthed in propounding her cause. In February 1962 she wrote in the *NZMJ*, 'It is well to remember that there is no food that cannot be a poison to some child. At the top of my list of poisons I put cow's milk.'[41]

For the unlucky mother of a baby or young child diagnosed by Alice as cow's milk allergic, life became extremely complicated. This was not the era of picking up an alternative at the local health food store. A recipe in Alice's papers for soya bean milk involved finely sifting soya bean flour, mixing it with sugar, salt and water, heating the mixture to boiling point in a double boiler, adding soya bean oil and thickening with arrowroot and dicalcium phosphate. This brew was then cooked for 45 minutes, stirring occasionally and adding water to allow for evaporation. Since a further typescript, on 'Milk Substitutes for Allergic Children', states that 'earlier attempts to feed babies on soya flour preparations nearly always produced quite severe diarrhoea and it was not possible to get satisfactory weight gains' (a technical problem that has since been overcome in commercial preparations), this was a tedious daily chore which produced questionable immediate results. A milk-free diet also meant no cream, cheese, butter, chocolates, toffees, ice cream or any preparation containing dried or condensed milk products, including buns, cakes, most meat sausages and some breads.

Alice's papers also include instructions for a 'homogenised meat mixture' (another cow's milk substitute), low-sucrose diets, cereal-free diets, fruit-free diets, low-leucine diets, diets for those suffering from phenylketonuria and food family lists, where allergy to one item indicated probable allergy to all. There were recipes using alternative ingredients and letters to local food manufacturers and retailers seeking details about the contents of products or proposing the manufacture of special items. For the lay person, it amounts to appalling evidence of the energy and determination needed to overcome the problems of food allergy sufferers. The discomfort and debilitation suffered by such people is also indicated by the fact that they regarded this undeniably difficult way of life as worthwhile. Some patients, though, did not agree and many medical professionals, including doctors, nurses and laboratory workers, thought Alice took this one too far – further than the evidence allowed. She had a slightly different attitude. In later life she wrote,

> I know I have been guilty of putting babies on diets eliminating milk and other foods when the child's distress has later proved to be due to

parental tension or to brain damage, but at least this gives one an excuse for maintaining an interest in the family and continuing support and observation. One might well say that prescription of a sedative for the child would provide an equal opportunity, but mothers demand something more than this. They will accept the sedative only if they consider that the doctor is also looking for a real cause of the child's distress.[42]

As Alice was aware, the care of children suffering from indeterminate but persistent complaints required particular responses in a doctor. Such cases could cause mothers not only acute personal distress but feelings of great frustration when medical professionals seemed not to be taking them seriously.[43] That Alice did added special lustre to her professional aura in many mothers' eyes. At the same time, since allergies were more common in children than adults, their treatment, which often extended over a considerable period of time, fitted in well with practice as a paediatrician and could lead to consultation in other areas of child health. In purely practical terms, though this is not how Alice would have looked at it, this was the stuff of which successful private practice was made.

The business skills Alice had already developed in her locum and partnership with Sayers, together with a natural prudence in economic matters, ensured her practice's financial success. Her basic attitude to money was a blend of frugality and generosity. Although she was inclined to practise economies in her personal expenditure, she was liberal in her dealings with people, or projects, she felt worthwhile. This was a long-standing characteristic. In 1944, when she wrote *Personal Relationships*, she donated profits from the sale of the book to the youth work of the YWCA.[44] Around the same time she complained to Faulkner, 'I do dislike extravagance in the daily routine.'[45] She made no secret of this, and few of her friends cannot recall some anecdote demonstrating her notions about necessary thrift. Alice could be generous about fees in cases of genuine hardship, but she was firm with those she believed could afford to pay. If accounts were not settled after correspondence, she was quite capable of threatening to put the matter in the hands of a collection agency.[46] By 1954 she felt financially secure enough to enter into a venture, along with three other specialists, which involved buying a house, Merivale, at 82 Symonds Street, and turning it into a suite of shared medical rooms.[47]

There was one aspect of her professional presence to which Alice paid comparatively little heed. As the pace of her working life quickened, she became less and less concerned with her appearance. This slide from grace had been hastened during the war years, when it was difficult for even the keenest follower of fashion to keep up appearances, and she was not unaware of how dreadful she often looked. 'There's no doubt that being busy all the time gets one into some slovenly habits,' she had written to Faulkner in June 1945. 'One neglects, of necessity certain things, one's wardrobe for example, & I sometimes wonder whether I'll be able to take an interest in my appearance again even when time does allow.'[48] There is also no doubt that, for some people, Alice's rather careless everyday appearance was especially noteworthy because she was a doctor, or rather a 'specialist'. Specialists were usually men, but they dressed impeccably. It was part of their aura. Elizabeth Hughes always dressed with understated smartness and authority. Alice was not devoid of any interest in her appearance. On formal occasions she could look so elegant that people who were used to seeing her in working gear were stunned. On the other hand, she often looked plain down at heel. For her admirers this became part of her appeal, her approachability, her 'difference'. For her detractors, it was just another of her shortcomings.

By the early 1960s, Alice had been a doctor for over 20 years, a specialist for 10, her private practice was established. She appeared as an 'expert' witness in court cases and was approached for her opinion in tussles over child custody. She was also one of a small group of local doctors available for advice as part of the early student health service at Auckland University.[49] As specialist paediatricians set up practice in provincial centres, the number of out-of-town patients who consulted her privately fell, but this was more than compensated for by Auckland's seemingly inexorable urban growth. Although the primary income earners in her patients' families covered a wide spectrum of occupations, they tended to be salaried or self-employed rather than waged workers.[50] In 1962 she was asked to give an opinion on the young son of the Governor-General, Lord Cobham. In the mid-1960s, when Merivale was bought by the University of Auckland, Alice moved into rented rooms at 88 Symonds Street, which she shared with a urologist, Ian Parton. All her working life Alice was ably supported, just as a male doctor would be, by her nurse-receptionists. Lola McKellar left in the late 1950s, to be replaced by a Viennese nurse, Sister C.A. Hanna.⁵¹ At 88 Symonds Street Alice shared a receptionist, Betty Neal.⁵² These women not only fielded her patients and performed day-to-day tasks around the rooms, but provided extra support, including occasional light meals when she was working and behind the scenes help with large functions at Denestone.

Alice's professional success distanced her to a degree from her fellow medical women. Despite her own belief that they had 'a real advantage' in the field of paediatrics, the area was attracting more men. When Alice attended the Medical Association's biennial conference in Auckland in February 1953, she was one of only 20 women among 500 men doctors.⁵³ Even within the NZMWA, there were concerns about lack of participation. During the 1950s the association's two branches were both struggling, despite a bid to gain publicity for the movement in the *NZMJ*.⁵⁴ With an official membership of 45 in 1959,⁵⁵ the Auckland branch attracted an average attendance of only 13 to meetings during the decade, and doctors who had graduated before 1940 kept its executive going.⁵⁶ Alice continued to give occasional papers and served as president in 1952, but even she seems to have been less committed than she had been during the 1940s. This must have been partly because of lack of time, but her atypical working role also limited her common professional interests with other members. In 1951, when the Paediatric Society was concerned about the possibility of Health Department intrusion into private practice, Alice raised the matter at the AKMWA general meeting. The attendance that evening totalled eight members and private practitioners were so poorly represented that it was decided to take no immediate action. The issue seems never to have arisen again.⁵⁷ This was not surprising. Any clashes between private practitioners and the Health Department must have placed medical women in an acutely embarrassing position, since for so many of them the regular hours offered in the department's employ were the only form of medical practice that would accommodate family commitments. There had been a much livelier reaction from the branch a month earlier when adjustments in Health Department salaries raised the spectre of a differential pay scale for men and women doctors working there.⁵⁸

The association's interests over the 1950s mirrored the marginal professional position of most women doctors and a narrowly focused feminist response to this. Medical politics were rarely discussed at AKMWA gatherings and women practitioners seldom participated in local NZBMA meetings.[59] On the infrequent occasions when wider issues arose, they evoked a conservative, if not a negative, reaction. In July 1950 the New Zealand Peace Council invited the association to send a representative to its meetings, and in 1958 requested a donation from the group.[60] On both occasions no action was taken, reflecting members' middle class and conservative origins at a time when 'peace' organisations were commonly seen as pro-Communist agencies. AKMWA members had a more comfortable relationship with the National Council of Women (NCW), the Federation of University Women and the Pan Pacific Women's Association, and their shared concerns about women's and children's health and welfare. But, even within conservative women's groups, women doctors occupied an unusual position. In 1958, when the aggregation of husbands' and wives' incomes for taxation purposes was upsetting employed AKMWA members, Elsie Davidge, one of their representatives at the NCW, cautioned them not to expect council support because many of its member organisations were against married women working.[61] Medical women were poised uneasily between professional structures, which demanded competition on equal terms, and the upholding of conservative social values, which required that they act like 'ladies', undemanding and always supporting their menfolk. Alice displayed this anomaly herself when, at the 1953 AKWMA annual meeting, she suggested that members might offer to help with morning and afternoon teas and occasional suppers for postgraduate courses.[62] This was a revealing gesture from a woman who had sought professional equality with her male peers.

During the 1950s, Alice's attention was principally directed towards nurturing paediatrics as a medical speciality. In 1946 she, Sammy Ludbrook and Elizabeth Hughes had constituted the organising committee that established the Paediatric Society of New Zealand.[63] Over the decade, principally because paediatricians were so thin on the ground, the executive remained in Auckland while membership was extended to any practitioner interested. The society's aims were wide-ranging, concerned not only with sick but also with well children, and not just with the child's body but also its psyche. A postgraduate educational programme was soon under way but establishing a place within child health structures was more of a problem, since the envisaged role was one of leadership and there were already established players in the field. Relations with the Plunket Society were eased by the fact that Plunket's medical directors, originally Helen Deem and, after her death, Neil Begg, also took a leading part in Paediatric Society affairs. Moreover, Plunket was a quasi-charitable, voluntary body whose lay membership welcomed the leadership of medical professionals. The state-run Health Department, with its school doctors, public health nurses and preschool clinics, was to prove more troublesome.

The Health Department had maintained a working relationship with private practitioners by confining the role of its medical personnel to diagnosis and referral. Any suggestion that Health Department doctors might be undertaking treatment was anathema to the NZBMA. When Auckland's medical officer of health announced in 1951 that he was establishing a Child Health Clinic, complete with consultant paediatrician, in the Department's city headquarters, Marinoto, the old bogey of a state health service raised its head. Alice was as inclined to this viewpoint as any. At a meeting arranged by the Paediatric Society to discuss the development with the new Director of Child Hygiene, Dr G.R. McLeod, on 10 July 1952, she complained that 'the policy adopted in the running of Marinoto strongly suggested that it represented the beginning of ... a full-time State salaried service'.[64] She was against the rapid expansion of the clinic and the use of the local media to publicise its activities,[65] though she had no objection to a small number of children being seen by a paediatrician employed by the department to provide educational opportunity for school medical officers, or to the Health Department instituting statistical research.[66] In 1959, when the department pressed for a larger role in child health services, criticising the Plunket Society's lack of accountability to the state, which was now heavily subsidising its activities, Alice again championed the role of the private practitioner. Together with the NZBMA president and the Wellington president of the College of General Practitioners (now promoting themselves as 'specialists' in family medicine), she presented, to a Consultative Committee on Pre-School Health Services,[67] submissions favouring the continuation of Plunket services and greater involvement of paediatricians and general practitioners in preschool preventive health.

Such episodes suggest that, at this time, Alice was at her most professionally conservative and yet in the early 1960s she would publicly turn her face against many of her peers. This apparent aberration is explained by Alice's theories about the responsibilities of the individual, which were twofold: first, to fully develop one's talents, and second, to use those developed talents to benefit society. During the 1940s and early 1950s she had concentrated on the first, establishing herself in the mould of classical professional success. By the late 1950s she was less comfortable in this position because she did not believe that the medical profession was taking its full share of social responsibility. This must have been particularly galling to her because several current developments were supporting the kinds of moves she most favoured. Many of the Medical Study Group's concerns had been addressed. Opportunities for postgraduate education within New Zealand had been expanded, hospital structures were increasingly departmentalised and psychiatry 'gradually but surely was being brought into its due relationship to general medicine'.[68] There was also a worldwide trend towards a broader approach to health issues. The influential postwar WHO placed new emphasis on the preventive aspects of environmental and social medicine and supported a team concept that included not only medical and paramedical personnel but also social workers, local and central government agencies, and voluntary groups.[69] The WHO had also broadened the definition of health to include 'a state of complete physical, mental, and social well-being, and not merely the absence of disease and infirmity',[70] and issued a Declaration of the Rights of the Child which included the right to be 'given the means requisite for its normal development, materially, morally and spiritually' and 'to be cared for with due respect for the family as an entity'.[71] In Alice's experience, however, New Zealand was not taking up the potential offered by these developments.

Over the 1950s, particular areas caused her increasing frustration. Alice's principal field of interest, paediatrics, did not attract the support she believed it deserved. By the time she retired from her fourth year as president of the Paediatric Society in 1960, there was not all that much to show for more than 10 years of effort. There was still no chair of child health at the Otago Medical School and the development of hospital services for children at Princess Mary had been grudging. In both instances, high hopes had been gradually eroded by deferred assurances and it was becoming hard to escape the feeling that these attitudes would persist. Alice's commitment to the development of paediatric services at Auckland Hospital dated back to the mid-1940s, when Sammy Ludbrook had envisaged

> a special Hospital for Children to create a service that would provide a post-graduate training centre that would raise the standard [of Paediatrics] throughout the Auckland Province and even throughout the Dominion.[72]

On his retirement she had become even more involved. During 1955 she was appointed to a subcommittee to look into the reorganisation of Auckland, Green Lane and Middlemore Hospitals and, together with other paediatric staff, set about formulating a proposal for future development that was presented to the board's standing committee for administration and future hospital planning in July 1956.

The theme, which remained consistent with Ludbrook's original plans, was centralisation of children's services at Auckland Hospital, taking in not only the whole of the Princess Mary but also the Infectious Diseases Block, with the development over the next five years of at least some specialist paediatric sections. The board's other hospitals need provide only emergency beds for children while Princess Mary would increase its wardspace and staff, and institute a cadet and postgraduate paediatric nursing programme and an undergraduate and postgraduate paediatric medical teaching unit, which could later be developed to professorial status. The social problems of hospitalised children were not to be overlooked, with plans for the accommodation of breastfeeding mothers and the development of school, kindergarten and occupational therapy facilities for inpatients.[73] This agenda cut right across other medical interests. After receiving a report from the Combined Medical Staff, which noted that some specialties did not like the idea of 'sequestrating children's beds from their present combined units', the board shelved the paediatricians' report,[74] and by the end of the decade was proceeding to erode the prospects of a centralised children's hospital establishing paediatric wards in other institutions.[75]

Even modest proposals to improve children's hospital experience proved unnecessarily difficult. During the early 1950s parents of patients in the children's wards at Auckland Hospital could not officially visit more than twice a week for half an hour, and in the isolation or babies' wards only at the discretion of the sister-in-charge.[76] Hospital authorities argued that such restrictions were necessary to avoid cross-infection and upsetting sick children, or, more precisely, the regimented ward routines to which they were subjected. The only exceptions to this practice nationally were infants scheduled for surgical repair of cleft palates by the husband and wife team of H.P. and C.M. Pickerill, but even in these cases sterile conditions were the main criteria. Patients were ideally nursed in separate rooms, principally by their mothers, so that they might be exposed to her germs only. The Pickerells' contention, that mother and baby were 'a biological entity, and to get results [they] must be treated as such',[77] was subverted by their request that foster-mothers be provided for the Maori babies on whom they operated since 'their mothers are in the majority of cases not suitable as nurses and give rise to considerable social difficulties'.[78] The movement towards more open parental visiting for hospitalised children, which Alice supported, was popularised as part of Bowlby's 'maternal deprivation' theories and cut right across such provisos.[79] In her review of Bowlby's work, Alice had referred to the damaging emotional effects of extended hospitalisation on young children and noted that 'daily visiting hours in children's wards . . . seems a simple measure that might well receive consideration in this country'.[80] Yet, despite requests for change, over most of the 1950s extended parent visiting remained dependent on the attitude of the paediatrician, or the ward sister, involved.[81] Parents admitted under pro-visiting paediatricians, such as Alice, were therefore at an advantage over those under more conservative doctors in the same hospital. It was not until late in the decade, and the publication of the Platt Report in Britain, which referred to the emotional needs of the child,[82] that hospital visiting hours at Princess Mary were officially extended to up to five hours daily.[83]

Despite her primary involvement in the physical care of sick children, it was the dismissal of progressive ideas about psychiatric care and mental and emotional health that finally exhausted Alice's patience with the medical establishment. In the early 1950s, the Paediatric Society had discussed setting up a 'child guidance' clinic in Auckland for children with behavioural problems. Alice, keen and fresh from her overseas experience, was nominated convenor of a subcommittee to investigate the matter,[84] but the initiative was pre-empted by Dr A.W.S. Thompson, the local medical officer of health, who proposed restructuring the contentious Child Health

Clinic to fill this vacuum. To avoid the stigma of 'men[tal] peculiarity', the clinic would retain its original name and operate on the 'medical basis – or rather, health basis which is ... desirable'.[85] The new facility held little more appeal for the Paediatric Society than Thompson's previous establishment, but its efforts to suggest anything better than the Child Health Clinic could provide were hamstrung because there were no child psychiatrists in New Zealand. The final report of its subcommittee could only further suggest making representations to the Department of Health to assist a suitable person to travel overseas for training.[86] The Child Health Clinic therefore continued to function in its new role under the existing leadership of paediatrician Grahame Fox who, on his own admission, had no training at all in child psychiatry,[87] and relied on seconded Education Department psychologists, the consultative services of K.R. Stallworthy of the Auckland Mental Hospital and the ubiquitous Eva Fischmann. By 1955, similar clinics had been established in Hamilton, Wellington and Christchurch, adding to tensions between the Health Department and the organised medical profession. Most doctors were prepared to accept the clinics as long as they followed 'ethical' channels of referral and dealt in areas not covered by existing medical practice. Others were more concerned that they were unable to perform adequately because of the lack of properly trained personnel. Over the mid-1950s Alice seems to have had a foot in both camps, but she was also driven by the deeper concern that all approaches to mental health services in New Zealand were simply not progressive enough.

The issue came to a head for her in 1957, when the Department of Health's Division of Mental Hygiene announced plans for a major rebuilding programme to expand their existing rural residential units for adults and children. This development was not going to sit comfortably with those who supported deinstitutionalisation. Within the medical profession (in its widest sense), such attitudes were held predominantly by paediatricians, private psychiatrists and psychotherapists, and members of the teaching staff in the newly established Department of Psychiatry at the medical school. Representatives of this interest group successfully gained NZBMA approval to set up a committee to report on alternatives which might be considered.[88] Alice, Neil Begg, Jim Watt, John Dobson and Peter Unwin represented the paediatric interest on the committee, where they were joined by Harold

Bourne, lecturer in psychiatry at the medical school, and psychiatrists Peter Cook and Wallace Ironside. Sir Charles Burns, an eminent physician, was its chairman. Members of the Mental Hygiene branch were invited to participate but declined,[89] although K.R. Stallworthy was co-opted on to a subcommittee set up by the Paediatric Society to look at this question.[90]

Unsurprisingly, given its membership, the NZBMA Mental Health Committee was highly critical of the Mental Hygiene Division's plans. In a lengthy report published in the *NZMJ*, it urged the creation of smaller units in urban areas closer to family support, with an emphasis on education and vocational training and the ultimate possibility of employment structured to the capacity of the individuals involved. The aim was development, not incarceration, 'a flowing lake as opposed to a stagnant pool', with psychiatric social workers providing support for patients and their families and improved training for all concerned.[91] A 1954 WHO report and the works of Bowlby and later theorists were cited to support the dangers of institutionalising children away from their families. The committee did not exempt the medical profession from being behind the times in this field, stating its 'hope of influencing in the first instance the general body of their own profession, and through them all other interested professions, departments, associations and persons'. Even Sir Charles Burns confessed that chairmanship of the committee had been a learning experience for him.[92] Publication of the report resulted in a bitter correspondence in the pages of the *NZMJ*. This would publicly signpost a new direction for Alice but to fully understand her motivation we must look beyond her purely professional concerns to the development of her social role as a woman doctor over these same years.

CHAPTER 7

Education for Life

> *To achieve human happiness as well as longevity,*
> *we must teach all we know to each generation so that*
> *it may build on the knowledge of those who have gone*
> *before.*[1]

Women doctors had traditionally interested themselves in women's and children's issues and Alice was no exception. But she was active within a particular context, sympathetic to a new wave of ideas that were only just beginning to have an impact and, by the early 1950s, were known to relatively few. This was not primarily a medical movement. The ground-breaking developments took place chiefly within educational circles and the key personnel were lay people from that background. Confident in their judgment, they knew how to organise, publicise and use networks and would be influential beyond their numbers. They were generally regarded by both the conservative middle class and most working class people as slightly eccentric; only those with receptive minds became involved. Alice responded at several levels. Their activities appealed not only to her interest in mental health, personal relationships and child and family health, but also to her belief in the power and importance of education in its widest sense. In later years she would describe this as adding a fourth 'R', 'Real Life', to 'Reading, Writing, 'Rithmetic'.[2] Moreover, their basic premise, that a child's early years provided the foundation for later psychological and social welfare, fitted comfortably alongside developments within paediatrics that were shifting beyond simply 'relieving the ills of childhood' to 'promoting good health [in the child] as the basis of healthy adulthood'.[3] For Alice, the nurturing of mental and emotional family health quickly became as necessary a component of preventive medicine as meeting physical health needs. This approach, shared by only a few of her professional peers, meant she established a special relationship with lay people of the same sympathies. It also led to a public role that would overshadow her more overtly feminist views as interest grew in these new parenting skills.

Alice's own initiation into the new theories can be precisely located in the early 1940s, because it is recorded in her detailed wartime correspondence to Faulkner. Before and during her first pregnancy, her ideas about child-raising had reflected current authoritarian models and the need for imposed 'discipline'. It was just before Lesley's birth that the term 'child psychology' began to appear in her letters, followed, a few weeks later, by the news that her educationalist uncle, Richard Lawson, had sent her 'a couple of little books . . . to assist in the upbringing of the child'.[4] Increasing references to 'the psychological approach' and a retreat from ideas such as feeding by the clock, corporal punishment and early potty training followed. By February 1944, Alice was criticising her Karitane nurse for lacking 'the necessary sympathy' in her approach to the baby.[5] At the same time she was recording her growing interest in aspects of mental health, the importance of sexual adjustment in marriage and her participation in the Psychiatric Society and NZFPA. In January 1945 she wrote to Faulkner,

> Believe me darling, the underlying motives in the management of children are all important . . . the only way we can help the future generations to make a better job of things is to allow them to make the best of their hereditary endowment instead of forcing them into conflict and subterfuges because we create emotional situations with which they are unable to deal. You know the value of satisfactory adjustments where sex is concerned, just enlarge yr. horizon a bit to embrace all of man's nature & take this psychological business seriously . . . . When I started off I didn't mean to ride my favourite hobby horse quite so far, but you so see what I'm getting at don't you?[6]

Alice now refused, on psychological grounds, to leave Lesley to cry for long periods and argued that her own 'overprotected' upbringing had left her ill-prepared to contend with a changing world.[7] From this time she was regarded as a 'permissive' parent – code for a follower of the new theories. As a toddler, Lesley explored house and garden with a freedom that made conservatives shudder, and submission, demure behaviour and quietness were not priorities. 'She'll be no wishy washy daughter,' Alice promised Faulkner.[8] Alice's commitment to the new ideal can also be seen in the emphasis she placed on her child's rights. She decried 'that abomination in the sight of the Lord, the possessive mother,'[9] and proposed that each year, on Lesley's birthday, she and Faulkner should evaluate not their child's progress but their own performance as parents.

> Do you think we can achieve the ideal of giving her all that is necessary now in love & material things & then stand back later on & leave her to make her own use of her life? Don't you agree that is what we should aim at? Shall we make it a rule that ea. birthday we should honestly review the situation and ask ourselves "are we claiming too much?"[10]

By 1950, Alice's increased professional status had added authority to her ideas and she was invited to contribute to *Homes and Families*, a booklet on parenting compiled by the Women's Committee of the National Council of Churches. The booklet, in itself evidence of the increasing seriousness with which lay people were approaching child-raising, was designed for study groups and young parents 'who, aware of the problems involved in the upbringing of a family, look for some help for their tasks'.[11] Alice was the only contributor who was a doctor. Her essay dealt not with diet and disease but with behavioural and emotional difficulties. Entitled 'Childhood Problems', it featured advice on bed-wetting, temper tantrums, lying, stealing, running away and, tucked into 'Miscellaneous', grizzling, masturbation, thumb-sucking and nail-biting. The educational genesis of her contribution was clear: readers were further directed to Susan Isaac's *The Nursery Years* and a New Education Fellowship monograph, *Play and Mental Health*. The concluding paragraphs reflected the psychological grounding of the entire piece.

> Parents must realize that the first five years of a child's life, far from being carefree, represent a succession of conflicts . . .

Some children have more difficulty than others because their own instinctive drives are more powerful. Some children are made difficult by a lack of security, or by parents who expect them to live up to a standard which is too high, or by those who fail to give them any consistent standard at all. It is probable that ideal parents would have children who presented no problems at all. We shall never know, for all parents are human.

When difficulties persist, or when parents become discouraged, the services of a good child psychiatrist should be sought. This should not be regarded as a confession of failure on the part of the parents, any more than seeking medical aid for physical ailments.[12]

This approach carried its own snares. Its acceptance of human fallibility, and consequent rejection of absolute standards of success or failure in parenting, was overwhelmed by the turgid psychological undertones. In the same publication an essay by Doris Low, which argued for the need for specific advice for young mothers, mentioned 'a statement by Dr Alice Bush – "No child is ever born bad. When trouble arises, it is not a naughty infant, but an incompetent mother that is the cause."'[13] References of this kind suggest that Alice was part of what later came to be seen as the medical profession's (and other 'experts") oppression of women during this decade. Loading mothers with almost total responsibility for the training and socialisation of their children, and linking the early childhood experience to future maladjustment, meant that women of the 1950s were handed not only a fulltime physical but also an unfair psychological burden. This is not an analysis into which Alice fits neatly. Although she did believe that a child's early years influenced its adult personality, saddling mothers with guilt was contrary to her concern for their own mental health. Conserving their physical health was equally important to her and she did not support Bowlby's (or anyone else's) extreme statements about selfless mothering. In *Maternal Care and Mental Health*, a section on the need for mothers to accompany their children to hospitals (and act in a nursing capacity there) did not question an assertion that mother-nurses needed 'little or no off-duty time, because the sleep requirements of a mother fall near to zero when her own child is acutely ill'.[14] In July 1959, when Alice appeared, as an individual, before the Auckland hearings of the Consultative Committee on Pre-School Health Services, she argued for the

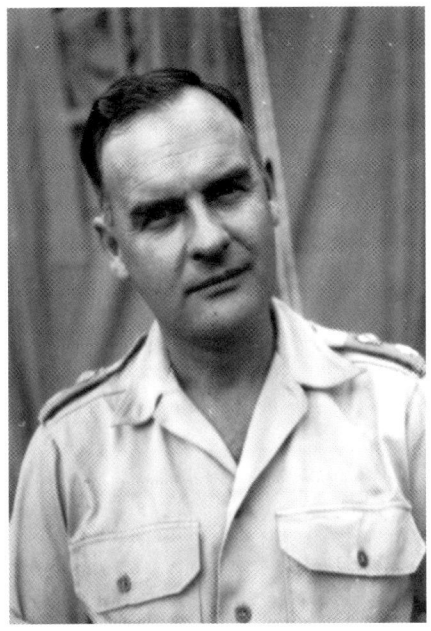

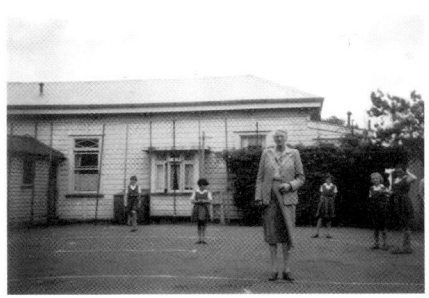

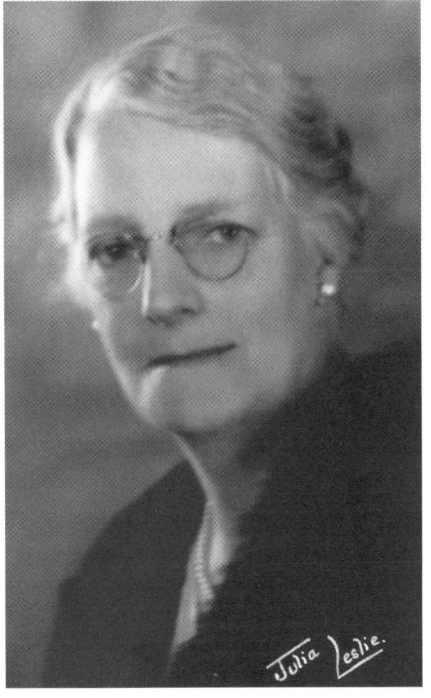

ABOVE: Dr E. G. (Ted, later Sir Edward) Sayers in the Middle East with the No. 1 New Zealand General Hospital in 1940 when Alice was his locum. They later became partners in practice. *Meg Bayley (née Sayers)*

ABOVE RIGHT: 'Major' Dorothy Hawkins of the Women's National Service Corps, in her other role as games mistress at Hill Top School. Taken in 1959, this photograph gives an indication of the school's small scale on its original site. *Hill Top School*

RIGHT: Marjorie Stanton in the late 1930s. By the time of Alice's marriage, her health had visibly deteriorated. *Julia Leslie. Courtesy Patricia Rogers.*

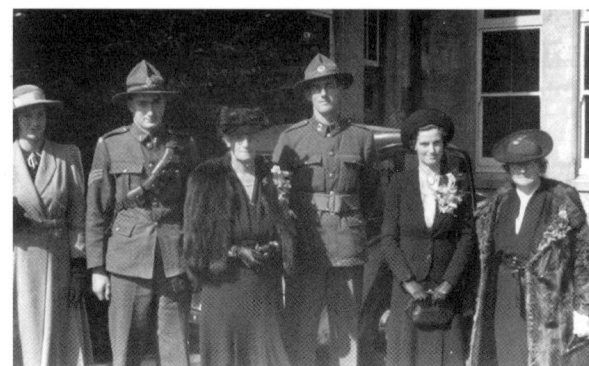

TOP RIGHT: The family at Denestone on Alice's wedding day, 17 August 1940. From left: Aileen, Allenby, Marjorie, Patricia's husband, Dacre Fox Rogers, Patricia and Faulkner's mother, Muriel Hamilton. *Royal Photos. Courtesy Christine Moorhouse*

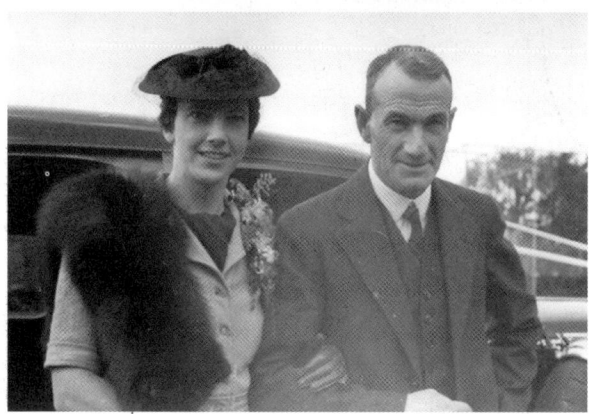

CENTRE RIGHT: Alice and her father arrive at the Diocesan School chapel. *Christine Moorhouse*

BELOW: After the ceremony. Despite Faulkner's controlled demeanour, he was a bundle of nerves. *Peter Bush*

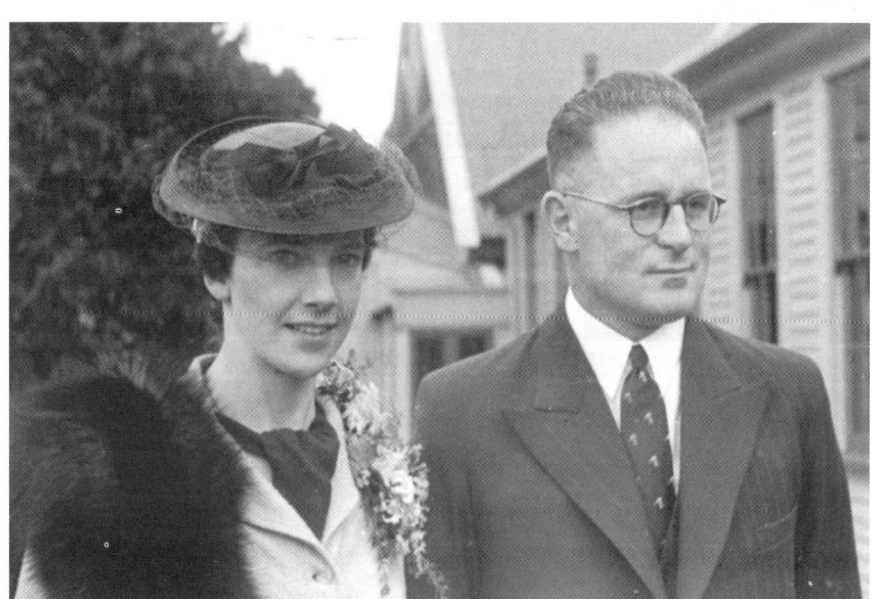

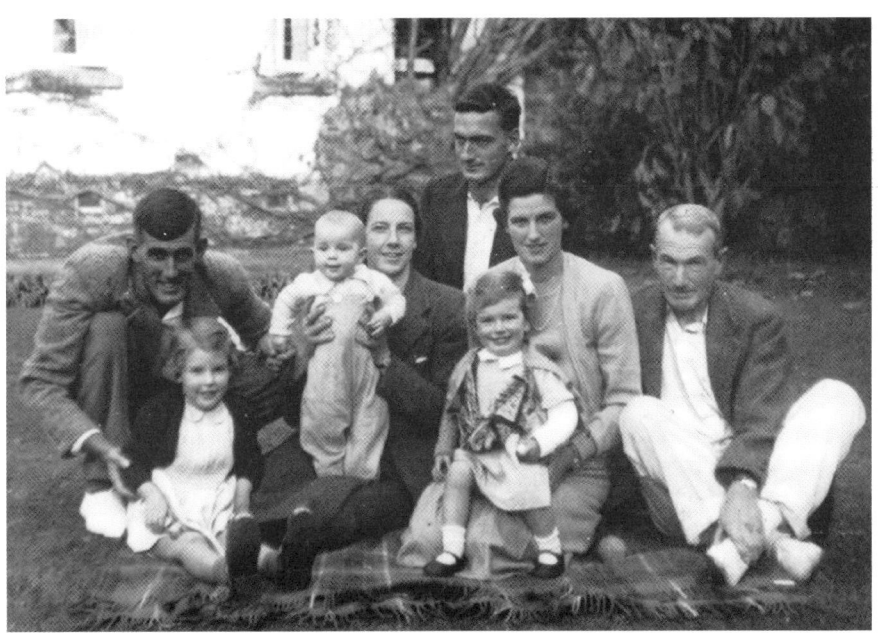

ABOVE: The war family at Denestone, 1944. From left: Dacre Fox Rogers, Gillian Rogers, proud mother Alice, holding Lesley, Allenby Stanton, Margaret Rogers, Patricia Rogers, Joseph Stanton. *Christine Moorhouse*

LEFT: Alice taking home movies of Lesley to send to Faulkner in Italy. *Christine Moorhouse*

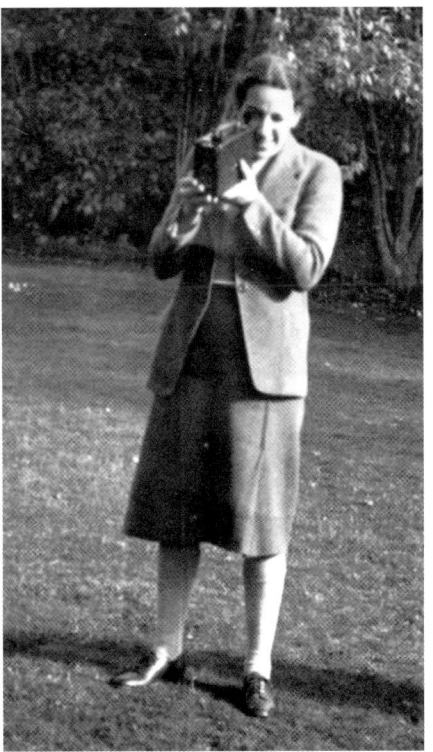

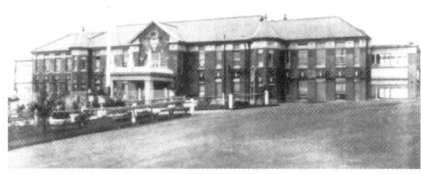

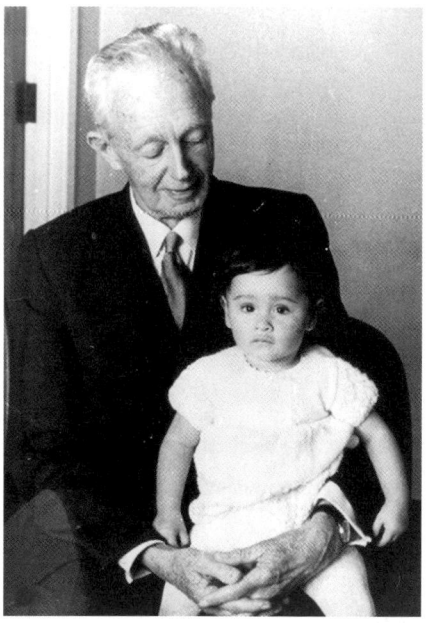

ABOVE: The original Princess Mary Hospital for Children. Seen here in its heyday, just after World War I, it was still serving as the principal accommodation for sick children at Auckland Hospital when Alice joined the staff in September 1944.

RIGHT: Dr S. L. (Sammy) Ludbrook, regarded as the 'father' of paediatrics in Auckland. Alice began her hospital career as his assistant.
Richard Ludbrook

BELOW: Alice and Lesley, New Year's Day, 1945. *Douglas Whillams (MC)*

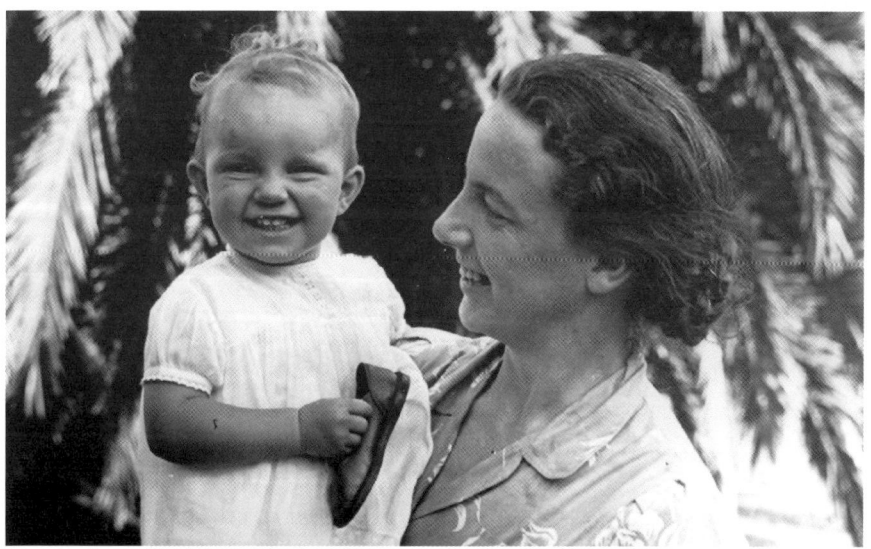

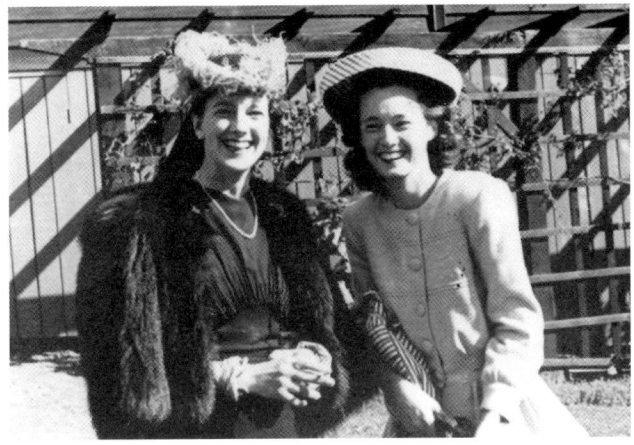

ABOVE: Alice (on left) at her glamorous best, attending a family wedding in Te Aroha, March 1945. *Christine Moorhouse*

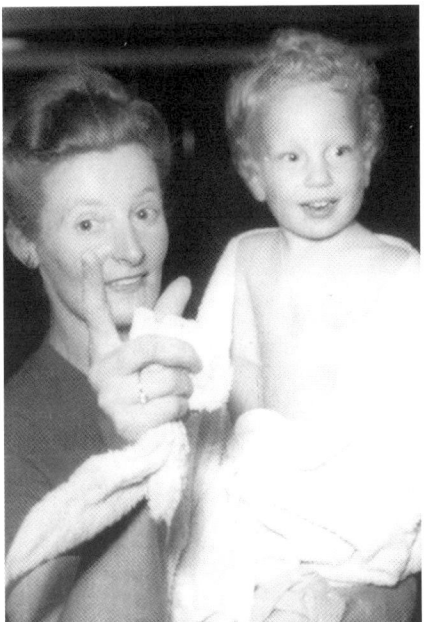

LEFT: Alice's son, Peter, with Karitane nurse Lola McKellar, on the return trip from England in 1949. When Alice set up her specialist practice the following year, Lola became her first nurse receptionist. *Christine Moorhouse*

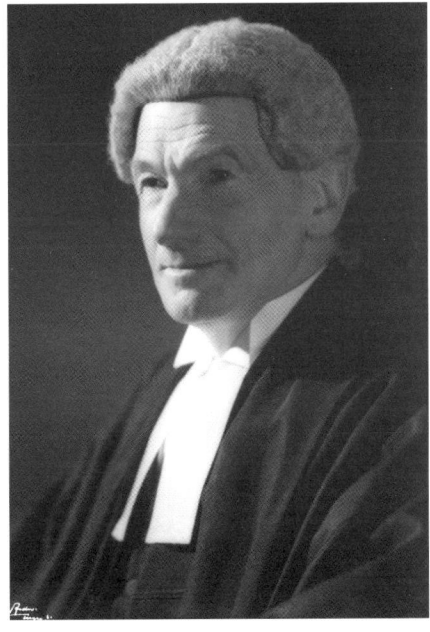

RIGHT: During Alice's absence overseas, Joseph had been appointed to the High Court bench. *Patricia Rogers*

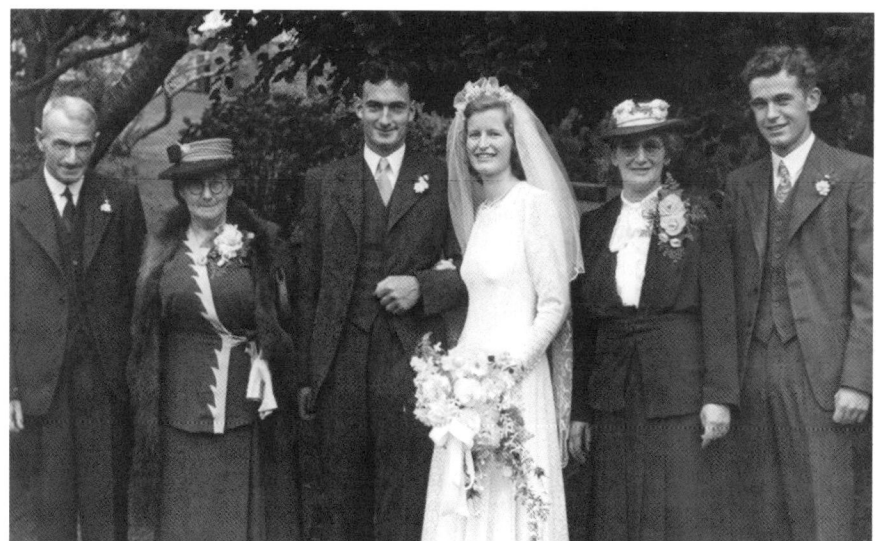

ABOVE: Alice's brother Allenby and his bride, Isabel Macky. Joseph stands on the far left, beside his sister, 'Aunty Betty', with whom Alice could confidently leave supervision of the domestic scene while her children were young. *John Lesnie. Courtesy Patricia Rogers*

RIGHT: Alice and her second daughter, Christine, in 1952. *Christine Moorhouse*

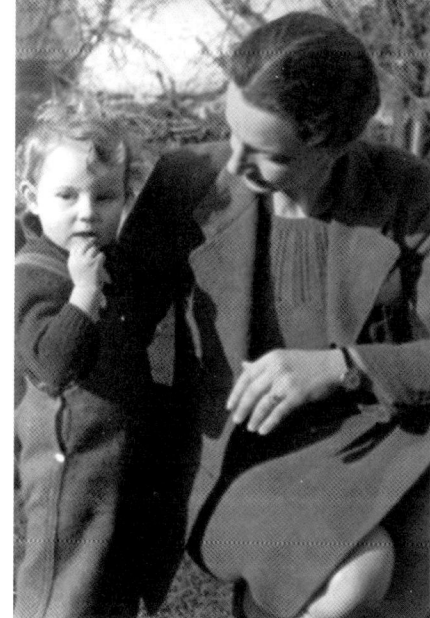

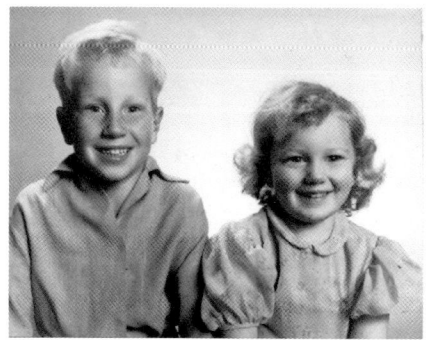

LEFT: Peter and Christine. *Aileen Odell*

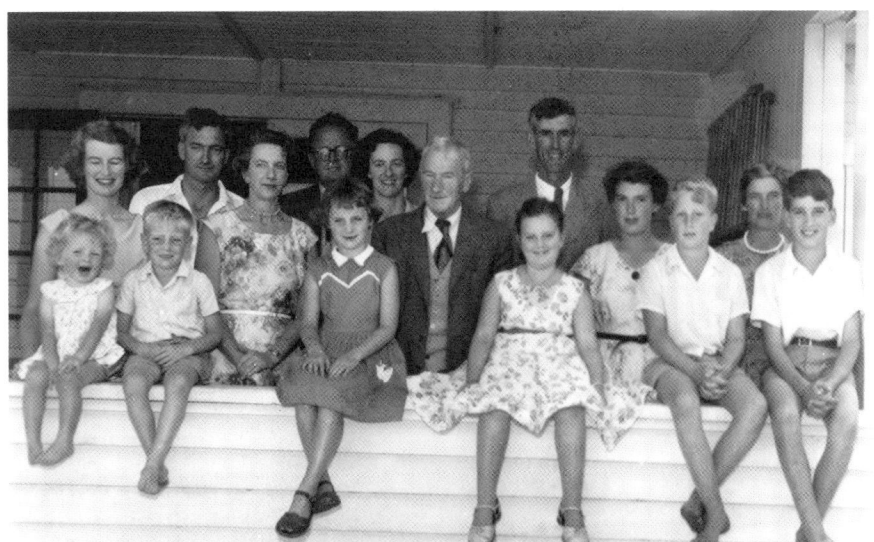

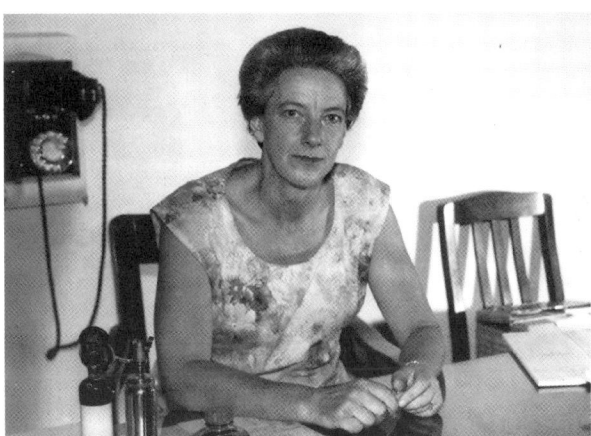

ABOVE: The family celebrate Joseph's knighthood at Deep Creek, January 1957. From left, at back: Isabel and Allenby Stanton, Alice and Faulkner Bush, Aileen Odell, Sir Joseph, Dacre Fox Rogers, Margaret Rogers, Patricia Rogers. Front: Josephine, Dennis and Kate Stanton, Christine and Peter Bush, John Rogers. *Patricia Rogers*

LEFT: Alice at her desk, Merivale. *Christine Moorhouse*

BOTTOM: Alice (on right) and fellow paediatricians in the 1950s, including, on left, Dr (later Professor) James Watt and Dr J. D. Matthews. Dr Elsie Gibbons stands in the centre of the group. *Christine Moorhouse*

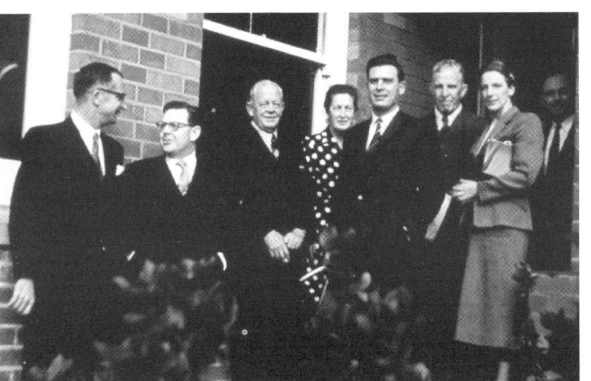

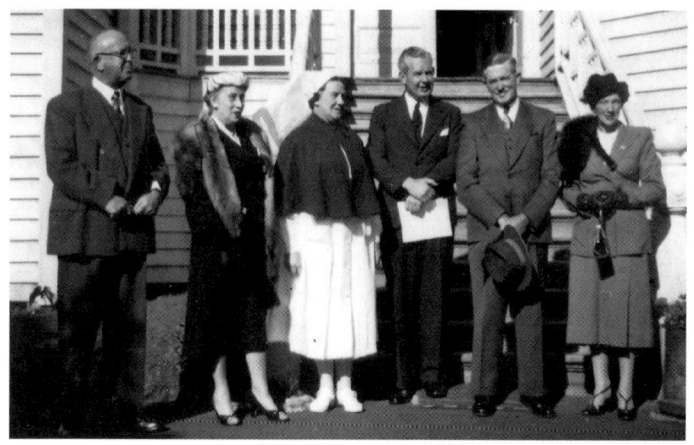

ABOVE: Alice's appointment to the Karitane Hospital brought her into contact with a wide range of people. Here, in the mid-1950s, she stands on the right of a group which includes (second from left) Mrs Dolly Paykel, president of the Auckland Plunket Society, and (second and third from right) the Minister of Health, Hon. J. R. Hanan, and Dr, later Sir Neil, Begg. *Christine Moorhouse*

RIGHT: On the same steps with a group of Karitane nurses, the wife of the Governor-General, Lady Norrie, Sister Collinge of the Mothercraft Unit, and Mrs Horton of the Plunket Society. *Tui Faram*

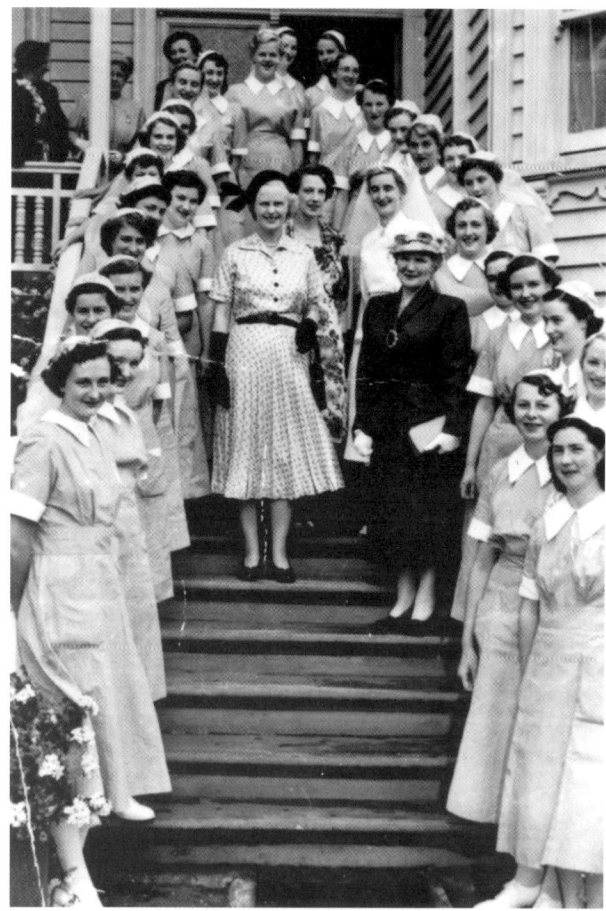

retention of Karitane Hospitals as a service to mothers who needed care as much as babies.

> The mothers of young children are the most important people in the community. On their ability to cope with their children depends the future of all that we value. Without good mothering the children grow up to be bad citizens. Money spent on roads, industries, transport, and all other services can bear fruit only if the mother and the family can function, and therefore when the mother cannot cope she must have relief, she must be rested and restored so that she can manage once again.[15]

Despite her commitment and energy, Alice was never an official 'expert' on parenting, a creator of orthodoxy in the way that medical directors of the Plunket Society tended to be. Her inclination to examine new ideas and adopt those she thought worthwhile ensured an open-minded approach. She also spread her message more immediately: speaking to small groups, advising parents who consulted her and writing short articles for publications whose readership could never be compared with that of the Plunket handbooks. She developed a relaxed, personal style that encouraged parents to select, from a variety of sources, the techniques they considered might work best for them. 'There must be variety in family life,' she argued in 1964. 'The recipes for rearing children are not quite like those for making cakes but there are some ingredients you may like to try in varying combinations.'[16] Underlying this flexible approach, however, were some important and constant essentials.

Alice recognised the influence of both nature (genetic inheritance) and nurture (the environment of childhood), but she believed the interaction between the two was the most important factor in deciding 'the sort of adult which a child will become.'[17] The role of parents during the first five years was central, providing the guidance and emotional sustenance that would see their children emerging into the wider world with sufficient self-confidence to meet its greater challenges. Children deprived of this early security and guidance were in danger of becoming 'sick members' of society, unable to forgo the immediate gratification of anti-social urges which, given different handling, they would have left behind in infancy. Unless there was some change, these children would repeat their learned experience with the following generation, creating a 'vicious cycle'. Punishment after the event was profitless. Change could come only through prevention and the recognition that the welfare of children was a communal responsibility on which money and time needed to be spent. The first essential was support for parents, who needed 'help not blame'.[18]

It was this perspective, and her inclination to action over theory, which lay behind Alice's devotion to programmes that promoted the development of parenting skills. Her faith in the educational process to achieve these ends was almost absolute. Only 'the most neurotic of parents' could not, she believed, be taught techniques of successful child-rearing. Even the absence of deep parental love should not be an insuperable barrier to success.[19] A primary target was parental authoritarianism and the imposition of standards that disregarded the child's social or emotional development. To break this pattern of expectation, parents had to be informed about the needs of their children and shown how to use that knowledge fruitfully. But though Alice respected the child's rights, introduced the child's perspective and encouraged the child's freedom to experience, learn and grow, she did not seek to make parents nothing more than acquiescent dogsbodies. Rather they were to regard themselves as the senior and more responsible partners in the development of a relationship based on mutual respect, so that their children would 'grow up with a recognition that persons are important and kindness and gentleness virtues to be cultivated'.[20]

Alice did not restrict the concept of partnership, nor the improving powers of education, to parents alone. It was also important that 'all who deal with parents and children .... [including] doctors ... magistrates, probation officers, child welfare officers, teachers and lawyers', should be 'prepared to keep going back to school'. Armed with the 'techniques of repairing the personality',[21] they should then encourage and support parents without undermining their confidence. In 1963 she warned, 'The worst thing that anyone can do to a mother is to make her afraid of her baby. By anyone, I mean all those people who feel that they have a right to instruct a mother about what she should do with her baby.'[22] At a general practitioners' seminar a few years later, Alice defined the particular task of the doctor as teaching 'each mother that the person who is going to know the most about her baby is the mother herself, if she studies it in an intelligent way. Basically what we need to do is to support mothers in becoming experts in their own families.'²³ She followed a similar line of reasoning in a review of Dr Claire Isbister's *Living with Children*. Although she believed that Dr Isbister, as a distinguished paediatrician and a wife and mother, was 'better qualified than most' to offer advice, she counselled readers not to accept everything she said. Alice criticised the book's sometimes vague definitions and several of its suggestions, but praised Isbister's easy, friendly style which recognised the experience of mothers and left them free to exercise their judgment. Such an approach, Alice argued, had 'more value than a less personal more authoritative treatise which would demand a choice between complete acceptance or rejection'. She thought it a good starting point for inexperienced parents and worth reading for 'the old hand because wise women know no greater pleasure than making the acquaintance of another wise woman'.²⁴

The most coherent collection of Alice's ideas on child-raising is found in a series of articles in the *New Zealand Family Doctor*, a 'health education' magazine published during the early 1960s by Wilson & Horton in conjunction with the Auckland Division of the NZBMA. In deference to medical ethics, Alice wrote as 'Mary Wood', but her articles demonstrated all her favoured themes, including the need to think carefully about the requirements of parenthood before a child was conceived.²⁵ References to the development of the social virtues of industry, economic prudence, self-discipline and respect for private property,²⁶ were acceptable to the most conservative reader. But extending aims beyond the purely material and the means by which these wider ends could be achieved were harder to swallow. Alice identified 'the really important things' in life as 'Happiness – Contentment – Making the most of what talents one has – Loving one's neighbour – Being happy in the give and take of relationships with other people', qualities 'of goodness' which depended 'so much on the environment [of childhood]'.²⁷ All forms of domination by adults, parental or within the marriage relationship, were abhorrent, including dogmatism, inflexibility, demands for instant obedience, the habitual raising of voices or the more subtle 'disguised cruelty' of teasing. Corporal punishment, because of its potential to 'create an attitude to violence which makes it an acceptable form of behaviour to achieve what one wants',²⁸ was absolutely untenable. Her 'Mary Wood' articles and other writings explicitly discouraged physically disciplining children and she was quite capable of approaching complete strangers she saw smacking a child in public and entering into heated discussion with them.[29]

Believing that 'real discipline is self discipline',[30] Alice argued that any form of punishment during the preschool years was fruitless because the child could not yet discriminate between right and wrong.[31] Love, not fear, should be the guiding force, with the expression of disappointment the only acceptable means of correction.[32] The primary objective should be to establish a good relationship by providing for children's happiness and satisfaction. She urged parents to constantly present their children with a positive self-image and reprimanded nurses at the Karitane Hospital for referring to their charges as 'naughty' or as 'a tiger'.[33] Unnecessary tension within the home could be avoided by creating a special area where children could play safely and happily without imperilling precious possessions,[34] but they should not be cocooned, since experience was essential to the learning process. 'Don't tell him that he will fall off if he climbs on the chair,' Alice cautioned, 'let him learn from a small bump that if he falls it hurts.'[35] She rejected a rigid approach to toilet training; this, and similar attitudes to masturbation, created feelings of fear and shame about the sexual organs which 'will have some effect on its [the child's] sexual life as it gets older'.[36] Even the phrase 'toilet training' was a 'misnomer' she suggested – it should be called 'toilet opportunity'.[37] Handled with love and understanding, she assured parents, most children would embark on their school years ready and willing to accede to reasonable requests. And this was the time when they should ensure that their children behaved acceptably, not, as it seemed to Alice, give up and hand responsibility over to the schools.[38]

In measuring how revolutionary these ideas were in their time, it is important to remember that few parents of this era had been brought up as liberally as Alice – and she now considered that even her own experience had been too restrictive. Firm control of even very young children was widely considered a virtue, corporal punishment a parental right and early toilet training the hallmark of many a mother's success. Alice's ideas challenged all these notions. Moreover, raising children a generation before had been strictly women's work. Now, she declared, 'a man has to be prepared to sacrifice some of the pleasures to which he is accustomed, not just dutifully, but happily. A good father no less than a good mother feels that his chief pleasure in life is to be derived from providing for his children and being with them.'[39] Men who were not so inclined were equally responsible for any social problems resulting from poor parenting. Because this was so often the case, it came as no surprise to Alice 'that delinquency is increasing and that the divorce rate is now one in 10, and every year brings an increase in the number of people requiring care in mental hospitals'.[40] No kind of household authoritarianism gained her favour. Mothers, urged in the past to impeccable standards of family hygiene and organisation, were encouraged to loosen up in their dealings with their children.

> Many a conscientious mother has felt it is an unfair world which makes her children show little appreciation of the virtues clearly displayed in her well-kept house, with its pile of clean linen, and tins well filled with cakes and biscuits, while her neighbour remains much more popular in spite of her untidy house, and the bread and syrup she gives the children when they come home from school.
> Indeed this feckless woman wastes hours just playing with the children. If you were a child, which sort of loving would you choose?[41]

This was not the only time when Alice suggested that parents should view themselves from their child's perspective. 'Take time off now and then,' she encouraged, 'to play families, but you be the child and let your offspring be the parent – sometimes mother, sometimes father. See if you can interpret what your child thinks parents are like.'[42] Adults had to understand that children learned by example. Alice was fond of handing out a tract, 'Children learn what they live', and hung a framed copy of it in her waiting room.

> If a child lives with criticism, He learns to condemn.
> If a child lives with hostility, He learns to fight.
> If a child lives with ridicule, He learns to be shy.
> If a child lives with shame, He learns to feel guilty.
>
> If a child lives with tolerance, He learns to be patient.
> If a child lives with encouragement, He learns confidence.
> If a child lives with praise, He learns to appreciate.
> If a child lives with fairness, He learns justice.
> If a child lives with security, He learns to have faith.
> If a child lives with approval, He learns to like himself.

> If a child lives with acceptance and friendship,
> He learns to find love in the world.[43]

Under these circumstances, parental self-examination was part and parcel of child-raising. 'Are you the sort of person who lacks the willpower to stop smoking,' she quizzed, or who yelled at the family, or ate too much, or moaned when mother-in-law came to stay, or endlessly criticised others, or rejoiced in putting one across the Inland Revenue Department? Parents must not be hypocrites: 'No fair-minded parents would punish a child for failure to achieve a standard which they had found too difficult'.[44] This was obviously not a road for the faint-hearted, but Alice's supportive and down-to-earth approach was appealing. At the same time, the social and economic security provided by the welfare state had promoted not only generally higher living and educational standards but also individual confidence and faith in the future, so that the receptive audience was widening.

Alice had by now mastered the relaxed use of language that humanised her texts. It was a technique she often used, even when dealing with professional people. In an *NZMJ* article, 'The Doctor and the Delinquent', she described sibling rivalry from the child's viewpoint.

> A newcomer in the family is viewed in much the same way as a wife would view a beautiful blond [sic] who had designs on her husband – with fear and hatred. The assurance that she would be a help with the housework and a good companion would help very little to ease the initial shock that she was to share her own beloved. She would like to wring her neck.[45]

It may not have been the quintessence of scientific demonstration, but everyone got the message. Getting the message across was Alice's priority and she realised that her articles and talks reached only those who were interested enough to seek information. She refused a suggestion made to her during the early 1970s, when the youthfulness of many parents was becoming a concern, that she should write a simple guide to child care for younger people because

> I don't feel that any amount of talking or writing will bring about a change. Only if the joys of interaction between adults and little children

are demonstrated to the young will they be able to approach parenthood with the proper sense of responsibility and with the practical knowledge necessary to establish a good positive relationship with their young from the earliest months.[46]

Participation of both boy and girl pupils in creches set up in intermediate schools, a concept she had long favoured,[47] became a minor crusade for her at this time. But the notion that it was the example of a harmonious home environment, where parents had time for each individual child, which would provide the best chance for the parental education of future generations took Alice into even more contentious territory.

Women doctors had long been regarded as acceptable agents to instruct adolescent girls and young women about reproduction, even though the immediate family's right to control access to this sort of information was deemed to be almost sacrosanct. They had the scientific knowledge, an appropriately maternal aura and a middle class background which usually ensured that they would not stray outside the conservative norms of respectable society. Alice's challenge was her conviction that such instruction should begin very early in life, and that sexuality should be divorced from feelings of repression and guilt to ensure future sexual concord and fulfilment between husband and wife.

Alice had begun her career in sex education quietly enough, as a speaker to small groups, but two major social crises widened her audience considerably. The first had been the war; the second was anxiety about the behaviour of adolescents (reclassified as 'teenagers') during the mid-1950s. Revelations of sexual activity among high school children in Lower Hutt, some below the age of consent, provided the spur for wide public debate. Since control of sexuality was closely linked to the moral fibre of the community, the reaction was one of panic. The government set up a special committee, chaired by prominent Wellington solicitor, O.C. Mazengarb, to enquire into 'moral delinquency' among children and adolescents. Members of the public whose appetites had been whetted by the 'Sensational Press Reports'[48] that accompanied the original court proceedings had a veritable banquet of racy copy to digest over the months the hearings were held in Wellington, Christchurch and Auckland. The committee heard 145 witnesses and read 120 submissions from individuals and groups ranging from the Communist

Party to the Council of Christian Education.⁴⁹ It soon became clear to the discerning that the Hutt Valley disclosures were only the tip of the iceberg. Evidence from the Auckland hearings suggested that the 'Problem of Juvenile Immorality' in the northern city was the 'Most Alarming in the Dominion'.⁵⁰

Alice did not appear before the Mazengarb Committee and only one group with which she was actively involved, the Paediatric Society, offered submissions. These, presented by Elizabeth Hughes, made recommendations that were fairly low-key considering the temper of the times; good home and school conditions, 'sensible well-informed parents', adequate but 'not over-organised' leisure time and not 'too much money in the child's hands'. Specific behavioural problems could be dealt with by referral from the family doctor to an appropriate clinic or organisation.⁵¹ The report of the committee of inquiry, popularly known as the Mazengarb Report, lacked the same equanimity. It quoted graphic accounts from the English and Australian press of 'sex cults' among the young and 'wild teenage sex orgies' involving 'bodgies' and 'widgies' in Australia, and drew attention to the notorious Parker Hulme case, in which two teenage Christchurch girls had planned and carried out the murder of one of their mothers.⁵² Witnesses, and the committee itself, came up with plenty of reasons for social breakdown, from the collapse of community and family life and religious principles to the degrading influence of 'playway' education, affluence, modern music, comics and other popular literature. It was more difficult to come up with solutions. In a bid to overcome obvious parental failure to give their children proper guidelines for correct sexual behaviour, some form of sex education for adolescents was deemed necessary. Although opposed to classroom instruction by teachers, the committee did favour a modified form of sex education through schools. Mother and daughter and father and son evenings, addressed by suitable speakers and sponsored by the new Federation of Parent-Teacher and Home and School Associations, could benefit both pupils and parents.⁵³ The federation was already producing some helpful pamphlets.⁵⁴

Alice was a member of the advisory panel behind this project, probably the first wide-scale presentation to the New Zealand public of her favoured approach to sexuality for young people. The rest of the panel consisted of educationalists, psychologists and doctors employed by the Health Department; Alice was the only private practitioner. The panel was headed by A.S. Partridge of the Auckland Federation of Parent-Teacher Associations and the Auckland branch of the NZFPA had a hand in some of the preliminary work.[55] Future supporters of Parents' Centres had also probably been involved during the previous 12 months 'of field work addressing gatherings of Parents and Mothers-to-be on Sex Education'.[56] The stated aim of the pamphlets was 'to assist parents to educate their children in simple, straightforward terms about questions relating to sex, and to encourage in the younger generation a healthy, wholesome, and informed attitude towards this important subject'.[57] There were five titles in the series, each directed at a particular audience: parents, the young child, parents of adolescents, the adolescent boy and the adolescent girl. Even the most conservative would have favoured the pamphlets' suggestions that 'self-control' was essential for the enjoyment of sexual activity 'in a civilised way at the proper time' within the context of marriage and family life, and that children needed to be protected from the 'dangers' and possible 'shameful' use of sex. Misgivings arose only when the pamphlet writers' ideas about achieving 'self control' became clearer, and their substantially different definitions of 'dangerous' and 'shameful' sexual activity.

The first indications of an alternative perspective came from the principal themes, that knowledge was the best defence against unhappy sexual experiences and that a person with 'a healthy mind' would think of sex as 'a perfectly natural, normal, and desirable part of life'. Here was a definite threat to the idea that, in sexual matters, ignorance and repression equalled innocence. The challenge was confirmed by suggestions that, from 'earliest infancy', children should be accustomed to seeing their parents' naked bodies in bathroom and bedroom, that questions about reproduction should be answered immediately and honestly in suitable language and that 'Silly tales about babies being brought in the doctor's bag or bought at the store' would not do. Conservative readers became even more uneasy when parents were advised not to allow 'exaggerated and unreasonable feelings of horror or disgust to complicate the position' if they found their child 'doing things he should not'. Minor 'forms of sexual play' between children were very common and did 'not mean any vicious, unnatural, or dangerous tendencies. They suggested normality rather than abnormality.' There was also 'good evidence' that masturbation was commonly performed by 'almost all males and many females' and that no harm would come of it. Even when 'others ... enticed children into sharing a sexual experience', parents should remember that their own reaction could be much more damaging than the experience itself. Moreover, respecting the secular spirit of the Education Act,[58] there was only one religious reference in the pamphlets and that pointed out that sex had been 'created by God, and was one of the things He looked at when He "Saw everything he had made and behold it was very good"'.

The result was a fanfare of disapproval from conservative quarters. The Roman Catholic primate, Archbishop James Liston, issued a critical message to be read at all masses,[59] and the Minister of Health found himself having to send mollifying letters to the Catholic Women's League and the New Zealand Inter-Church Council on Public Affairs.[60] At the same time, supporters of the pamphlets criticised the initial print run of only 10,000 copies compared with the 300,000 copies of the Mazengarb Report that were to be circulated throughout New Zealand.[61] The pamphlets were to outrun their critics. They remained a popular resource, were reissued several times (with suitable updating) and were still being 'distributed widely' by the Health Department in 1969.[62] Wherever they went, Alice's name appeared on the cover along with other members of the advisory panel. There is no doubt that she was wholly in favour of their more open approach. Dealing honestly with children in every area of life was central to her philosophy. In 1959 she defended the organised visit of a group of schoolgirls to a murder trial, arguing that 'Children must learn about life as it is, not as we should like it to be'.[63] In 1962 she wrote in the *NZMJ* that a child 'was never too young to be told the truth about sex, science or sociology, even when the whole truth would be too much at one time'.[64] The right to sexual knowledge was a vital element in her relationship with the NZFPA. Together with their personnel in the North and South Islands, Alice was involved in the earliest mother and daughter evenings. She also spoke to other groups in various venues, including addresses to male students at the Engineering School of the University of Auckland.[65]

What her audiences heard was a message that consistently advocated an informed approach to sexuality. In speech notes dating from the early 1960s, Alice identified monogamous sex within marriage as an ideal but one that most young people would have difficulty in achieving; a 'mistake' might be a regarded as a 'loss', but not an irrecoverable one leading to oppressive feelings of guilt. In this area, as in any other, parents must offer positive ideals to their children, 'not just a series of negatives', take time to listen and recognise their difficulties and accept that the teenage years would probably be 'stormy'. They must also provide adequate knowledge. Even contraception and venereal disease could be discussed in simple terms with older children; you could not 'tell too much of the truth'.[66] The presentation of new, 'progressive' ways to sustain such older values as a stable family life made Alice popular with both sponsoring groups and the public at large. By 1968, mother and daughter evenings had become so popular that one such function at the Auckland YWCA, where Alice was the scheduled speaker, attracted a queue three to four deep spilling out to the street. Alice was smuggled through a rear door while an estimated 600 teenagers and mothers were turned away with assurances that the programme would be repeated in the near future.[67]

Despite her popularity, Alice was not one to rest on her laurels. She continued to push boundaries. In 1967, when the New Zealand Educational Institute proposed the introduction of 'family life education' to the senior school curriculum, she argued, in a letter to the *Herald*, that this would mean 'too little will be done too late'. Nothing less than 'a dynamic programme . . . commencing at Standard I and carried right through to Form II can be expected to make a worthwhile contribution toward the arrest of the present vicious circle of immaturity, immorality and insecurity for children'.[68] Even to maintain of the 'ideals of chastity before marriage and fidelity within it', the notion of young children receiving 'family life education' was more than some could take. One horrified correspondent responded,

> Dr Bush maintains that the need is for a positive morality and information about the facts of life before the age of 10 years. Must we then assume that [this] . . . involves sexual detail? . . . If [opposition to] such a view involved being labelled puritanical, then we should embrace it. How much finer to have our little New Zealanders known as children of God than as men of the world.[69]

In fact Alice believed that children should be fully informed about 'the facts of life' even before they reached school age. Addressing a seminar of general practitioners the same year, she argued,

> I feel that every child before he or she goes to school, should know not only where babies come from, but how they got there. When I put to mothers that they should be able to explain the father's part in conception to their 4 and 5 year olds, their immediate answer is that they might start experimenting. My reply is that this is when they should start experimenting. Sexual play between children of 5 to 7 is a normal and almost necessary part of growing up. . . . Some parents mightn't be able to give approval to this sort of thing and to them my advice is – don't supervise your children too closely.[70]

Underpinning Alice's increasing public profile in both sex education and child-raising was her belief that theory was valueless unless acted upon. In 1940 she had written to Faulkner

> I just want us to be two real people who will be always trying to translate into practical everyday life the principles of human conduct, that we know to be sound . . . to practice [sic] rather than to preach and to fight the good fight without forgetting what St Paul says in the 13th chap. of Corinthians.[71]

This theme was recalled every now and then in their later letters in the context of the futility of 'faith without works'. It was the 'faith', however, which provided the impetus for action and for Alice the 'faith' was the entire package of psychologically 'sound', properly informed and freely practised personal relationships that would provide the richest possible individual and family life in the postwar world. By the late 1950s it was clear to her that lay groups were more committed to advancing, and acting upon, these new ideas than her own profession. While the Paediatric Society and the Health Department haggled over the provision of services for emotionally disturbed children at the Child Health Clinic, the Family Guidance Centre had been providing counselling since the mid-1940s. Early Parents' Centre supporters had been central to the campaign for extended visiting hours for children in hospitals. They also provided what Alice considered were very good antenatal courses, including preparation for parenting. In the same year that the medical profession rejected the NZBMA Mental Health Committee report, Parents' Centres supporters had formed a public education body, the Mental Health Association, to promote progressive ideas.[72] Within a sometimes hostile public environment,

NZFPA members sought to provide access to knowledge about birth control and sex education. Their latest move, founded on the belief that contraception was 'a foundation stone of every other branch of welfare work done on behalf of the family',[73] had been to establish family planning clinics in the four main centres. The activities of these groups were hampered not only by limited facilities and funding but by a lack of recognition and backing from medical professionals.

Even Alice had not been centrally involved in their day-to-day concerns over most of the 1950s. Her role had been that of a supporter, adviser, speaker, vice-president or patron, offices that called for only occasional contributions of time and money. But although it was a rather loose and informal working relationship, it was extremely valuable to the groups concerned because they received so little encouragement and, when specific problems arose, Alice could be relied upon. The kind of support she provided varied. It could be as basic as the willingness to recognise inadequacies in her profession, as she had in 1943, when the national executive of the NZFPA discussed the best strategy for gaining the co-operation of doctors in a proposed campaign for painless (anaesthetised) childbirth.

> Dr Cole was inclined to defend her profession but Dr Bush, who has been considerably mellowed by motherhood, frankly admitted that most doctors knew nothing of women in labour since they only came in at the finish when the chloroform was given. She said that in her Dunedin training she learnt very little about childbirth and would have felt very diffident about doing maternity work equipped only with the knowledge she gained during her training. She had never seen a woman in labour except the final stage.[74]

Or she could act more positively, as a bridge between these groups and medical structures, a task often complicated by the fervent idealism of frustrated lay activists. During the 1953 hospital visiting debate, she upheld future Parents' Centre members' efforts to educate both the public and the hospital authorities in favour of increased visiting hours in the children's wards and agreed that the management of surgical problems in children could be improved. But she cautioned that their suggestion that no child should be admitted to hospital without 'passing a board of experts' was impractical, while the idea that hospitals should provide accommodation for the entire family was 'quite fantastic, and seriously detracts from the value of the argument as a whole'. Instead, she proposed hospital accommodation for mothers supported by a subsidised domiciliary nursing service for the care of other children at home.[75]

This was a comparatively low level of participation compared with the commitment and activities of lay people, but it was considerably more than most doctors were willing to give. They saw these groups as a challenge to their status as the one true source of health care. Professional purists would have been suspicious of many of Alice's activities. The NZBMA insisted that its members obtained permission before they could speak in public or be named in the print media; such appearances were regarded as a form of advertising. Alice had long believed that this attitude was at odds with what she saw as the profession's social obligations.[76] The same reasoning lay behind her willingness to be publicly associated with many lay groups. 'If the doctors are too busy these days,' she had written to Faulkner in December 1944, 'to sponsor the education of the public in medical matters, we must at least lend our approval to others who have the time.'[77] By the late 1950s she was increasingly of this mind. She was a vice-president of the NZFPA and the Auckland branch of the Mental Health Association and had accepted an invitation to act as a medical adviser to the Auckland Parents' Hospitals Committee which,[78] in May 1959, became the Auckland Parents' Centre.[79]

The appointment of medical advisers to Parents' Centres arose out of the organisation's bid to gain official NZBMA acceptance for its antenatal classes. The NZFPA was making the same move in respect of its clinic service, where employment of professional staff was central to its aim of providing reliable and 'scientific' contraception. They wanted no confusion of their services with the 'back-street' or 'under the counter' operations that had been the historical alternatives to birth control advice from private medical practitioners in New Zealand. The model was provided by the British Family Planning Association, where patients were seen by a registered medical practitioner, assisted by a registered nurse and a receptionist.[80] Until now both Parents' Centres and the NZFPA had carried on their enterprises in a very small way, using sympathetic doctors prepared to lend their name or a few hours of their time, even though no formal approach had been made to the medical association. The confrontation that developed between these groups and the NZBMA would provide an irresistible challenge to Alice's anti-authoritarianism and her sense of fair play which, together with her dedication to the beliefs and aims she shared with these groups, would push her to the forefront of events. Developments, though, were well under way before she entered the fray. The doctor who put the match to the fuse that ignited this flare-up was not Alice but Harvey Carey, Professor of Obstetrics and Gynaecology and Medical Director of National Women's Hospital in Auckland.

CHAPTER 8

Taking a Stand

> *The medical profession must review their undertaking of a service to the people in the light of recent advances.*[1]

During the 1950s Harvey Carey had established links with Parents' Centres, the NZFPA and Marriage Guidance.[2] He was also pursuing modifications of established birthing practices and promoting rooming-in to combat cross-infection in maternity hospitals.[3] These moves were not supported by his more conservative colleagues and Carey's vigour and outspokenness meant he was well on his way to becoming a controversial figure within academic and professional circles.[4] During 1957 he began to prompt Parents' Centres to federate. Apparently he advanced this idea,

> so that we [Parents' Centres] can take part in top level conferences etc on maternal welfare and be a strong united body which will influence public opinion . . . . He [Carey] feels that his work at a top level is hampered continually because to date there is no strong body backing his progressive ideas from below. The Health Department and hospital boards evidently say they can't move until public opinion allows them to do so.[5]

Although this was scarcely an altruistic proposition on Carey's part it held obvious advantages for a group that was keen to expand its own role. As Parents' Centres' Helen Brew expressed it, 'he feels he could use us — and we think we can use him!'[6] During 1957 and 1958 Parents' Centres federated, appointed national medical and educational advisory councils and applied for recognition as an 'ethical medical auxiliary' along lines Carey suggested. On 10 December 1958 the NZBMA council ruled that it considered co-operation with Parents' Centres to be ethically correct.[7]

Carey, a vice-president of the NZFPA since 1956,[8] had also begun to encourage their national executive, known as the Standing Committee and based since June 1958 in Christchurch, to seek formal recognition from the NZBMA. On a visit to the South Island in November 1958, he apparently implied that Auckland was already committed to such a course.[9] NZFPA members were under no illusions that support from the medical profession for their activities was limited. The association's history had been dominated by unsuccessful attempts to have contraceptive services provided within established health structures. It was continued failure to achieve this aim that had led the NZFPA to establish its own clinics. There was also a fundamental philosophical difference between the two groups concerning contraception. Where the medical profession had tended to relate its use to basic health and population issues, the NZFPA had extended its advantages to social and psychological need. Yet ethical recognition of Parents' Centres, which shared so many of the NZFPA's values and whose relationship with the medical profession had also been contentious, seemed to indicate a change in attitude, or at least in the balance of power. At the beginning of December 1958, the NZFPA's dominion president Phyllis Zeff, a recent migrant to New Zealand with experience in the British organisation, wrote to the general secretary of the NZBMA enquiring 'what measures should be taken by us to place matters on a satisfactory footing, as we are anxious to establish a good relationship on ethical lines between your Association and ours'.[10]

When news of Zeff's approach to the NZBMA reached the Auckland branch, the reaction was one of disquiet. In January 1959 Glenys Lowe, the branch secretary, wrote to Alice as a 'friendly' doctor asking her for advice, disclaiming Carey's intimations that they favoured approaching the NZBMA and expressing concern that the current move would fail.[11] Although Alice had 'retired' from medical politics, she was well placed to offer guidance. She was aware, as many lay people were not, of the profession's continuing concerns about any incursions into the realm of the private practitioner. Because it had its origins in the establishment of the social security system, this attitude had hardened recently with the election of another Labour government. While the NZBMA was considering the services offered by Parents' Centres and the NZFPA, they were also critically examining the establishment of industrial health clinics, the proposed registration of chiropractors and the activities of school medical officers and Child Health Clinics. Even paediatric spokespeople trying to establish periodical examinations of well preschool children were faced with NZBMA objections to 'clinic' work in the form of private practitioners undertaking sessional employment with the Health Department.[12] Many practitioners saw the answer to these problems in strict adherence to professional ethics, which included established structures of referral and rigid rules about publicity.[13] Alice knew just how high were the hurdles which the NZFPA needed to overcome, despite its relatively low level of activity: publicising its services through speakers and the print media, employing doctors in clinics on a sessional basis, providing an alternative service to private practitioners and accepting self-referred patients. Her forebodings were borne out when, in the middle of 1959, an NZBMA council meeting refused ethical recognition of the NZFPA until the matter had been considered by NZBMA divisions and 'appropriate [medical] Societies'.[14]

Alice's immediate reaction was to take up the NZFPA cause within professional structures. When she proposed recognition of the association at an NZBMA Auckland branch meeting on 2 September, not only was the move rejected but the ethical status already granted to Parents' Centres was withdrawn, despite some concern that this would place the NZBMA 'in a very poor light . . . unless very concrete reasons for so doing could be made public'.[15] When Alice relayed this news to the NZFPA's medical adviser in Christchurch, Dr Vivienne Croxford, she was told that there was scant hope of success in that division either.[16] On 9 September, following advice from the council of the Obstetric and Gynaecological Society, the NZBMA council officially denied ethical recognition of the NZFPA and withdrew it from Parents' Centres.[17] The NZFPA Standing Committee, uncomfortably aware that events were spinning out of its control, had sought the backing of several leading medical people in the South Island. Although some professed personal sympathy with the association's aims and objectives, and 'stressed that [NZ]BMA recognition is imperative',[18] none was prepared to take up its cause. Dunedin and Christchurch clinic doctors and vice-presidents, all in private practice, felt it wise to keep a low profile.[19] The increasing tension of the situation helped to bring to a head existing internal disputes within the NZFPA concerning advice on subfertility, participation in a cervical smear programme being developed by Carey and clinic advertising, all of which could be seen as direct challenges to private practitioners. As a result, relations between the Auckland and Christchurch branches became severely strained.[20] In October Alice received a letter from Phyllis Zeff containing several enclosures and asking for her assistance.[21]

It was not in Alice's nature to stand back and await developments, to bow to the course of events. She was not only concerned with the rejection of the NZFPA and Parents' Centres, she was also angry about the critical reaction to the NZBMA Mental Health Committee's report. Both actions constituted a dismissal of the importance of nurturing and maintaining mental health, which for her had become central to the welfare, not just of individuals and families, but also of society at large. She made this link quite clearly in a stinging letter of rebuke that she shot off to the *NZMJ*. Headed 'Mental Ill Health and the British Medical Association', it attacked the profession for its lack of responsibility, concluding,

> Is the medical profession today fulfilling its obligations towards prevention of mental ill health?
> I would venture to suggest that it is not and is indeed guilty of obstructive rather than constructive action in this field. At its last meeting the Council of the Association expressed official disapproval of the two community efforts towards education for more successful family living, the Family Planning Association and the Parents' Centres. I presume they have something better to offer and I trust that the general body of the profession will shortly be informed of a constructive policy towards a preventive mental health service in New Zealand.[22]

Despite the 'presumption' in her letter, she knew her profession had little to offer to replace the services the NZFPA and Parents' Centres were providing. The ideas that sustained these groups were only just beginning to gain a foothold within medical ranks and, if recent experiences were anything to go by, it was very unlikely they would be widely taken up in the near future. Alice also believed, as many of her colleagues did not, that both lay groups were capable of providing quality services. They were not 'cranks' but willing and able people who had already proved they could work comfortably with like-minded doctors. Alice had the standing and experience to deal with the intricacies of medical politics and her letter to the *NZMJ* had demonstrated that she was prepared to go further than other medical professionals to promote the NZFPA cause. It must have been obvious, if not to her then to many in the NZFPA, that she was their best chance of saving the day.

The disinclination of other practitioners to become publicly involved was intensified when, in the February 1960 *NZMJ*, the Medical Association's Branch Ethical Committee ruled on specific points arising from participation in NZFPA and Parents' Centres' activities. Practitioners were warned of the unprofessional nature of the NZFPA and that its activities came 'very close to covering' (the term used when work was carried out by doctors on behalf of or, more pertinently at the direction of, unqualified lay people).[23] NZBMA members could belong to, or bear office in, such societies as individuals, but their names should not appear on headed notepaper (the names of Alice, Harvey Carey and Vivienne Croxford all appeared as vice-presidents on the NZFPA letterhead at the time). To accept employment with such groups was ill-advised; to refer patients to them rather than to their own colleagues was 'unethical'.[24] The NZFPA's clinic services were particularly vulnerable to the effects of this ruling. The association was committed to a doctor service, and in 1960 it was estimated that 97 per cent of all eligible medical practitioners in New Zealand belonged to the NZBMA.[25]

By openly aligning herself with the NZFPA, Alice was placing herself at odds with her professional organisation as she had not done since the 1940s when she was a member of the Medical Study Group. Together with Dr Ruth Black, who had worked at the Auckland clinic since 1955,[26] she began lobbying 'friends' and 'liberally minded doctors' in a campaign to allay the fears of private practitioners.[27] A circular letter pointed out that NZFPA clinics provided a supplementary service for women who might not be able to pay for private consultations, or had particular problems finding a suitable contraceptive or with the 'personal or religious convictions' of their own doctor. 'Every woman,' the circular maintained, 'is entitled to the knowledge of how to plan her family' and withholding this knowledge could lead to unnecessary surgical sterilisation or illegal abortion. Practitioners were urged to support the NZFPA at divisional meetings and by correspondence to the *NZMJ*.[28] There appears to have been virtually no response to the latter appeal. Only two letters appeared in the *NZMJ*, and both were from women doctors already working in NZFPA clinics.[29] The most lengthy and detailed, signed by the Auckland clinic doctors, suggested that the Branch Ethical Committee's recommendations showed little knowledge of the organisation and running of NZFPA clinics. Great emphasis was laid on NZFPA's British affiliate and that body's support from conservative and medical circles. The letter also stressed mandatory conformity to the same clinic standards with responsibility for medical concerns solely in the hands of registered medical practitioners. The NZFPA would, the letter concluded, 'continue to function here as it does elsewhere and surely it is better if it does so under the supervision and with the cooperation of medical practitioners'.[30]

This was becoming a rigorous campaign for NZFPA personnel, and internal disunity did not help. As the 1960 NZFPA biennial June conference approached, it became obvious that Auckland wanted the Standing Committee back, despite the fact that Christchurch had been asked in 1958 to accept the responsibility for at least two terms. Auckland members may have lost faith in Carey as a medical champion, but Alice was providing an attractive alternative. Early in March 1960 Glenys Lowe wrote to Phyllis Zeff and Judy Lunn, the dominion secretary,

> One piece of advice [that] seems to be unanimous from all those au fait with B.M.A. politics is to keep out of Prof. Carey's way. In fact one acquaintance has even suggested that our stock would rise considerably in the medical world if we openly quarrelled! I hardly think we should go to these lengths but I do think we shall need to be extra careful just now.

She went on to describe how Alice was being encouraged, and seemed willing, to become more involved in NZFPA activities.

> Dr Black mentioned to Dr Bush that Auckland has suggested that V.P.s be asked to future conferences. Dr Bush was distinctly interested. She regards this Conference as probably the most important in our History

and will make every effort to be present if invited – she does not expect financial help either. I am particularly thrilled at the interest she is showing. She is the daughter of Sir Joseph (late Mr Justice) Stanton. Her Brother [Allenby] is Hon. Solicitor to several social organisations. Best of all she is politically acceptable [compared to Carey] to B.M.A. both in and outside Auckland.[31]

By May the battle lines were drawn. Auckland nominated Alice as dominion president, following her hasty election to the Auckland branch committee.[32] This could hardly fail to upset Christchurch personnel. They also wanted to take Alice on board, but as convenor of a new national Medical Advisory Committee, a role that their own doctor, obstetrician Vivienne Croxford, no longer felt she could fill.[33] They did not want to give up the Standing Committee and they resisted the idea of a doctor as dominion president.[34] They nominated Phyllis Zeff for a further term, implying that this was more than a simple alternative choice by advising members that they understood that Alice was prepared to take up the presidency for only a year. Then another conference would be needed and it would be 'very unlikely that the present Dominion Officers will be prepared to take over for 2 years from that time'.[35] It was probably true that Alice did not intend to become a permanent fixture as NZFPA president, but it was unlikely she would have been unwilling to conform to the usual term of office. Auckland responded by circulating biographical notes about Alice to all branches, accompanied by a disclaimer of any intention of a special short-term presidency.

> It may be inferred from our letter to Standing Committee of May 4th that Auckland was only putting forward nominations because of the present position re B.M.A. and not seeking to retain the Standing Committee. Obviously Dr Bush is a busy woman, and naturally Auckland members would do all they could to help her, but there has been no suggestion that Dr Bush be nominated as a figure-head.[36]

This was the unhappy state of affairs as delegates gathered at Wallis House in Lower Hutt for the fifth NZFPA biennial conference. Thirteen delegates and 13 observers from six branches attended, along with three vice-presidents, although of these only Alice stayed at Wallis House.[37] There is no record of the behind the scenes lobbying that must have taken place but the outcome was clear enough. The

Auckland nominees were elected and the Standing Committee reverted to the city. Warm tributes were paid to the retiring officers. Phyllis Zeff, who remained the association's representative at the NCW, was invited to become a vice-president and Judy Lunn to become South Island liaison officer, as well as continuing to be the New Zealand representative on the governing body of the International Planned Parenthood Federation (IPPF).[38] It was agreed that, in future, the Standing Committee should rotate between branches. Although no set period was laid down, four years was reckoned to be a reasonable term for any one branch.[39] Doctors' names were removed from the association's letterhead and Phyllis Zeff moved that the Medical Advisory Committee be ratified, with Alice as chairman and convenor.[40] Although this might all have been technically satisfying to the Auckland lobby, it must also have been obvious that there was a lot of fence mending and bridge building to be done.

The demands of conciliation were not difficult for Alice, who was genuinely at one with the association's lay workers. Her recent involvement with the NZFPA may have been peripheral but her personal experience of the group went back to 1943 and she knew that they had nurtured the association and ensured its survival throughout its wilderness years. Although she had become president as part of the NZFPA's strategy to maintain its clinics, she never saw these as a complete service. It was the clinical focus of the medical establishment, and its relative lack of interest in the emotional, psychological and preventive aspects of health, which had made the postwar voluntary family welfare movements attractive to her. Over the 1960s she made it clear that she did not believe in lay workers simply providing a support service for the association's medical staff. They had their own important and continuing role to play in the field of motivation and education.[41] But her greatest asset in her relations with lay people lay in the fact that she did not act as they anticipated a doctor, particularly a specialist, would. The Christchurch delegates who had not met her before the conference were 'very pleasantly surprised' by her easy manner. They did not find her 'rather arrogant', but 'outgoing, straight from the shoulder', and they 'admired her although [they] did not always agree with her'.[42]

Her disinclination to aspire to the loftier altitudes of professional supremacy did not simply reflect Alice's attitudes towards lay people. Although she was committed to professional excellence, and could be very short with those whose performance she felt did not measure up, her participation in the higher regions of the NZBMA was spasmodic, a marginal role that arose from personal choice. In 1958 she declined nomination to the NZBMA council's executive committee.[43] Her male associates, even Douglas Robb, were more attracted to these activities. In 1961, recently knighted, Robb was elected president of the British Medical Association, the NZBMA's parent body, when its annual general meeting took the form of a Commonwealth conference in Auckland. It was enough to raise the hackles of some older medical practitioners, who remembered his earlier, anti-establishment campaigns.[44] Over the early 1960s, men of Alice's own age and experience were also rising in these ranks. Paediatricians Neil Begg and Jim Watt both served on the NZBMA council's executive committee,[45] and on the Central Specialists' Committee.[46] In 1964 Neil Begg was elected chairman of the NZBMA council,[47] and Jim Watt became the first professor of child health at Otago University in 1967. Like Alice, they supported lay groups, but their approach and their interests were different. Neil Begg was concerned mainly with the Plunket Society, a relatively conservative organisation. Jim Watt supported Parents' Centres, but principally from behind the scenes. Alice was to take up leadership of the NZFPA cause both within professional structures and in the public arena.

At the 1960 NZFPA conference, Alice had listened to criticisms of NZBMA attitudes from Phyllis Zeff and from NZFPA doctors who had experience in Britain, and who could not understand why British doctors' freedom, to work for the FPA or not as they pleased, could not be replicated in New Zealand. After making it quite clear where her sympathies lay, describing the NZBMA as 'suffering from an inferiority complex and that they feared that doctors would lose patients', Alice agreed that co-operation between the two bodies must be pursued. She proposed that the Auckland branch of the Medical Association might be persuaded to recommend to the council the setting up of a committee 'to explore methods of cooperating with organisations, such as NZFPA, which [were] working for the benefit of happy family living'.[48] At the close of the conference, Alice issued a press release confirming her new commitment:

> For very many years I have been a member of the Family Planning Association and I feel that it has now reached a stage in its development

when its clinics are an accepted part of New Zealand life. As the medical work of the Association has now become an integral part of its work, a happy cooperation with the British Medical Association has become important. I have accepted the position of President because I think this will enable me to act as a liaison officer between the Family Planning Association and the British Medical Association.[49]

Acting as 'a liaison officer', or channel of communication, between lay groups and her profession was not a new role for Alice, but never had their differences been so firmly and officially entrenched. She had already explained to conference delegates that gaining ethical recognition would mean directly challenging the opinion of the Branch Ethical Committee, which had been expressed through its chairman, Dr J.P.S. Jamieson. Born and educated in Scotland, Dr Jamieson was an institution in the NZBMA. He had led medical opposition to the original provisions of the Social Security Act and been honoured within the profession by the rare award of the Gold Medal of the BMA.[50] Friend and foe alike attested to the strength of his personality, a redoubtable blend of tenacity and dominance, 'rock fast on matters of principle'.[51] Now in his 70s, and in failing health, he was certainly not alone in opposing recognition of the NZFPA but his unique standing placed him in a particularly strong position to influence events. Moreover, there was still sufficient vocal community opposition to the NZFPA to lend his views wider authority. When a report of the 1960 conference, including Alice's statement, appeared in the Wellington press, it stimulated 'Parents of a Large Family' to respond:

> It pains one to see the medical profession involved. We thought the Hippocratic oath was concerned with the preservation of life, not its calculated inhibition. We would be surprised if orthodox B.M.A. opinion gave its benediction to the Family Planning Association. If the planning association wants to see some homes with "healthy parents and children" without the "strains, stresses, and fears of modern life," let them open their eyes and see some of the happy, unplanned large families about.[52]

Alice, with the help of other 'friendly' doctors, initiated the campaign to set aside the Ethical Committee's findings by enlisting the support of the NZMWA members at a meeting held at the home of Dr Grace Pinkerton, wife of Harvey Carey.[53] A few weeks later, armed with their vote of confidence in the NZFPA, she addressed a well-attended Auckland NZBMA division meeting, where she argued that the Ethical Committee had made a 'wrong decision' because it had been given incomplete information. She proposed that the NZBMA should recognise the NZFPA, 'or at least ... approve of the cooperation of its members with the Association', emphasising that doctors did not work under lay direction there but were alone responsible for medical matters. The meeting's cautious reaction revealed the serious implications of a challenge to the Ethical Committee's findings. Sympathy for a 'miscarriage of justice' was modified by an observation that any request to the committee to reverse its decision would need to be 'extremely carefully considered', perhaps for several weeks. It was only after further wrangling that most of those present finally agreed to support Alice's proposal

> ... that the subject of the Freedom of the Profession to cooperate with the Family Planning Association should be referred back to the Branch Ethical Committee for reconsideration in the light of information which was not previously made available to it.[54]

It was hardly the 'woman's right' argument with which she had originally planned to approach the meeting,[55] but it was an alternative that offered a realistic chance of keeping the clinics open. An appeal based on 'professional freedom' placed the campaign in a wider context, reaching beyond Alice's own liberal sentiments, or even the current issue. Professional freedom was a cornerstone of the medical world. It had formed the chief defence against the threat of state authority which Dr Jamieson had himself led in the past, while that very year the incoming NZBMA president had placed the doctor 'in the forefront of the fight for freedom, for the principles of democracy'.[56] It was enough to get a majority vote in Auckland and by mid-August a lengthy letter supporting the same argument and signed by Alice as dominion president of the NZFPA, was being circulated among other NZBMA branches.[57]

When Alice attended the September NZBMA council meeting in Wellington, to present the Auckland division's remit seeking a re-examination of the NZFPA case, her personal agenda once again widened. Parents' Centre supporters in Auckland had quietly continued with their activities since their own recognition had been withdrawn, a strategy favoured by Alice, who had advised that 'the proper thing for the parents centres to do is to carry on as if the BMA had not made a fool of itself'.[58] Nevertheless, discretion was the order of the day. Antenatal classes had been established in Mount Eden for patients attending local private obstetric hospitals with sympathetic matrons. They accepted only women referred by their own doctors, who were advised that Alice was willing to 'speak to our work'.[59] Despite these precautions, the NZBMA received a complaint that Parents' Centres were distributing an old pamphlet in which they claimed recognition by the association. After discussing the matter, the NZBMA council decided to set up an investigative subcommittee. Alice was invited to be a member, along with Jim Watt, Neil Begg, Wellington obstetrician W.M.E. Tweed, and the current NZBMA president, D.C. Low. The council also agreed to refer the NZFPA's case back to the Ethical Committee 'for reconsideration in the light of further information which can be presented'.[60]

For the rest of the year the Ethical Committee reconsidered NZFPA activities, while the NZBMA council turned its attention to organising the Commonwealth BMA meeting to be held in Auckland in February 1961, generally anticipated as a highlight of the profession's existence in New Zealand. At the same time, the NZFPA wrote to individual practitioners nationwide, in the hope of gaining more support for its case,[61] while Alice canvassed Auckland doctors for their 'factual' experiences with Parents' Centres.[62] She also prepared 'The Doctor and the Delinquent' for publication in the *NZMJ*. The link made in the title may have puzzled some, but it was crystal clear to those familiar with the promise of wide social benefits from improved early childhood experience and the need, stressed in her text, for increased co-operation between medical and other professionals and lay groups to combat problems such as delinquency. Parents' Centres, Nursery Play Centres, the Marriage Guidance Council and the NZFPA, were suggested as particular groups requiring 'assistance and encouragement from the medical profession'.[63] By the time 'The Doctor and the Delinquent' appeared, the Ethical Committee's latest report had been circulated to the NZBMA divisions, although, unlike the first one, it seems never to have been published.

If Alice had supposed that arguments for professional freedom might have swayed Dr Jamieson, she was very much mistaken. The issue was not addressed; indeed both the profession and the NZFPA were admonished:

> If the F.P.A. would turn its attention from lay, propagandist methods to purely medical clinics under medical control, under gynaecologists of merit, accepting only cases referred by doctors, our objections would disappear. And if the profession would undertake its duties in this aspect of work with care and efficiency, the F.P.A. would cease to exist.[64]

The report went on to argue that, in providing contraception, only the patient's health and life should be taken into account. Reasons 'of convenience and indulgence' were 'not admissible'. These were exactly the attitudes family planners had spent more than 20 years trying to overcome. There was no recognition at all of the social or psychological benefits which were, and would remain for Alice's lifetime, the distinguishing feature of the association's philosophy and formed the basis of her enduring relationship with it.[65] Accepting the impasse, she wrote to the general secretary of the NZBMA, 'asking for top level discussions'.[66] As a result, a special NZBMA sub-committee, composed of three members of the current executive, was set up to re-examine the NZFPA case. Around the same time Alice and Ruth Black achieved a majority vote in favour of NZFPA activities from the Auckland branch of the Obstetrical and Gynaecological Society.[67] Then, with Glenys Lowe, they met the NZBMA subcommittee that had already examined the existing files.

The resulting report, presented to the council in mid-June 1961, rejected the Ethical Committee's findings as 'too sweeping and too strict'. After a point by point disputation, and references to the changing climate of opinion on birth control and sexuality within marriage, it concluded that it should not be considered unethical 'for a member of the New Zealand Branch of the British Medical Association to accept employment at one of the Family Planning Association's clinics as at present constituted'.[68] In September, after the Ethical Committee and all divisions had been given the opportunity to comment on it, the 'general question' was deferred for a year, but the paragraph that declared it 'ethical' for NZBMA members to accept employment in NZFPA clinics was carried.[69] This was clearly a compromise. It reflected not only the considerable personal influence of Dr Jamieson, but also the still significant strength of the opinions he represented.

The subcommittee appointed to report on Parents' Centre activities (of which Alice was a member) also presented its report in mid-June. Although this upheld the belief that 'antenatal education and preparation for parenthood in its broadest sense' should be under medical supervision, it also argued for freedom of choice. Not only should a practitioner be able to direct patients 'to the classes he thinks will benefit them most', but 'both patient and doctor have a right to express their preference as to the classes to be attended'. If Parents' Centres worked 'under medical control and provided a service acceptable to both patient and doctor they should be regarded as a suitable alternative to hospital antenatal classes, as should any other body meeting the same criteria'.[70] Just how difficult it had been to get this report through had been indicated by its passage at the Auckland divisional meeting a week earlier. Only after 'considerable discussion' and several avowals of the federation's desire to 'work under medical supervision', was grudging approval won for its continued activity in this field. When Alice, seconded by Harvey Carey, moved 'That this Division approves the recognition of the Federation of Parents' Centres provided there is absolute certainty of Medical Control' – surely sufficiently strong language to satisfy the most reluctant professionals – the vote was carried only by 12 to 9, with 7 abstentions. The NZFPA had fared little better with support for its recognition running at 10 to six.[71]

These were tenuous successes at best, and Alice clearly felt the need to follow them up. From this time she focused increasingly on pursuing both professional and public acceptance of the importance of mental and emotional family health and the support of organisations which, in various ways, sustained them. At the end of 1961 she began working as a consultant at the Auckland Child Health Clinic, a venture she certainly did not undertake for personal advancement since the vacancy was that of an assistant paediatrician and the post was upgraded when she was appointed.[72] The attraction was the clinic's work with children's emotional and behavioural problems and the need to address the lack of properly qualified personnel. During her tenure Alice actively sought a child psychiatrist to head the clinic. When Dr R.J. Methven, a New Zealander who had undertaken further study in Melbourne, took up the position in the mid-1960s, she maintained her interest by continuing at the clinic at reduced hours, performing preliminary general examinations for which she considered a psychiatrist's time 'too valuable'.[73]

Working at the Child Health Clinic confirmed for Alice the value of her favoured interdisciplinary team approach and reinforced her ideas about the proper use of psychiatry and psychology, which had nothing to do with professional mystique. In a 1965 book review she praised the fact that 'Psychiatric theory here ceases to be an esoteric cult understandable only to the elite, who speak a different language from most of us, and becomes a practical guide to the understanding of everyday problems of home, school and community'.[74] Nevertheless, for the general public, psychiatric theory was surrounded by esoteric barriers, both practical and linguistic. When, in July 1961, Alice, in the correspondence columns of the *Herald*, argued for family planning and instruction in parentcraft by counsellors within the context of modifying the 'urges of the Id' by cultivating the 'Super ego', the predominant reaction was one of bewilderment.[75]

Parents' Centres could count on her support in a variety of roles. She spoke at conferences and meetings, acted as an editorial adviser for their magazine, made herself available for consultation on any administrative or medical point, maintained mutual sympathies in the needs of hospitalised children and sustained links with their mental health offshoot. In 1967 she became a member of the federation's Educational Advisory Council.[76] Alice was similarly committed to the Family Guidance Centre. She was a long-standing member of the Advisory Committee, gave financial support and lectures and offered her home for meetings.[77] In many ways, this was the organisation nearest her heart. In 1968, when she made her last will, she nominated the centre as the beneficiary of her residual estate, should her immediate family predecease her.[78] But the NZFPA was to demand much more of her time and attention, not just because she was continually re-elected president for the remainder of her life, but because national and international issues over the 1960s made the association's work relevant in a way it had not been before. The shift was already under way at the time of the NZBMA crisis, although its practical effects became noticeable only over the following years. Within the association Alice was active at several levels. As dominion president, she chaired the Standing Committee meetings and acted as a public figurehead. For a short time she headed the Medical Advisory Committee. She provided copy for *Choice*, and also worked regularly in the Auckland clinic. This was another extension of her medical practice clearly not undertaken for financial or professional reasons. The payment of NZFPA clinic doctors was a moot point at the time and Alice was already earning a good living in her practice. Neither did her clinic work add to her professional status in paediatrics and allergies. On the other hand, she was strongly committed to providing access to contraception and clinic doctors were in such short supply that, even towards the end of her life, she often covered in branches temporarily without one, in addition to her own regular clinic commitment. Clinic work also meant that she could keep up with the practicalities of changing contraceptive techniques, now coming thick and fast.

Oral contraception, better known as the Pill, had just become available in New Zealand when she took up the presidency. It signalled the true medicalisation of birth control. Unlike the old barrier methods, which could be supplied over the counter and efficiently fitted by any experienced person, hormonal contraceptives were prescription drugs, available in New Zealand only through registered medical practitioners. General practitioners began to take up 'family planning' as they had never done before. It demonstrated, Alice remarked at the NZFPA's 1964 conference, 'their willingness to give their patients the means to plan their families by a method within their competence'.[79] So ready was their acceptance of this new regime that the NZFPA Medical Advisory Committee suggested that no further new clinics would be needed and that the association's future lay in its educational role.[80] Alice did not believe this meant the association should stand still; rather, new branches should be set up in areas where clinics were not required, solely for educational work.[81] The NZFPA did not actively push oral contraception. Occlusive devices continued to be offered to new patients and couples already successfully managing these were not advised to change. Nevertheless women were attracted by a method that promised convenience and efficiency and by 1965 increasing numbers coming to NZFPA clinics were asking for the Pill.[82]

The development of new methods of contraception appealed to the progressive element in Alice's nature. In 1964, when Edith Summerskill, now sitting in the House of Lords, had described women taking oral contraceptives as just 'guinea pigs', Alice had positively bridled. 'It is not possible,' she wrote to the press, 'to say what will be the condition, 20 years from now, of people taking new antibiotics, antihypertensives, or indeed any new treatment prescribed for their immediate safety or comfort.' She suggested the alternative of seeing 'pill-takers' as 'adventurers willing to take some risk in the pursuit of a better life for themselves and their families. There are few of us who would subscribe to the banning of motor cars, yet if there is a risk attached to the taking of "the pill" it is infinitesimal compared with the risk of using the road.'[83] Entries in Alice's personal diary suggest that she was taking the Pill around this time.[84] As an NZFPA doctor, she kept herself informed of the latest information on its effects and was under no illusions that it was necessarily for everyone.[85] In her view, all forms of contraception had shortcomings but these had to be balanced against the alternative risks of an unwanted or complicated pregnancy or abortion, and the improved social, physical and mental health of all family members that she believed resulted from 'spaced' pregnancies. This was also to be her approach to the later development of inter-uterine devices (IUDs) and the three-monthly injectable contraceptive Depo-Provera.[86]

The youth and sexual revolution of the 1960s not only increased the demand for contraception but proved a particular difficulty for the NZFPA, which had based its arguments on the need for birth control within the context of sustaining marriage and family life. Personally, Alice was inclined to balance idealism with realism. During the first half of the 1960s she had a reputation for being approachable in her private practice when young, unmarried women were seeking contraceptive advice.[87] Later in the decade she advised parents upset by the 'liberated' lifestyle of their young to be open about their concern, but if this had no effect they should make sure that their daughters could get the Pill, 'buying time' and avoiding pregnancy.[88] When, in 1966 and long after the death of Dr Jamieson, the NZBMA Ethical Committee issued a statement asserting that 'the supply or prescription by medical practitioners of contraceptives to unmarried persons, thereby facilitating extra-marital relationships, is not in keeping with the highest ideals of the medical profession',[89] Alice responded by questioning the assumption that extramarital sexuality created unstable marriages and arguing that the ruling was, yet again, an infringement on the right of practitioners to prescribe as they thought fit.[90] As NZFPA president she needed to take a more moderate position, testing the ground for public acceptance of any extension of the association's services by speaking as 'an individual'.[91] It was not until 1970, within the context of a rising extranuptial pregnancy rate, often involving very young mothers, and the hotly contested demands for increased access to abortion, that it seemed politic to ask in the press just where the 'interests of the family' might begin and end and whether these might not 'be best served by extending FPA services to the unmarried'.[92] At an NZFPA seminar in September 1971, Alice extended the debate by referring to the fact that it was illegal in New Zealand to instruct those under 16 years of age in the use of contraceptives, or to advertise contraceptives to anyone under 21. Were these laws 'in the best interests of the community', she asked, or 'a remnant of a sociological outlook which is now completely out of date'?[93] Her remarks emphasised the speed of social change, since the law was a relatively recent one, an offshoot of the Mazengarb inquiry first encoded in the Police Offences Act (1954),[94] and amended by increasing the monetary penalties fourfold as late as 1967.

In pursuing such causes, the NZFPA defended itself from criticism from outside (and inside) its ranks by following the path that had proved successful in establishing its clinics: basing the provision of contraceptive services on the individual right, and therefore the individual responsibility, of doctors willing to assist their patients in this way. This line was successfully followed in 1970, when access to contraception for the unmarried became official policy, by describing 'the form of advice given' as 'a medical decision'.[95] Contraception for those under 16 was more complex, not a moral but a legal question, although Alice argued in the *NZMJ* in July 1973 that it was really no more culpable on the doctor's part than supplying antibiotics to a woman suffering from the effects of a septic abortion.[96] The same year the NZFPA's submissions supporting repeal of the Police Offences Act were presented to the Statutes Revision Committee by, and under the names of, Alice and Ruth Black. They argued that the legislation was inadequate in the face of social change, that it no longer served the purpose for which it was designed and that it had become 'a restriction of the freedom of responsible professional workers who are deeply concerned about the welfare of the children of today and tomorrow'.[97] Over the years of her presidency, however, Alice's chief concerns were directed not towards those who were asking for contraception but those who, in her opinion, most needed this boon to individual and family life and social progress, and were not getting it.

CHAPTER 9

Going to the Needy

> *So far the only organisation attempting to see the benefits of scientific fertility control are available to those who need them most, but are least able to ask for them, is the Family Planning Association. We have a great deal of responsibility and a tremendous task ahead of us, and very little time.*[1]

Alice believed that those at the lower end of the socio-economic scale, struggling with housing, education and health, their problems compounded by large families, were candidates for the benefits of birth control. In 1960s New Zealand these criteria were most likely to fit Maori. Like most urban dwellers, Alice had become aware of this fact only after the Second World War, when Maori began to move to the towns and cities, particularly Auckland, in search of work. Usually lacking the education and training for any but unskilled jobs, they tended to live in the poorest housing areas, unfamiliar with urban amenities and without the customary support provided by the extended family and traditional food sources. At the same time, their birth rate was soaring. Between 1936 and 1961 the Maori population had increased by 103 per cent, while the non-Maori increase over the same period was 50.07 per cent, including migration.[2]

Even before Alice had become president, the NZFPA had been eager to include Maori among their clientele,[3] but it was her experience as a paediatrician that gave an extra edge to her own concern. Maori infant mortality in 1959 was over two and a half times that of Pakeha,[4] preschoolers died of respiratory tract diseases at five to six times the Pakeha rate, school-aged children died, disturbingly often as the result of accidental injuries, at a rate nearly three times higher than their non-Maori peers.[5] Since a 'disproportionate number' of Maori children were admitted to public hospitals for treatment,[6] Alice saw many at Princess Mary, the Karitane Hospital and the Child Health Clinic. Too frequently they were suffering from accidents, diseases arising from their home environment, or emotional problems that restricted their ability to make the most of urban educational or social opportunities. From this perspective, family planning seemed not only essential to any social and economic progress for Maori but also an important facet of preventive medicine.

Alice could not have become involved in a more contentious area. Dealing with another race and culture within the context of reproduction was fraught with difficulty; resonances of eugenic thought could become uncomfortably apparent. At its worst, eugenics had linked evolutionary progress, or the lack of it, to genetic inheritance, often along racial lines. This approach had been taken to its ultimate conclusion in the concentration camps of Nazi Germany, but it had also been an arrow in the quiver of early birth controllers and the Eurocentric notion of 'more' or 'less developed' societies had historically underpinned New Zealand's official race relations policy. Because it was more concerned with nurture than nature, the family planning movement had modified these theories but echoes of earlier doctrines still tended to emerge occasionally. The NZFPA's emphasis on 'responsible' planned parenthood also lent a moralistic tone to their pronouncements when spokespeople described as 'irresponsible' those struggling to bring up children but not practising family planning. Alice herself was prone to these tendencies. Modification of attitudes, even within individuals, is a complex process and her disposition towards evolutionary change combined elements of old and new. In an attempt to avoid off-putting dogmatism in the NZFPA's dealings with new clients during 1964, she had warned that too rigid an approach

> has the longterm result of putting evolution into reverse, it assists intelligent, responsible, often ambitious small families, sometimes very small families but takes no cognizance whatever of the far greater number of reasonably good citizens who nevertheless are inclined to take

life as it comes and feel that anything too meticulous is more trouble than it is worth. The long term result of this policy is a steady increase in the less responsible, less able, less intelligent citizens and this must eventually spell disaster to a democracy.[7]

Alice's public support of contraception or voluntary sterilisation for intellectually handicapped people in particular circumstances[8] intensified this impression.

These factors, together with the use of IUDs and Depo-Provera, would later open the entire scheme of taking family planning to Maori and Polynesian women to the same kind of criticism directed at international birth control programmes. They were seen as exercises in cultural imperialism, stained by racism and imposed, in their own interests, by the rich and powerful to the individual and communal detriment of the poor and powerless. Although Alice's leadership role and total commitment to family planning would place her within this framework, she did not share this world view. The social and political climate in which she worked favoured the integration of Maori into a Pakeha lifestyle. Alice came into conflict with this general consensus because she believed that government policy was denying Maori women access to the services they needed, which offended her liberal notions of equal opportunity for all. For her, this exclusion constituted 'racial discrimination'.[9] Central to her stance was her conviction that family planning was not an end in itself but a means to an end. In 1970, when the Minister of Maori Affairs, Duncan MacIntyre, was impressed with the fall in fertility rates of Maori women over 24 years of age,[10] Alice disagreed.

> I didn't find any comfort in his figures at all. It is the young Maori mother with her four or five children under five who is producing the material out of which our schools are failing to make satisfactory students. . . . Mr MacIntyre says that he doesn't feel that it would be proper to direct a campaign specifically at Maori mothers. I would of course agree with him. All mothers and particularly the underprivileged, whether brown or white, should get information and motivation for responsible parenthood.[11]

Nevertheless, the need to work through Maori agencies, already recognised by bureaucracy in the early 1960s, did lead Alice to approach them in a directed way.

Early in Alice's presidency there had already been several encouraging developments. At the NZFPA conference in June 1962 she gave a special welcome to J.K. Hunn, Secretary of Maori Affairs and a major influence on government policy at the time, and spoke of the part the association could play 'in offering to the Maoris equality with Europeans in opportunity for family planning'.[12] Coincidentally the Auckland clinic was on the move, shifting from middle class Remuera to Pitt Street, nearer the inner city, where many Maori and immigrant Pacific Island families lived. The strong educational bias of many of the association's personnel resulted in contacts with sympathetic Maori. In September a Maori Adult Education tutor attended a Standing Committee meeting to advise on 'the Maori situation as regards Family Planning' and to invite an NZFPA representative to a Young Maori Leaders' Conference to be held at Ruatoria the following Labour Weekend.[13]

When Alice went to the Ruatoria conference on behalf of NZFPA, it was the first time she had come close to the essentials of Maori life. What she saw confirmed her view that Maori women wanted access to birth control. At both Ruatoria and Tikitiki they formed the most receptive part of her audience, and a remit 'That the Maori people should take steps to bring to Maori mothers information about family planning' was passed. Two doctors in the area were already doing some contraceptive work and it was arranged that the NZFPA would send them supplies of the Pill. One difficulty made itself obvious. Maori elders and Maori men generally were not keen on the idea of birth control.[14] The historical origins of this attitude had been expressed by Bishop Wiremu Panapa in 1959, at the seventh annual conference of the Maori Women's Welfare League (MWWL). He looked back to the turn of the century when Maori were believed to be a 'dying race',

> faced with the problem of total extinction. In 1907 we were down to 42,000 ... on the turn of the second half of the century we numbered 151,000. That is a miracle! ... It is the miracle of the Maori race.... This tremendous increase in the Maori people should be the glory of our Nation, must be the glory of our Nation.[15]

For the Maori women of Ruatoria, having babies had less to do with national glory than with the trials of daily living. They complained that their men did little around the house or with their children.[16]

But the desire to overcome the depopulation resulting from the disease and poverty that had accompanied colonisation added to the tensions already being experienced by newly urbanised Maori women.

Although there seemed to be a demand, the NZFPA made scant progress in its attempts to meet the contraceptive needs of urban Maori women over the next two years. Setting up an informal clinic in school buildings accessible to Maori,[17] and not charging those who could not afford to pay,[18] did not bring the response for which they had hoped. Alice also experienced personal frustrations. In 1962 she had asked for a ruling on giving contraceptive advice, or referring to the NZFPA, parents of patients attending the Child Health Clinic whom she believed would benefit from such services. She was informed that 'general policy' was to refer these cases back to their own doctor.[19] As a hospital paediatrician, Alice knew that Maori women tended not to consult general practitioners. Their point of contact was the public health nurse, the frontline worker who visited homes and provided primary health care. Alice was to remember this when, in 1964, she represented the New Zealand National Council of Churches at a Consultation on Responsible Parenthood in Bangkok, part of the expanding round of activities she was undertaking as president of the NZFPA. The conference's conclusion, that the churches in the East Asian area should 'take active steps' to see that parents knew about family planning and 'where to find the right services',[20] provided the sort of link between Christian duty, perceived need and activism that Alice could not resist. The conference proceedings also provided an example of the effectiveness of using an existing health service.[21] In 1971 she recalled how she had

> listened to Dr Kinch of Sweden explaining how, in the Sweden–Ceylon project, education for family planning could be accomplished by the medical officers and infant welfare nurses as part of their preventive health programme. From that day I have looked forward to the time when this could become a possibility in New Zealand, because I could see no other way of taking the great benefits of a free choice of family size to all members of our society.[22]

Placing family planning services within public health structures would mean a complete reversal of established New Zealand policy.

The state had long been reluctant to become involved in what was considered a politically sensitive, and nationally disadvantageous, area. Even under National, which favoured assistance to voluntary organisations over the development of the public health sector,[23] the NZFPA had never received direct financial government support.

And attitudes had not changed by the 1960s. While Alice was in Wellington for the NZFPA's 1964 conference, she called on the Minister of Health, D.N. McKay,[24] with some specific suggestions for overcoming financial or social barriers to family planning services. These included the education of public health nurses in family planning techniques, social security payments for medical services relating to birth control and reducing the price of oral contraceptives by subsidy or the removal of duty. She also suggested that hospital boards might set up clinics in rural areas to supervise patients requiring IUDs, and that family planning information could be distributed through the Health Education Branch. After some consideration, the minister informed Alice that her ideas could not be implemented. The Maori Health Committee (created as a result of the major government incentive for Maori development in the 1960s, the Hunn Report) had already considered family planning and had been unable to reach agreement over it. This, McKay suggested, reflected 'the divergent views over this matter in the community', and since bodies such as the Medical Association or other community groups had expressed no opinion on the matter, the minister 'could hardly consider involving the Department of Health in the way you suggest'. Similarly, the absence of an approach by the Hospital Boards' Association made him reluctant to impose upon them the duty of providing clinics. Family planning, the minister concluded, was 'more properly – and probably more efficiently – handled by a voluntary body than by a tax supported agency'.[25]

If the minister thought this would be an end to the matter, he did not know Alice. While he had been mulling over his response the debate had entered the public arena through press reports of her speeches to various NZFPA gatherings and a personal letter to the *New Zealand Herald*, in which she linked access to family planning information through the public health system to the hope of any fulfilment of Maori aspirations 'in educational standards, or any other aspect of modern living'.[26] During her Wellington visit, Alice had also called on Ralph Hanan, the Minister of Maori Affairs, and found a more receptive audience for her ideas. Hanan's staff had arranged a meeting with the executive of the MWWL, without whose co-operation and support, the minister had advised, no approach regarding family planning could succeed.[27] Here Alice's path would be smoothed by the fact that the league welcomed Pakeha women as members and encouraged liaison with Pakeha organisations. It also had an underlying philosophical affinity with the NZFPA. League policies included improving the socio-economic position of Maori through education and health care, and empowering Maori women. Alice had already become friendly with the mayoress of Auckland, Thelma Robinson, a league supporter,[28] and by August she herself was a member of the Arohina group in Auckland.[29] When Alice met the MWWL executive the following month, her ability to work alongside lay women bridged any cultural divide and discussion was 'lively and often entertaining'. Members undertook to initiate the topic in their home areas and it was hoped that Alice might be able to address an MWWL conference. The League president, Ruiha Sage, would also be present at the December meeting of the Maori Health Committee, when Alice would speak in favour of family planning.[30]

This would be a rather more testing experience since, apart from Mrs Sage, the committee was composed wholly of men. But Alice had probably been considerably empowered by studying a Ministry of Maori Affairs backgrounding document, 'For a Better Understanding of the Maori', which described traditional Maori values and social organisation. It referred to contemporary child-rearing composed largely of 'indulgence and inconsistent disciplinary control', and children lacking 'help guidance or encouragement in their educational and vocational aspirations'.[31] It noted that the 'golden period' of childhood, in which a child was 'the centre of attention', lasted only until the birth of the next baby, and that community or kinship pressures, such as adoption by childless relatives, often broke 'the normal strong mother (or parent)/child relationship'.[32] Here was almost every social contingency for which Alice believed family planning could provide a solution and within this context, she told the Maori Health Committee, race was irrelevant.

> What I have to say is just as true for the European families as for the Maori. Parents are only human whatever their race and a mother and father have only two pairs of hands and there are only twenty-four hours

in the day and the strongest mother must have sleep and she will be easier to live with if she can get some recreation.[33]

Alice did not condemn large families and was unconcerned about the increasing ratio of Polynesian peoples in New Zealand, either as a result of natural increase or immigration.[34] Her interest was in 'the quality of family life', establishing good parent–child relations and preparing children to become successful adults, 'using the word success in a wide sense'. From this perspective, she argued, the well 'spaced' family held particular advantages for Maori, allowing them to make social and economic advances while preserving 'a specific attitude to life and their own code of values'.

> I have seen Maori boys at the Child Health Clinic, handsome, of fine physique, one would think a young Rangatira, but both school work and a psychological test indicate a learning capacity below the average of the community as a whole and the story is usually one of living with a series of different relatives practically from birth. History shows that the Maori is capable of imagination and of initiative and of learning about ideas, the small proportion who cope with the higher standards of academic education is attributable to family instability. The Maori who was born with the talent to be a lawyer, a doctor, a scientist, ends up driving a tractor because as a child he was deprived of his mother, not because she was a rejecting person, but because she had other babies whose needs seemed more urgent. Other kinds of educational handicap are obvious, lack of supervision of homework, lack of privacy in a crowded home where the children attending secondary school really need peace and quiet for concentration.[35]

Alice had already emphasised the health advantages of family planning, identifying herself early on as a paediatrician whose professional experience with Maori children formed the basis of her concern. She confirmed this by suggesting that, if a mobile family planning clinic for rural areas were to be considered, it should also provide immunisation, dental examinations and cervical smears, serving family welfare 'of which family spacing is only one part'.[36]

Elements of Alice's address could be seen as evidence of cultural insensitivity, or even ignorance, but she was well aware of the contentious nature of some of her assertions. Her primary concern was with the realities of urban life for Maori. Although 'For a

Better Understanding of the Maori' was explicit on the tradition of shared parenting, she would argue that this practice was less likely to work outside a rural setting.[37] On this particular occasion, perhaps because she was speaking to a captive audience of 20 men, she spent some time on another controversial area: male 'antagonism to the idea' of family planning. She professed herself unsure about how much of this resulted from 'a failure to understand that modern methods of birth control involve no restriction or interference with the marriage relationship'. Maori fathers did not, she conceded, come to meetings, but the 'few with whom I have had personal discussions have been easy to persuade'.[38] For this reason, she suggested that education, an area in which the NZFPA would gladly co-operate by running seminars for Maori Welfare workers, was the most practical starting point[39] – and immediately demonstrated this approach by treating those present to a rundown on current recommended contraceptive techniques.

Alice's address surely ruffled a few feathers but the results were further evidence of her powers of persuasion. After 'lengthy discussion', the committee agreed to officially ask the Health Department to institute a health education programme on family care which included family spacing. Because of its 'social and political aspects', however, the Minister of Health should sanction the idea before its form was considered by a subcommittee.[40] Alice and Ruth Black went on to achieve a similar success at the quarterly meeting of the NZBMA Auckland Division, despite an attempt to subvert their efforts with an 'amendment' that the NZBMA should express its concern about the marked fall in the birth rate and do what it could to check this decline. Also passed was a remit proposing that information on fertility control be included in the health education programme and that public health nurses be permitted to discuss with 'under-privileged' mothers the 'help they could have from their family doctor'.[41] Under Alice's patronage, the remit progressed, by way of the NZBMA Council and the Director-General of Health, to the Minister of Health.[42] The following July the dominion conference of the MWWL supported similar moves.[43] The matter was now in the department's hands.

Alice could not resist a little crowing about the apparent success of this campaign. In a *Choice* article entitled 'Winds of Change', she referred to an intensification of international interest in fertility control, claiming that in New Zealand 'we have had a revolution also'. She demonstrated this by comparing the 1959 NZBMA Ethical Committee report on the NZFPA and the latest council remit to the Minister of Health.[44] This was taking optimism to its extreme. Over the next two years the Health Department was to be bombarded with submissions from opposition groups,[45] while the National government remained loath to alter its established position.[46] As the 1966 election approached, the situation was still unresolved. When the opposition Labour Party professed itself in favour of change,[47] this was apparently enough to turn a lifelong political conservative into a public critic of National. Alice, as NZFPA President, wrote to the newspapers:

> The National party has stated that it is neither necessary nor desirable for family planning information to be included in the health education programme of the Health Department. This makes a travesty of their claims to offer equal opportunity for advancement and education for all people.... [and denies some mothers] one of the most valued freedoms of the 20th Century, the freedom to plan their families in accordance with their resources. Persistence with this policy will perpetuate for another generation the existence within our own shores of an underprivileged group, with a high birth rate, a high infant mortality, a lower expectation of life and a lower standard of education than the rest of the community.[48]

In December of that year the new Director-General of Health, Dr Douglas Kennedy, finally presented a draft policy statement to the Minister of Health.[49] Departmental officers were to give general contraceptive information when requested. They could refer patients to their family doctor for further advice or give the address, telephone number and hours of the nearest NZFPA clinic if that was what the patient preferred. Where there was a language, cultural or similar difficulty, a note of introduction could be provided. The patient could also be asked, at a later and appropriate time, if any further help was required.[50] This approach was too passive for Alice. In June 1967, at a meeting of the national executive of the NCW, she pushed for a letter to the Minister of Health insisting that the department should adopt a 'more positive' policy.[51] The following month the Director-General of Health was informed of a similar resolution from the triennial conference of the New Zealand Federation of University Women. Kennedy assured both organisations that there was sufficient leeway in the department's directive to allow essential information to get through without departmental officers intruding on what was still an individual choice.[52]

Family planners were not so sure. They continued to pursue the policy of 'going to the needy'. In Auckland attention was now focused on the sprawling state house suburbs to the south of the city, which had become the latest home of the poor and relatively powerless. In Otara, residents were attempting to foster community spirit. A temporary urban marae had been established, with the Otara Maori Committee acting as a co-ordinating body. In December 1967, the committee invited Alice, as president of the NZFPA, to speak to a meeting of elders about family planning. After representatives of the Auckland branch of the association had been welcomed, their hosts listened courteously and attentively while she spoke. She followed familiar themes, stressing the spacing of children according to individual needs and arguing that planned pregnancies meant better health for mothers and children. Maori women who looked after themselves made better mothers than Pakeha, she asserted, but those who neglected their health did not. She referred to the relatively high mortality rates of Maori children and the economic and emotional strains of unplanned families.

When, after the formalities were over, Alice's views were challenged, she handled the situation with equanimity. This was a world with which she was becoming more familiar. In February 1965 she had participated in another marae-based health course at Te Araroa,[53] her verbal skills were already finely honed, she was never averse to a good debate and she had just enough spark to command respect. The elders spoke of their love of children and of large families, of 'Maori Aroha', which they believed was God's gift to them. How could Alice explain the achievements of men like Te Rangi Hiroa, Sir Peter Buck, who came from large families? There would be more such scholars, she responded, if families were smaller. Although NZFPA members supported her arguments for family planning, it was Alice who directly challenged the men. In her summing up she 'questioned whether some Maori men were not flaunting their pride in large families, at the expense of their own children'. When a speaker quoted the Old Testament, referring to God's promise to Abraham that his children would be 'as the stars from Heaven', Alice countered with a biblical quotation of her own. As a paediatrician, she said, she would refer to the New Testament bidding, 'better to have a millstone tied around your neck and be thrown into the depths of the ocean, than to cause the feet of a little one to falter'. This verbal interplay may well have swung the balance in her favour. It appealed to Maori far more than being talked to, and the closing mood of the meeting appears to have been very congenial. After Alice had thanked the committee 'for its courtesy and honesty' informal discussion continued over supper.

According to Colleen King's account, the group left with repeated invitations to return ringing in their ears. When they did, in January 1968, the family planners were 'amazed by a complete change of feeling.' They were told of the 'great impact' the previous meeting had made; those who had come 'to scoff remained to pray'. Although the Pill was still treated with reservation, the principle of family planning had been accepted. Alice was presented with 'a beautiful bouquet, and was honoured by being named as an honorary Tohunga of the Otara tribe. (... laughingly translated ... as "witch doctor"!).' Since she was due to leave for overseas, 'Now is the Hour' was sung in Maori and English and Alice was asked to return when her travelling was done.[54]

Over 1969, the NZFPA produced special pamphlets for Maori and Pacific Islands people, the Auckland branch held a series of meetings with Maori leaders to try to learn more about 'Maori thought in order to equip ourselves better to help Maori mothers', a clinic was opened in South Auckland,[55] and the media was used to maintain pressure to involve Health Department workers in family planning.[56] The campaign did not go unchallenged. In May 1970 a further claim by Alice that a change in Health Department policy regarding family planning would contribute to Maori educational achievement[57] was publicly criticised in the correspondence columns of the press by Stella Casey (later Dame Stella). Mrs Casey was a well known woman in her own right, active in the NCW and respected for her liberal views. She argued that Alice's approach was offensive to 'all those who happen to have been born to closely spaced families of young mothers, as if this fact automatically precludes educational achievement' and believed it to be 'particularly offensive to Maori New Zealanders with its implied solution of "no Maoris – no problem".' She went on to call for increased government expenditure in education and the accommodation of Maori culture and language within educational structures.[58] Alice responded by pointing out that 'spacing children does not necessarily mean smaller families' while 'the use of language should be learned on mother's knee by the two year old', an experience unlikely to occur where there might be 'two younger ones to care for'.[59] The debate demonstrated that, as careful as Alice and family planners might be to argue for 'spaced' rather than 'smaller' Maori families, eugenicist implications were always waiting in the wings when contraception was suggested for 'other' groups in society. There was, however, a subtext to this particular exchange; Stella Casey was also a Roman Catholic and prominent in the church's Catholic Women's League.[60]

One obstacle to state involvement in family planning had always been a concern to avoid offending Roman Catholics, who abided by their church's ruling that all acts of sexual intercourse should take place within marriage and be open to the transmission of life. Barrier methods of contraception were forbidden. The only way for Catholic couples to avoid pregnancy was to abstain from intercourse at the time when conception was likely to occur.[61] This 'rhythm' method, as it was known, presupposed a regular menstrual cycle and an agreeable husband, assets not every Catholic woman possessed. Although family planners considered it a particularly poor approach, unreliable and inhibiting upon sexual relations between married couples, they included rhythm among the choices they offered clients, to avoid accusations of an anti-Catholic bias. Not all Roman Catholics were happy with this method either. The advent of oral contraception, which allowed women to control their fertility efficiently and, if necessary, secretly, held major implications for the Catholic church. This was complicated by the fact that many doctors found the Pill useful for women who suffered from irregularities in the menstrual cycle and in some pathological conditions brought about by endocrine imbalance.

By 1964 it was being argued that Catholic women might use the Pill for medical purposes and also to regulate their menstrual cycle so that they could successfully practise periodic continence. The temporary sterility involved was permitted as an 'evil effect tolerated but not directly intended'.[62] The overall result was one of confusion, and the Pope set up a Commission on Family Planning, which created a climate of optimism and hope for change.[63] As Alice reported from an Economic Commission for Asia and the Far East (ECAFE) conference in Wellington in 1965, 'Roman Catholic delegates from Asia could be divided into those who waited hopefully for good news from Rome, and those who felt that they could wait no longer'.[64] By 1966, family planners were aware that the Vatican intended no major modification of its stand on birth control,[65] but many of the church's members appear to have anticipated otherwise. Such was the accumulated pressure for change that in 1968, when the Pope issued his encyclical *Humanae Vitae*, which condemned all 'artificial' means of contraception as opening the way to 'marital infidelity, immorality, loss of respect for women and even political danger', the reaction was critical.[66]

Choice devoted almost an entire issue to *Humanae Vitae*, including the opposing views of Archbishop Liston and a spokesman for the Anglican church, the Right Reverend G.R. Monteith. A lengthy statement from Alice also appeared, which pondered on the implications of the encyclical for the NZFPA and its clients.

> We are not bound by any loyalty to the Pope, [but] it behoves us to study the Encyclical in toto because it is the opinion of a man who presumably has been given his present position of authority because he was judged wise and perceptive, but we feel free to believe the he may be mistaken even as an interpreter of the doctrine of his Church. . . . We know that many Roman Catholic couples will continue to use all methods of birth control as they have in the past. . . . Our duty is plain, we must continue to dispense correct scientific information about human reproduction and its control. . . . The Pope has spoken to all the world of the Roman Catholic view of marriage. There is need for the Protestants to be equally vocal about their attitude and the community services which should be developed to sustain the health of non-Catholic families.[67]

Alice also expressed concern about the effect the Pope's ruling would have on Catholic doctors who were approached by non-Catholic patients for contraceptive advice other than the rhythm method. This was not simple speculation on her part. In 1965 she had received a letter complaining that all three doctors practising in the Hawke's Bay town of Waipukurau were Catholic and that none would give alternative contraceptive advice. A few women had unsuccessfully lobbied for the establishment of a birth control clinic at the local hospital. They now wondered if it might be possible to establish an NZFPA clinic there.[68] Alice had complained to the local NZBMA branch but, three and a half years later, the situation remained unresolved.[69] At the time of the encyclical,

Catholic leaders emphasised that prescribing the Pill for birth control purposes was not a matter for the individual conscience of Catholic doctors.[70] It could still be prescribed for other reasons, and the church was encouraging research to establish the time of ovulation more accurately.[71]

Alice argued that the Catholic church's stand would penalise those most in need of contraceptive advice, 'the underprivileged, the uneducated, and those of limited understanding'. The idea that 'any doctor would deliberately refuse information pertaining to the health and happiness of a family because of his religious principles would be quite outside their comprehension'. These were people of low self-esteem, and little confidence. They could not sustain the courage to go from one doctor to another. In a 'protestant country' a woman was entitled to 'this form of preventive medical service and its availability should not be dependent on the religion of her medical practitioner or the nurse who supervises the care of her children'. She objected to 'a specific problem which arises out of the very nature of a minority' being projected on to members of the majority, something not permitted in the cases of vivisection, blood transfusions or vaccination.[72] In her presidential address to the NZFPA conference in November 1968, she again referred to this kind of imposition, warning that the association might need to reconsider its established policy of giving general practitioners primacy in the provision of family planning. 'A Roman Catholic judge or lawyer,' she argued, 'may not conduct the affairs of clients as if divorce were not valid in law.' All doctors had a legal responsibility to give correct information to patients or guide them to the appropriate consultation.[73]

Alice also had this difference of opinion with Neil Begg, medical adviser to the Plunket Society. On the face of it they had much in common. Both were Protestants and paediatricians who championed child welfare and preventive medicine, but they differed over whether contraception could be regarded as part of this approach. Plunket had been founded in the early years of the century when there were widespread fears of 'racial suicide' linked to a declining New Zealand birth rate and contraception was regarded as a threat to the state, the family and social morality.[74] Over 50 years later, Begg was still condemning contraception in New Zealand on the grounds of social and moral destructiveness, although, as chairman of the NZBMA council during the 1960s, he had instituted an ill-fated scheme to fund a 'birth control bus' to provide contraceptive services in rural Fiji, urging contributions of £1 per head from members in the correspondence column of the *NZMJ*.[75] Begg's attitude was a particular worry to Alice, and the NZFPA, because Plunket was New Zealand's major voluntary infant welfare agency and they were keen to nurture contacts with it. These attempts had often been successful at an unofficial level and NZFPA speakers were welcomed by many Plunket Mothers' Clubs, but the society remained officially opposed to the provision of contraceptive information as part of its services.

By the early 1970s, the involvement of public health nurses, who acted as infant welfare nurses in areas not covered by Plunket, in distributing family planning information seemed to call for a re-evaluation of relations between the NZFPA and the society. Negotiations began with Plunket's nursing director so that its nurses might gain some basic contraceptive knowledge and be aware of sources of further information.[76] The fragility of this enterprise was demonstrated with the publication of an anti-contraception article by Neil Begg in the April 1972 edition of *Plunket News*,[77] and the decision by Plunket's conference the same year that information about contraception should not be included in its mothercraft classes and should be provided by Plunket nurses only on request.[78] For Alice, this was a backward-looking act when everyone should be looking forward. She drafted a long letter to Plunket's president, regretting her own previous support for the society's nurses as childcare specialists, and suggesting that she must now advocate public health nurses as 'better trained and more suitable' advisers in family health and welfare for those in greatest need. Family planning was part of 'the welfare of the family as a whole', and the only way to effectively educate underprivileged mothers was on a 'person to person basis by the nurse who advises on the positive aspects of child care'. She ended by suggesting that

> Heavily subsidised as it is by Government funds, the Plunket Society has a duty to provide a comprehensive service of child care, without distinction of class or creed.
>
> As a doctor who works for the Plunket Society [at the Karitane Hospital], I will have difficulty in explaining to friends and colleagues why the Society has not kept in touch with community needs while New Zealand progresses rapidly toward a multi-racial society with all the problems of big cities, ignorance and social upheaval.[79]

Alice could make this claim only because the goal of involving the state in the provision of contraceptive services had been achieved. In April 1971 the Maternal and Child Health branch of the Public Health Division had been renamed the Family Health Branch and family planning had been added to its functions.[80] A list of 'Advisory or Related Agencies' included the NZFPA's recently constituted National Medical Advisory Council, which Alice supported but on which she did not serve,[81] and the Paediatric Society of New Zealand.[82] In October the Director-General of Health, Douglas Kennedy, formally announced a revised policy on the provision of family planning services, placed within the context of changed community attitudes to fertility control and the New Zealand government's recent support for international population activities. Although general practitioners were still acknowledged as the primary source of family planning advice, it was recognised that they were inclined to limit their practice to prescribing oral contraceptives. The NZFPA, in contrast, could advise on all methods and, in certain circumstances, charged no fee. Health Department staff might choose not to be involved, but those who did could now discuss family planning where it might be seen as an 'important health measure', including, in particular cases, adolescents, young adults and single mothers. In-service training would include formal courses open to general practitioners and NZFPA staff. Doctors who worked for the Health Department could spend some of their time working in NZFPA clinics or take sex education classes in schools. Departmental, and even hospital board, premises could be made available for family planning clinics in areas where these needs were served in no other way.[83]

Although wider trends (including a rapidly rising extra-nuptial birth rate and a developing abortion debate) and senior Health Department personnel whose personal views about contraception were very much in tune with her own (particularly Drs Joan Mackay, Douglas Kennedy and Elsie Davidge) had undoubtedly been influential, Alice had played a significant role in this achievement. When it was announced on 14 December 1971 that the NZFPA was to receive a government grant of $10,500 during 1972,[84] she was in a mood to celebrate, even though the grant would in fact add to the work of association personnel. At a meeting held at Denestone and attended by representatives from the Christchurch, Hutt Valley, Dunedin, Hamilton, Whangarei and

Wellington branches, Alice, as chairperson, posed the central question, 'How much shall we rely on the grant and how independent do we want to be in this matter?' The meeting prudently decided that the association should remain as independent as possible, but also expand and professionalise. At the end of the evening Alice produced a supper of strawberries and 'real champagne – a donation from my wine and spirit merchant'.[85] Media coverage conveyed a spirit that amounted almost to euphoria, celebrating the end of 'two decades of official disapproval' for the association and plans for new clinics to serve 'every part of the country'.[86] The November issue of *Choice* carried a message from Alice, which welcomed the end of 'an era of inequality and opportunity and racial discrimination in our land', where 'access to knowledge will no longer be confined to those who read magazines, go to meetings, or have an extra special family doctor. It will be available to all.' But, despite her ebullience, she struck an enigmatic note with a quotation from Shelley with which she had, uncharacteristically, prefaced her thoughts. Entitled 'Looking Back', it ran

> We look before and after
> And ponder what is not
> Our sincerest laughter
> With some pain is fraught.[87]

CHAPTER 10

Widening Horizons

> *As our new horizon . . . let us resolve to make this transition from domestic to international stature a reality throughout the whole association. . . . By service to others we shall surely gain strength and competence for dealing more effectively with our problems at home.*[1]

Alice's mixed feelings in 1971 were largely the result of frustrations in another area to which her role as NZFPA president had introduced her: the international population movement. This was an issue which, until the 1960s, had seldom entered New Zealanders' public consciousness beyond the use of theories of possible Asian expansionism (the 'yellow peril') to promote pronatalist policies. There is no evidence that Alice had any particular interest in the topic before this time. The NZFPA, however, had links with the international birth control movement from its formation. Indeed, during its early years the association received more moral and practical support from overseas in the form of funding, printed material and encouragement than it did within New Zealand. Over the 1950s, the NZFPA had formalised this relationship by becoming a member of the International Planned Parenthood Federation (IPPF). In 1964, when reorganisation of the federation gave regions greater autonomy, the NZFPA's involvement increased, partly because Australia did not become active in the IPPF until late in the decade. At that time, therefore, New Zealand was the only 'developed' member country in the South-east Asia and Oceania Region (SEAOR) of the IPPF. When invitations to regional meetings, with all expenses paid, began to come the way of the NZFPA, the consequences for its members were profound. Still struggling to establish their cause in their own country, they became active participants in an international organisation whose influence and status would increase phenomenally over the decade, as population control gained the open support of mainstream conservatives in the Western world.[2] These developments not only took Alice along with them, they inspired within her a wider vision. Her faith in the power not only of birth control, but of all that she believed accompanied it to acheive social and economic advancement, reached its peak in this context.

Alice's entry on to the international stage came in July 1962, when a request from the medical officer of health in Rarotonga for assistance in introducing family planning to the Cook Islands was forwarded to her as NZFPA president.[3] Hers was not a groundbreaking exercise. Ena Compton, founding nurse of the Auckland clinic, had twice visited Pacific islands during the 1950s, teaching and discussing contraceptive techniques. She had been funded by the IPPF and similar arrangements were now made for Alice.[4] When she sailed for Rarotonga on the *Moana Roa*, after applying for 18 days' special leave from her hospital duties,[5] there is no indication that she had any grand scheme in mind. Her decision to take 12-year-old Christine with her suggests that she saw the venture more as a happy blend of good works and an opportunity to spend some time with her daughter. But the situation she encountered in the Cook Islands presented the combination of human need and professional challenge that Alice found particularly appealing. Here was a country with a poor cash economy, a limited land mass and an extremely high birth rate. This was the first time that Alice had worked in an unfamiliar setting and culture, but she was sufficiently practical, and had enough of the missionary in her personality, to adapt Western contraception for use in this new situation. She quickly realised that early use of the Pill was not desirable because it interfered with lactation and the maintenance of breastfeeding was crucial. There were practically no dairy cows to provide fresh milk and dried milk was too expensive for most families. Alice therefore advocated fitting new mothers with diaphragms one month after delivery, with regular checks over the following three months; it was not an infallible technique, but better than nothing. When the baby was weaned, the mother might elect to go on to oral contraceptives or stay with the diaphragm.

Since the price of commercially marketed oral contraceptives was beyond family budgets, Alice proposed making up a series of stilboestral and progestogen tablets placed under clear tape with seven placebo tablets in sequence to make pill-taking continuous. She estimated that these could be sold for around a sixth of the usual price, which should place them within the reach of all. She also understood, when she ran into resistance from the local men, that their hostility was culturally based. 'To be the father of many children,' she reported, 'is to enjoy prestige with little responsibility.' For this reason she centred her hopes on the local health nurses, themselves Island women with children and 'enthusiastic to make available to all mothers the advantages of family spacing'. They were trained to fit diaphragms, which would be made available at cost price through the hospital dispensary. Alice also demonstrated a range of alternative contraceptive techniques, including condoms and other occlusive devices in combination with a spermicide, and discussed the 'safe period'. In Rarotonga she noted the presence of 'a large migratory group of families who have come in from the outer islands and are awaiting a passage to New Zealand'.[6] After this trip Pacific Island women living in New Zealand became a concern of the NZFPA.[7]

The Rarotongan trip was satisfying but it was the next opportunity to travel abroad as NZFPA president that really broadened Alice's physical and philosophical horizons and became, in Alice's own eyes, the source of her commitment to taking 'the benefits of scientific fertility control ... to those who need them the most'.[8] In late 1963 the New Zealand National Council of Churches (NCC) invited her to represent them at a Consultation on Responsible Parenthood to be held in association with the General Assembly of the East Asian Christian Conference in Bangkok in March 1964. Although the Standing Committee was keen for her to go, the fact that this was not an IPPF project made finance a problem. The NCC was willing to arrange accommodation but unable to contribute to the substantial travel costs involved, and the Standing Committee did not believe that this was an exercise on which they should spend

New Zealand funds. The association therefore approached 'certain [unnamed] business houses and individuals who might have an interest in assisting the finance of the project'.[9] Around £400 was collected and Alice proposed meeting any shortfall by having her clinic attendance fees paid into a special fund which, in future, would be used by the Auckland branch committee to help with the overseas travel and accommodation expenses of NZFPA representatives.[10] For Alice, the involvement of an organised religious group fully authorised the evangelistic appeal of family planning activism. On her return home she categorised the venture as an opportunity 'to be able to say "Thank you" to the many [Protestant] Christian churchmen and laymen who have given us [the NZFPA] such valuable support' and referred to the establishment of an NZFPA sub-branch in Taumarunui as 'a good example of missionary activity'.[11] But the Bangkok conference was to prove more important as a watershed for Alice herself.

In her 50th year she was a neophyte solo traveller in exotic South-east Asia, an area that had only recently entered the official orbit of New Zealand affairs because of its apparent military and political significance as a corridor for Communist advances. Alice had travelled relatively little internationally, but her natural energy and effervescent curiosity had made her an active tourist when opportunities arose. Flying by way of Sydney and Darwin, she spent nearly three days in Hong Kong. Two mornings were given over to visiting hospitals and there was some socialising in the evenings. In between, Alice was out and about, ostensibly shopping but also, most often, as she described it, 'enjoying to look and watch the people'. She was fascinated with glimpses of a lifestyle so different from her own. It seemed to her that whole families lived virtually on the street. She judged the children to be 'a bit skinny' and observed that they worked hard, either in school or contributing to the family economy, but thought them 'wonderfully well behaved'. 'Happiness and the joy of living,' she sagely informed readers of *Choice* on her return, 'are not dependent on material possessions or on a particular way of life.'[12] Alice continued her keen observations in Thailand, seeing as much as she could on and off the tourist trail. She was escorted through temples and 'poked around' villages. Through a happy coincidence she was able to attend the wedding of a Thai woman doctor, Churi Indrampaya, who had spent time in New Zealand as a Colombo Plan student, and was accorded the privilege of pouring water over the hands of the bride and groom. She visited the country's old capital and took a tour through the floating markets and a silk factory, reporting back to Faulkner and the family, 'Have now seen ricefields, buffalos, sugar cane ... and many ruins' as well as having 'a real look at the homes of Bangkok & the way people live'. Calls at the Red Cross, the Children's and the Christian Bangkok hospitals horrified her but also confirmed the validity of her cause. 'They certainly need family planning here,' she wrote.[13]

In Bangkok, Alice not only attended conference proceedings but also visited two centres for Christian youth work, had supper with an American missionary family and took part in a panel discussion with a group of students on preparation for marriage.[14] She was stimulated and characteristically forthcoming. It was, she reported to Faulkner, 'very busy and quite exciting. Met some delightful people. Had a fair whack at speaking my mind & this seemed to be appreciated.'[15] By the time she came back she was able to present the entire experience to *Choice* readers as one of particular significance, both for her and for them. Although she acknowledged fears of expansionism prompted by population growth, Alice concerned herself chiefly with elements of the conference debate that were more compatible with her, and their, personal inclinations. The emphasis of the gathering had been

> very much on the importance of the individual family rather than on population statistics, and the importance of maintenance of human dignity and giving each individual child a chance to grow and develop fully was the motive behind the move for "responsible parenthood"....
> When education for family planning is associated with positive education in child care and family welfare it is acceptable to parents and frees them from superstition and even from the tyranny of age-old traditions which have become obsolete in a mechanised world.[16]

For Alice and her NZFPA contemporaries, it was this focus on individual family, individual child, which held the key to involvement in the international population movement. The Standing Committee had supported the NCC's invitation in the belief that it would 'underline the importance of "family living" in Asian Countries'.[17] When Auckland NZFPA worker Ethel Biddle (together with Ruth Black) first officially represented the association at a regional council meeting in Singapore in 1964, an occasion on which she was introduced to IPPF Secretary General Sir Colville Deverell, she described the experience as not at all formidable. For her, these were people whose values and ideas were simply 'family planning' writ large. When she entered the council room, she felt she had 'joined a family who were meeting to discuss mutual problems'.[18]

Alice's particular stance is most clearly illustrated in a paper that she prepared for a United Nations Children's Fund (UNICEF) conference held in Bangkok in September 1965, 'to consider the place of children and young people in national planning and development'. Alice was invited to represent the IPPF, she explained, because 'it [IPPF] is deeply concerned not only with population problems, but also with the welfare of children and individual families' and 'children are my concern'.[19] Addressed to the Committee of the Whole on Education for Agricultural Development, the paper did not contain a number-crunching exercise on the importance of birth control in relation to food production, but focused on the early childhood experience as an answer to the ultimate economic and social development of individuals, and thereby communities, even in Third World nations. Introducing herself as a paediatrician 'very much concerned with child development and education', Alice moved from pleas for assistance in the fields of social work training and family and child care to the adult farm worker's ability to adopt new agricultural techniques. Adaptability, she argued, depended on education but, even at primary level, this could be disrupted by failures and dropouts. The answer lay in the preschool years, when attitudes were acquired that persisted through to adulthood. 'I feel it is no exaggeration to say', she confirmed, 'that a good farmer is made or marred before his fifth birthday.' Governments could contribute by broadening health care to include mental health, running school courses in family living to prepare both sexes 'to undertake more responsibly the duties of parenthood' and by setting up preschool centres along the lines of the play centres currently being organised by the Maori Education Foundation in New Zealand. 'Fruitful concern on the part of a Government with the most important years of the child's life,' she confidently stated, 'will be repaid not only by increased agricultural production, but also by reduction of delinquency and crime and by modification of the attitudes which at present obstruct economic planning and population control.'[20]

This proposition may seem to require such a leap of cultural faith that the suggestion would sink without trace, especially since, when Alice arrived in Bangkok after a 12-hour flight delay, she discovered that hostilities between India and Pakistan had disrupted all air traffic and the conference had been cancelled. She put her name down for a flight to Singapore and in the meantime 'set about the task of justifying my expenses for IPPF'. The next few days were 'full of adventures', she told *Choice* readers, 'but I will tell of the positive side'.[21] This included a description of the local FPA clinic, its wares openly displayed to the public, and ideas about preschool education in the area. Apparently she was just as busy in Singapore, where the regional office of the IPPF had invited her to be their guest when passing through.[22] After Alice had gone home, the New Zealand High Commissioner there and Lex Gray, recently appointed Preschool Officer for the Maori Education Foundation in New Zealand, received letters from Ong Kah Kok, a deputy director of the People's Association of Singapore, seeking 'opportunities for members of our staff to visit New Zealand, study and working [*sic*] within the project [the play centres] so enthusiastically described by Dr Bush'. The People's Association was already trying to establish kindergartens in its 180 community centres, Ong Kah Kok explained, but the idea of play centres, with their element of parental involvement, seemed a promising new avenue.[23] Alice was pleased with her trip, which so easily might have been a non-event, and summed up her experiences on a note of optimism.

> In two crowded weeks I have met educationalists, doctors, nurses and administrators who are all aiming at giving the Asian child a better chance in life. In South-East Asia I believe that real progress is being made toward a happier, better fed, better educated family. We can only hope that the experience gained here can be applied toward the solution of the apparently insoluble problems of other parts of Asia.[24]

Alice might have been delivering an old message but her involvement in the international population movement presented her with a much wider, and more influential, audience. In March 1965, she travelled to Wellington to represent the IPPF at the 21st session of the Economic Commission for Asia and the Far East (ECAFE), another United Nations subcommittee. The conference delegates, from 40 countries and 16 non-governmental agencies, discussed topics including rural and community development, income distribution, employment, housing, social welfare, health, nutrition and social development.[25] Alice's address dealt with the effect of population growth in the region. The problem facing ECAFE countries, she argued, was a result of health measures which had lowered the death rate but left the birth rate unchanged so that much of the progress made in increased primary production and economic growth had been almost cancelled out by population growth.[26] In taking this path, she adopted an unfortunate phrase she probably picked up in Bangkok in 1964 and for which she was later publicly castigated: 'death control must be accompanied by birth control'.[27] This lesson, she reflected, had been learnt by the people of the Western world 'without assistance from leaders or teachers' over the 150 years following the Industrial Revolution, but their experience had been 'buffered by the opportunity to export surplus population to the great empty spaces of the world'. Contemporary Asia did not have these advantages of time and space, so 'the process must be speeded up by planned education', presenting the same problems as education for other purposes, such as better land use or agricultural practices. It required information, psychology and motivation, financial backing and technically trained personnel. The United States had promised financial aid and 'Extensive sociological surveys' had shown that 'if the common people were given freedom of choice in this matter they would solve the problem'. Only when the leaders of Asian countries were convinced that success was possible, and when information about fertility control became 'an integral part of all health services and education for living', would the 'lowering of the birth rate become a blessing and not a curse'.[28]

Like other NZFPA members, Alice found the atmosphere at these gatherings congenial. Before the ECAFE conference, she confessed she had wondered 'Would I be welcome?', but the mood of the meeting and the attention paid to population soon dispelled her fears.[29] The only sour note occurred after her return to Auckland. Her paper was fully reported in the *Star*,[30] but the *Herald* neglected to publicise the population issues raised at the conference until she wrote a critical letter to the editor.[31] Alice was not alone in her irritation concerning the lack of public debate in New Zealand about international population trends. In January 1965, Dr Erich Geiringer of Wellington, a radical immigrant doctor much out of favour with the professional establishment, wrote seeking her opinion on a scheme he had in mind involving 'a vigorous public appeal for money to aid the birth control activities of underdeveloped countries'. This was to be 'full scale, nationwide and permanent ... the effect of which should be not merely to collect money but to educate the public about the full gravity of this problem'.[32] Alice was naturally receptive to this idea. Her correspondence with Geiringer over 1965 reveals the value she had for him both as a source of information and as a figurehead, since he was keen to get 'establishment' names attached to his appeal.[33] Alice answered his questions about IPPF structures, attitudes and experience, suggested useful contacts and agreed to allow her name to be used first as a signatory then as a member of the advisory committee of what became known as the Appeal for Population Control (APC).[34] Alice's family connections were also instrumental in obtaining the support of Sir Edmund Hillary and his wife Louise for Geiringer's campaign,[35] and she personally recruited 'names' in Auckland.[36] By the time the first APC newsheet came out in September 1966, it listed 75 supporting signatories and included Alice among the speakers to address meetings of university and training college students.[37]

Geiringer's appeal was also publicised in *Choice*,[38] but there was a limit to the amount of time Alice could personally give to his project. In April 1966 she wrote,

> At present we get very little help from the press and I have not yet been able to persuade anybody to take an active part in organising a committee in this city. There are quite a number of people who will be willing to serve on it but a leader is yet to be found.
>
> I am leaving for Singapore on 2nd May and will be away practically all that month. If you know anybody in Auckland who would have the necessary drive and organising ability to act as a convenor for a committee here you go ahead and get them going. I would be able to supply names of people who might be willing to cooperate but I cannot commit myself to any actual campaigning, for I just do not have the time available.[39]

The APC's activities gradually diminished in the 1970s, although it was never officially terminated and was still receiving occasional donations in the late 1980s.[40] It was only one 'ginger group' among old and new organisations that were forming the huge groundswell of the population lobby in the later 1960s. In February 1966, *Choice* reported, 'The emphasis appears to have almost imperceptibly shifted from the question of whether to give help to the problem of how to provide it and to what extent.'[41]

The burgeoning international interest in world population saw local family planners entertaining IPPF notables in New Zealand. In June 1965 Dr Alan Guttmacher, chairman of the Medical Committee of the IPPF and president of the Planned Parenthood Federation of the United States (or should it be 'Mr World Population?' speculated *Choice*), spent three days in New Zealand, accompanied by his wife.[42] Accommodation was arranged by Dennis Bonham,[43] who had replaced Harvey Carey as professor of obstetrics and gynaecology at National Women's and who, like Carey, had friendly relations with the NZFPA. Bonham also organised a Saturday morning seminar at the hospital on 'modern conception control and world population problems'. That evening 'a V.I.P. cocktail party' was held at Denestone, where Dr Guttmacher spoke briefly on world population, comparing the annual increase in India with the total population of Australia. On Sunday Alice drove the visitors to Rotorua and on the way back, at the invitation of the local NZFPA, Dr Guttmacher spoke to a large audience in Hamilton; his address was recorded for the benefit of other branches. On Monday morning NZFPA doctors from Hamilton and Whangarei joined with Auckland medical staff for an informal discussion with Dr Guttmacher followed by luncheon at the home of Isabel Stanton, Alice's sister-in-law and president of the Auckland branch.[44] Guttmacher also made radio and television appearances during his short stay.[45]

If this visit aimed to stimulate interest in international population matters, it certainly succeeded in Alice's case. During a Standing Committee meeting a few weeks later she suggested, as a 'follow-up', that there seemed to be a

> fertile field in N.Z. for getting important people interested in all aspects of world population as opposed to just our domestic problems. I think it would be practical to institute an overseas Division within the NZFPA and I hope that all Branches will give this consideration and if they feel that it would be a good idea will have in mind the names of people who might be approached by an initial letter to form this Association.[46]

When there was no branch support, the Standing Committee began to consider asking about other groups that seemed to be concerned with the population 'problem'.[47] This was the time when Alice was most active in the APC. But the IPPF connection meant that the issue was not going to go away for the NZFPA and *Choice* continued to buzz with the latest news of the population lobby's activities. The IPPF was to double its budget to $US2 million in 1966, and again to $US4 million for 1967. Three-quarters of this money had been raised in the United States, so a 'guiding hand' had been extended 'into 106 nations with birth control assistance'.[48]

NZFPA personnel continued to travel overseas. In September 1965 Glenys Lowe had attended an IPPF council meeting in London, and Judy Lunn and Alice represented the NZFPA at a regional council meeting in Singapore in May 1966. For Alice this trip combined business with pleasure in more ways than one. As on her Rarotongan trip in 1962, she took Christine, now aged 16, with her. They left Auckland on 2 May, flying to Sydney then Manila, where they were shown around by Dr Gregorio Lim, president of the local FPA. His sightseeing tour included the slums and squatters' areas, an experience that Alice found 'certainly pretty shattering'. In the evening she and Christine were entertained at a restaurant by a group of local medical women.[49] They travelled to Hong Kong and experienced its variety before going on to Bangkok and Penang, where ancient grandeur contrasted with the 'filth & poverty that exists off the beaten track', something which had 'to be seen to be believed'.[50] In Singapore, Alice took a place on the Regional Medical Committee, which discussed various topics, including improving services and the exchange of information, bringing in 'people of standing', the chances of foetal deformity resulting from the use of IUDs or oral contraceptives, and the possible legalisation of tubal ligation and vasectomy.[51] She also joined Judy Lunn at the regional council meeting where she reported on the state of the association in New Zealand, including the lack of government involvement and 'population problems among the Maoris, particularly with mothers who had gone to live in cities or in highly industrialized centres where the standard of living is high'. The NZFPA needed films for health education purposes and was receiving 'great assistance' from Dennis Bonham, who had previously been president of a local Family Planning branch in Britain. An IUD clinic was operating in association with

National Women's Hospital and it was hoped to have some results available from this in the near future.[52]

Back in New Zealand, Alice was once again irritated by the inadequate press coverage of the international population issue. In her biennial report to the NZFPA conference, published in *Choice* shortly after her return, she stated

> Because of the absence of this problem in New Zealand there tends to be a conspiracy of silence over what is going on in the rest of the world. Some of our leading newspapers either ignore the situation or accord it little space; our politicians feel it is not their business. We believe that New Zealand is in a position to make some financial contributions to IPPF and to supply medical assistance in overseas programmes.[53]

Alice's enthusiasm on this occasion had been fuelled by the imminent arrival in New Zealand of Sir Colville Deverell, but local reaction to his visit demonstrated the lack of interest that so irked her. The prospect had sent a flurry of anticipation through the higher echelons of the NZFPA and a subcommittee had been set up to arrange an itinerary.[54] Civic receptions, meetings with Maori and other leaders, addresses to universities and public service clubs were planned.[55] As NZFPA president, Alice wrote personally to the Prime Minister, Keith Holyoake, as well as to the Minister of Health and the Director-General of Health, informing them of Sir Colville's availability to meet government representatives.[56] An extensive guest list was drawn up for a reception to be held at Denestone, including politicians, educationalists, medical, business, legal and religious leaders.[57] In many cases, the response was disappointing. R.G. McElroy, the Mayor of Auckland, could not fit in a civic reception for Sir Colville, but was willing to meet him for about 10 minutes at lunchtime.[58] The Governor-General's wife, Lady Fergusson, declined an invitation to open the NZFPA conference at which Sir Colville would be the featured speaker because she was 'very heavily committed to engagements'.[59] Nevertheless, for Alice the visit was an empowering and confirming experience.

> His coming seemed to set a seal on the change that has been occurring in NZFPA over the past two years; the change from a domestic organisation to one with a broader outlook and an international responsibility . . .

> Those members who have shared in the work of IPPF by attending conferences, preparing reports and answering correspondence have come to appreciate how much New Zealand is truly a part of Asia and how great is our responsibility to our developing neighbours to offer not only a share of our trade, our educational services and some material assistance, but also the need for this country to join with the other more favoured nations who have realised that the only way to put a bottom to the sieve is to assist with population control as well as famine relief.[60]

Alice might have been fervently in favour of such a move, but the New Zealand government remained reluctant to become involved in the population movement until international pressure made further resistance virtually impossible. At the end of 1967, Keith Holyoake wrote to the Secretary-General of the United Nations informing him of the government's decision to endorse the principles of the organisation's statement on population, already supported by the United States, Britain and Australia. A copy of this letter was also sent to John D. Rockefeller III, who had been interested enough to write to the prime minister, encouraging such a move.[61] *Choice* diplomatically described the government's action as particularly well timed, since 1968 had been designated Human Rights Year,[62] and access to information about family planning was declared a basic human right during that year.[63] But some disturbing aspects were beginning to emerge in the discourse surrounding 'family planning' for Third World peoples. By the late 1960s, there was increasing concentration on 'motivation'. Isabel Stanton, who had attended the 1969 regional council meeting as a rapporteur, reported her impression that the

> main concern seemed to be about how the necessary practice of Family Planning can be sold to Government Officials, medical schools, rural communities, etc. There were so many international organisations agreeing about the obvious need for Family Planning programmes and arguing about how best to encourage them. Indeed, international Bankers regard money lent for Family Planning Schemes as an investment, such schemes being essential and as important as any other form of development.
>
> I remember vividly the hammering the WHO representative received at one Working Group because his organisation will only go into a

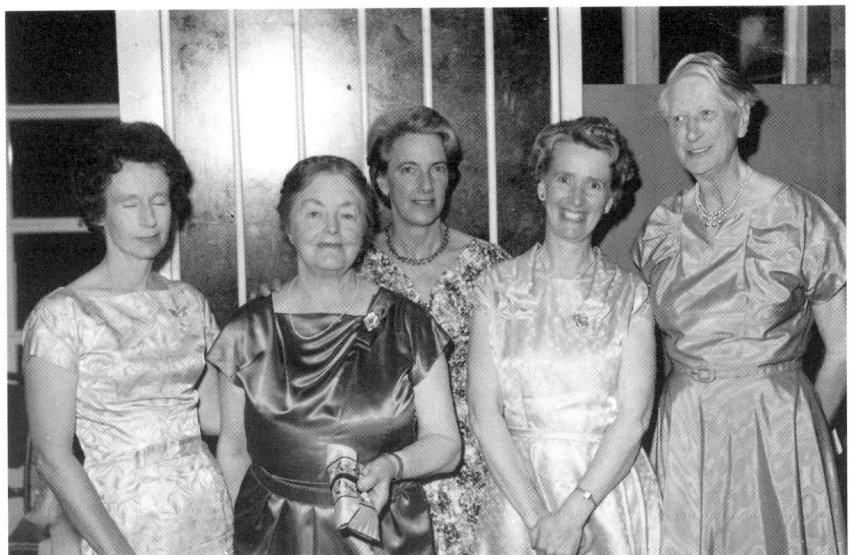

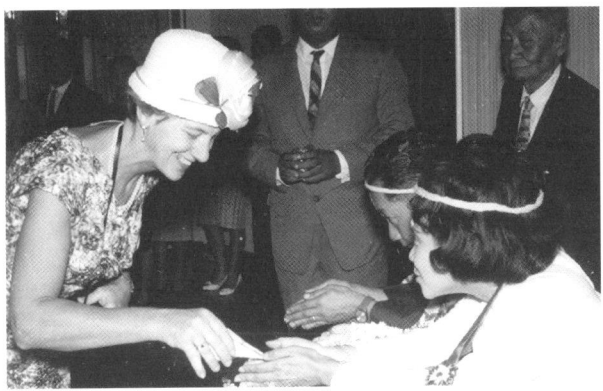

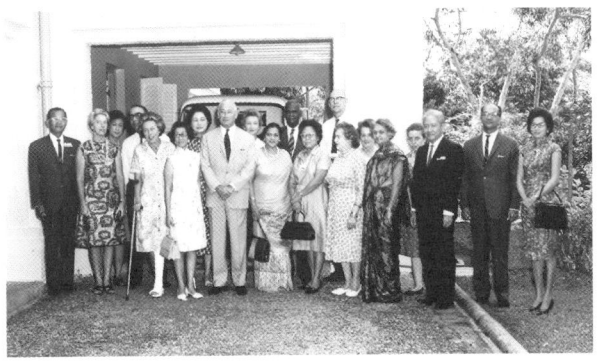

ABOVE: Alice at a Hill Top reunion around the time of the school's move from Khyber Pass Road to Blockhouse Bay. She is standing behind Miss Boult (second from left). Miss Hawkins is on the right. *Christine Moorhouse*

TOP LEFT: In Thailand, 1964. Alice pours water over the hands of Dr Churi Indrampaya and her husband following their wedding ceremony. *MC*

BOTTOM LEFT: IPPF SEAOR Conference, Singapore, 1966. Alice stands second from left. *Juan Photo Service. Courtesy Christine Moorhouse*

RIGHT: Alice (far right) with, from left, Dr Laurie Chute, Dr Ronald Caughey and his wife Catherine. As a result of this meeting, Alice worked with Dr Cecil Collins-Williams at the Hospital for Sick Children in Toronto in 1968. *Helen Evans Reid (MC)*

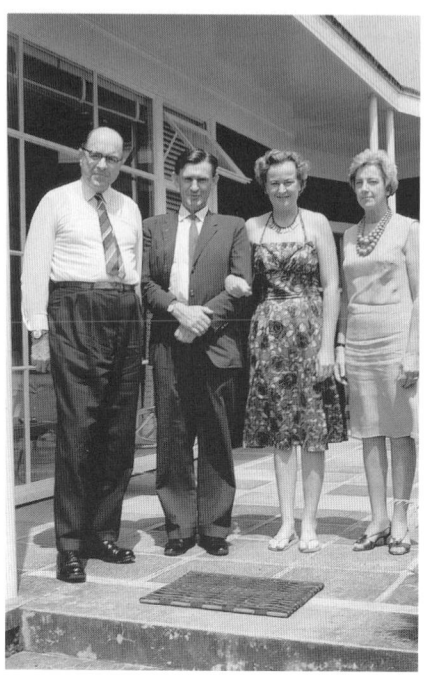

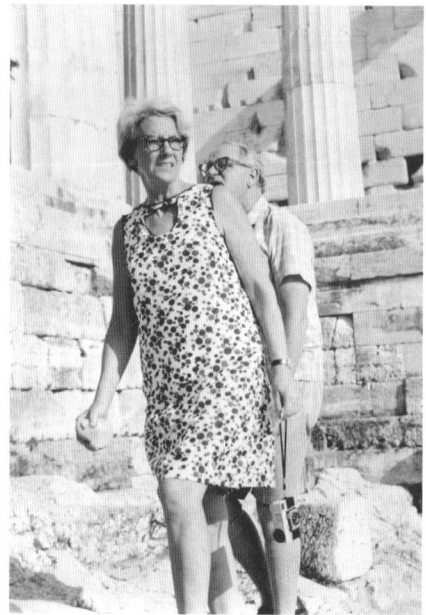

LEFT: After three months in Toronto, Alice and Faulkner travelled through the United States and Europe. They visited Greece on their way home in July. *Christine Moorhouse*

RIGHT: At the medical women's dinner, MANZ (formerly NZBMA) Conference, Auckland, February 1969. From left: Dr Margaret Maxwell, Dr Elizabeth Hughes, Alice, and Dr Margaret Gatman. *NZH*

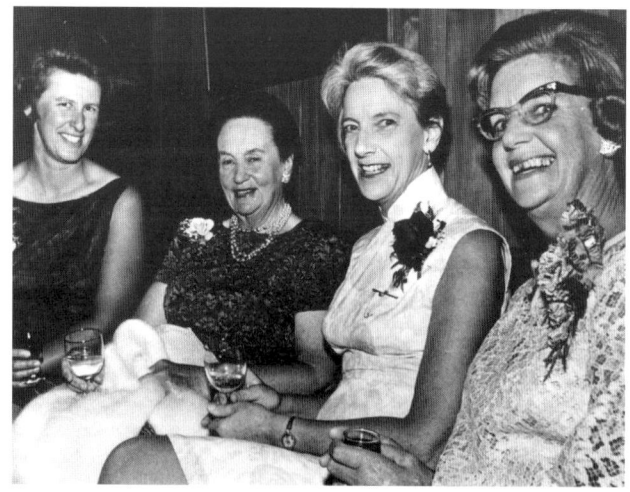

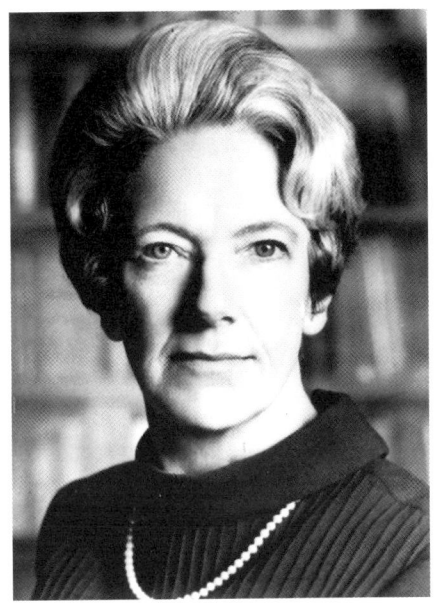

LEFT: By the late 1960s Alice was so frequently approached by the media for comment and an accompanying photograph that she sat for this formal portrait. *Aileen Odell*

BELOW: Alice meets the Queen, Princess Mary Hospital, March 1970. *Christine Moorhouse*

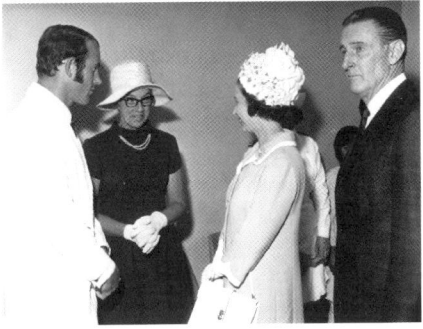

BELOW: This photograph of a Princess Mary ward shortly after Alice's death gives an indication of the conditions which concerned her. *NZH*

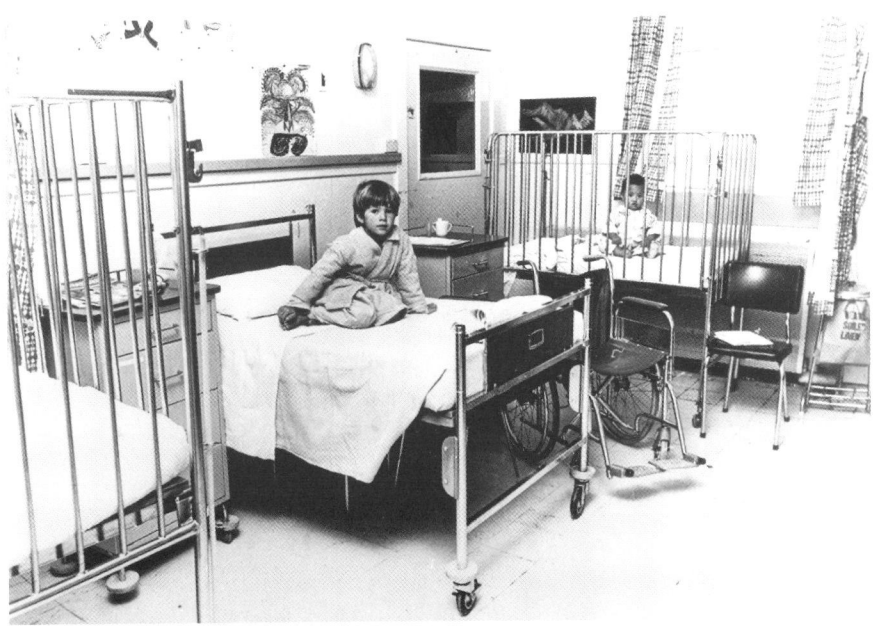

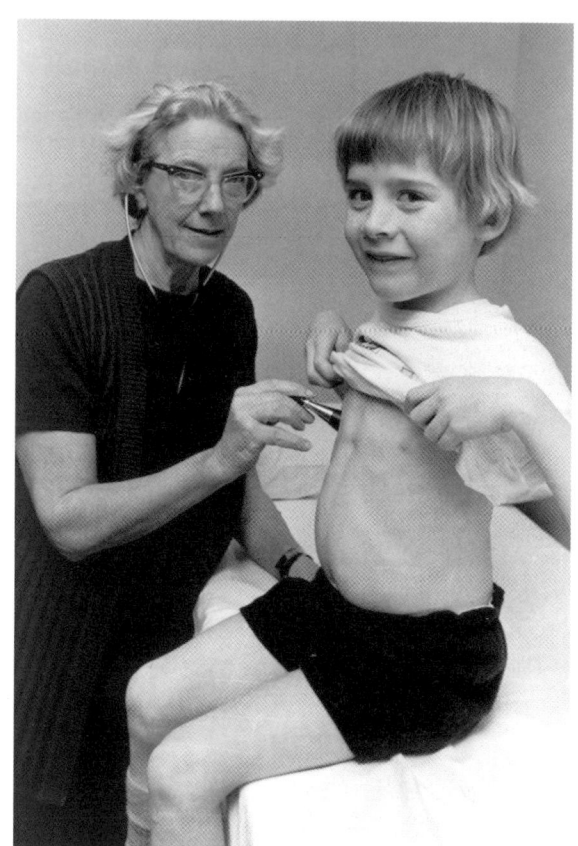

RIGHT: Alice in her public persona as an experienced and widely respected paediatrician of the early 1970s. *NZH*

BELOW: At an NCW National Executive meeting, October 1971, with Mrs Lt. Colonel Enid Weggery of the Salvation Army. *Holt Photography. Courtesy Enid Weggery (MC)*

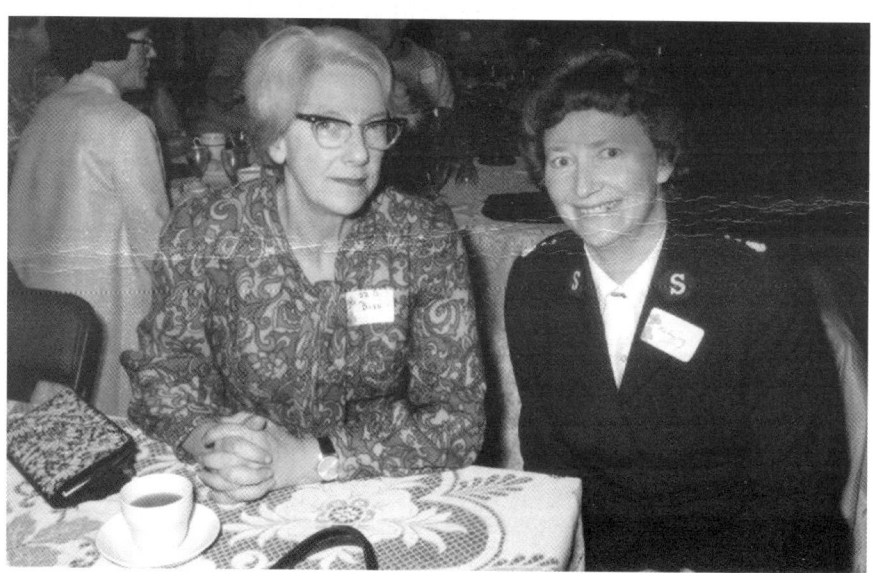

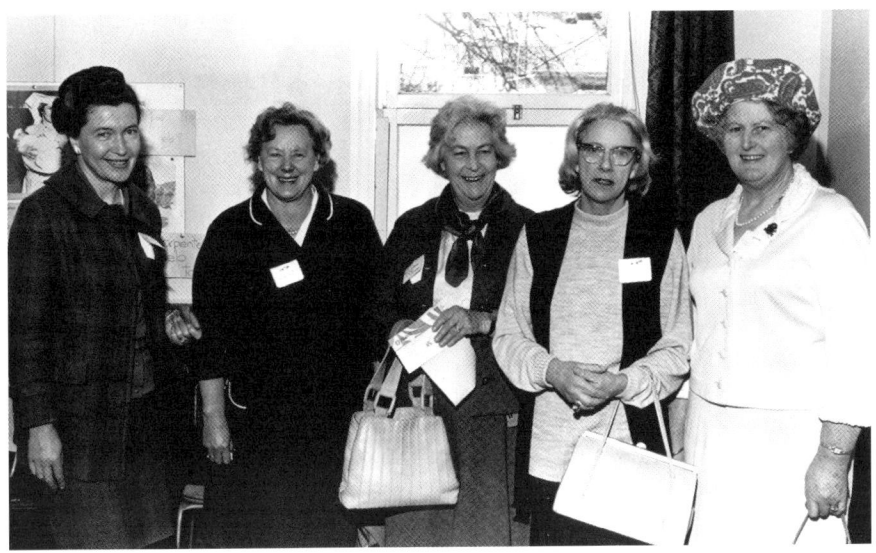

ABOVE: Alice, second from right, shows the strain of a demanding life, at the NCW national conference in 1972. *Geoffrey C. Wood Collection, Nelson Provincial Museum*

BELOW: Alice with, from left, Rt Rev. Bishop Eric Gowing, Sir Joseph Stanton and Faulkner, in the early 1960s, before the abortion debate had placed Alice and the Bishop in opposing camps. *Christine Moorhouse*

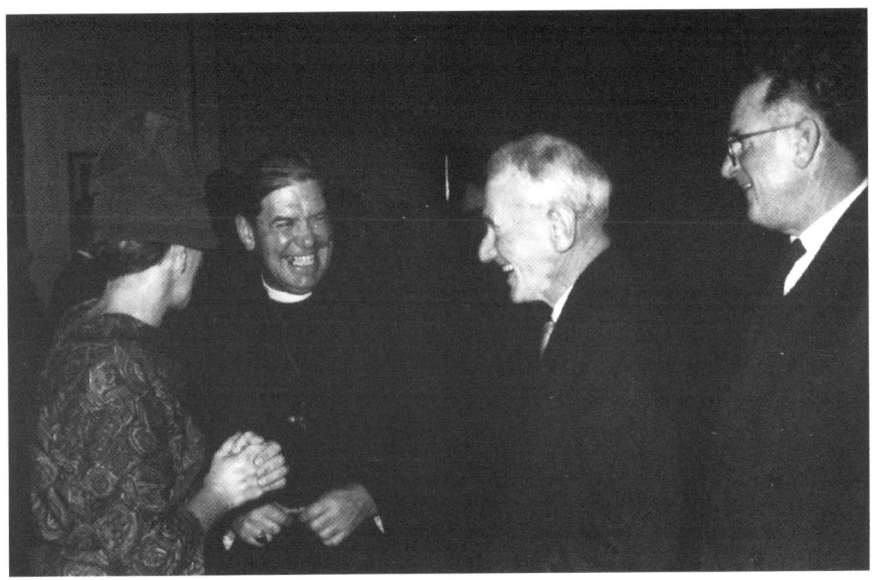

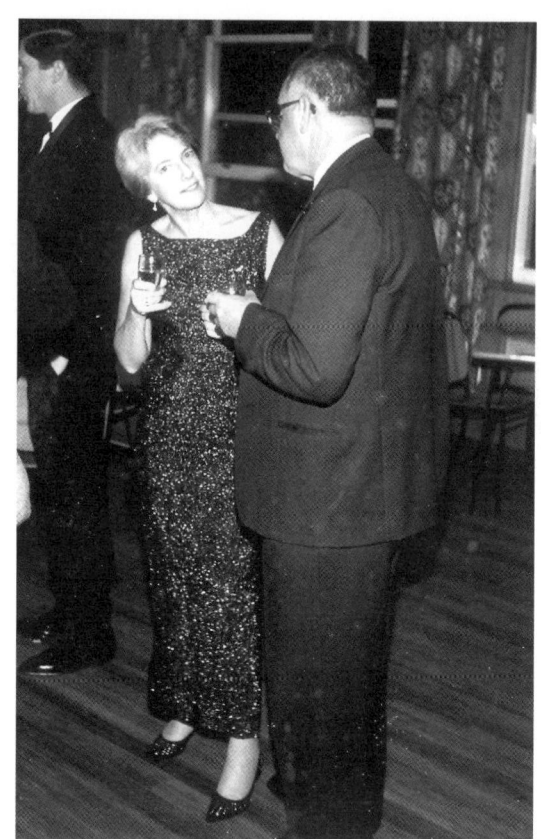

RIGHT: Alice steps out with Faulkner. She made the dress herself. *Peter Bush*

BELOW: Peter, Christine, Faulkner and Alice, enjoying a friend's wedding reception held, at Alice's invitation, at Denestone. *Ray Bridal Services. Courtesy Christine Moorhouse*

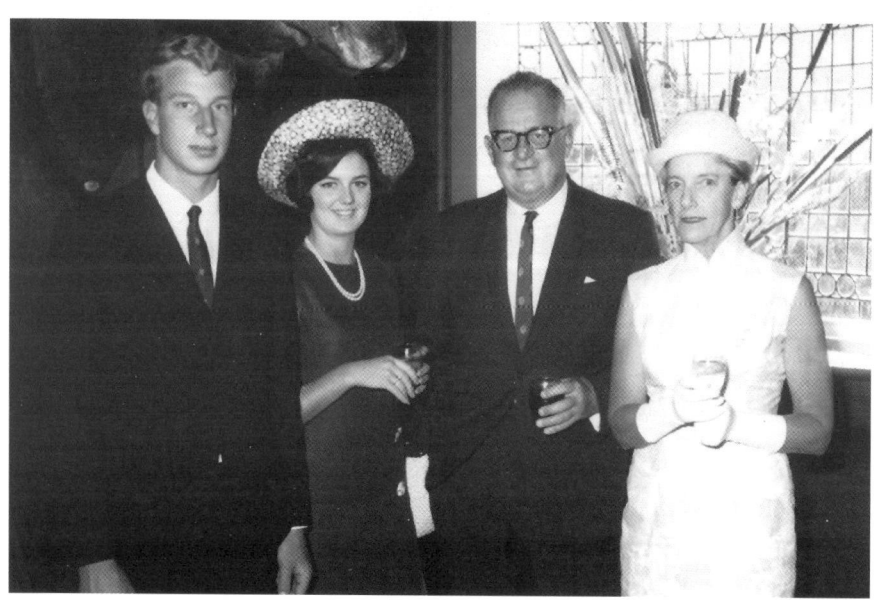

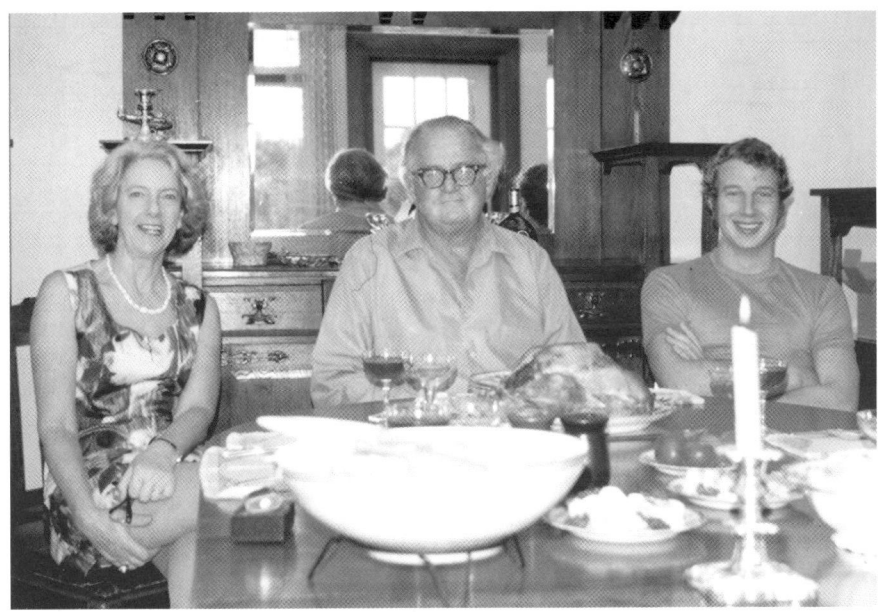

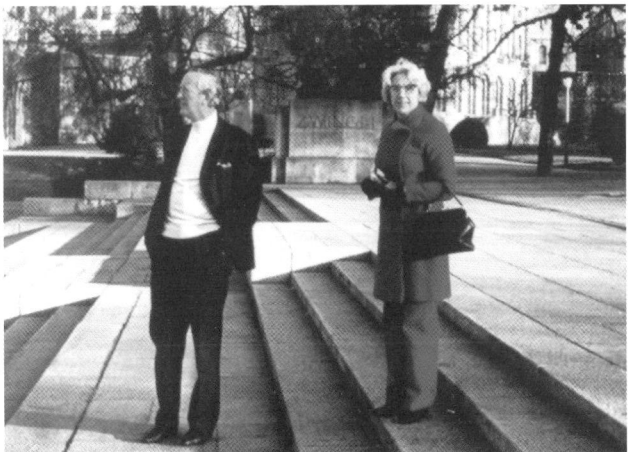

ABOVE: Christmas Day, Denestone, 1970, with Faulkner and Peter. Alice, radiant and proud on Christine's 21st birthday. *Christine Moorhouse*

LEFT: Alice with the Rev. Les Clements in Geneva, 1973, 33 years after she and Faulkner had unsuccessfully suggested he marry them in Taihape. *Christine Moorhouse*

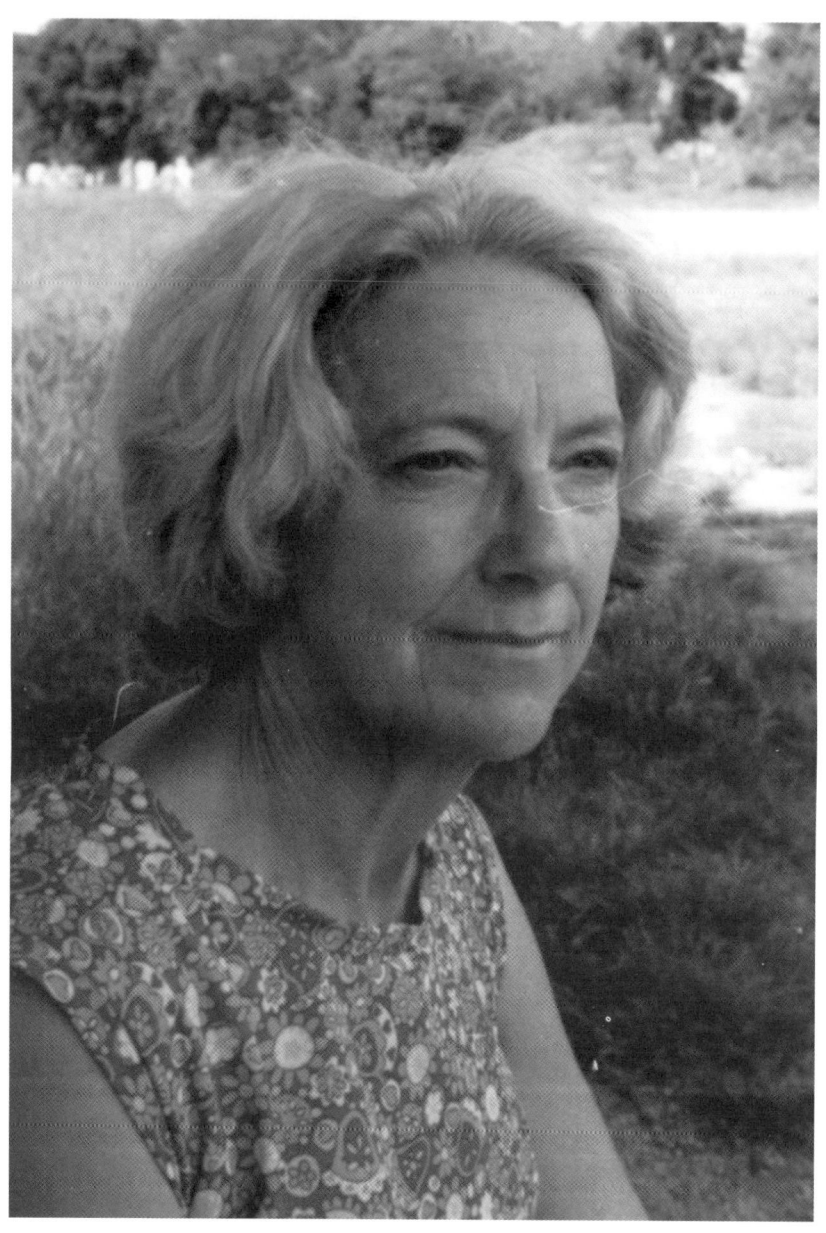

Alice's last holiday, with Christine in Mexico, October 1973. *Christine Moorhouse*

country when invited. "You offer your services for any other kind of epidemic," he was told.⁶⁴

The August 1969 issue of *Choice* contained a segment on 'Incentive Payments' as presented in an IPPF report. Although it was admitted that this approach had some disadvantages, including inadequate preparation and assurance of patients, side effects glossed over, IUDs removed and reinserted, choice of unsuitable methods and disputes over fees payments, several 'advantages' were also listed.⁶⁵

Dissension regarding the ethics of the population movement was to ferment within the NZFPA as another facet of the association's relationship to the IPPF took centre stage. The NZFPA was inclining toward asking for more financial help from the IPPF in order to expand services.⁶⁶ At the same time, the IPPF, which had already intimated that it favoured the NZFPA moving away from financial dependency, suggested the possibility of a loan of $10,000 'for the purpose of fund raising'. In March 1971 Warren Fuller, employed by the IPPF to visit potential donor countries, was dispatched to 'examine the practical aspects of the situation' in New Zealand.⁶⁷ Alice saw Fuller three days after his arrival, before she left the country to attend an IPPF conference in Baguio. He was then escorted around Auckland and Wellington by various NZFPA personnel and supporters before flying to the conference, where he reported that he believed that $100,000 could be raised annually in New Zealand if 'the special claims of IPPF were properly represented'.⁶⁸ Intimations that the NZFPA might become actively involved in fund-raising for the IPPF were softened in *Choice* by Ruth Black, who reported that, 'Those clinics struggling to cope with the indigents may be pleased to hear that funds raised for IPPF in a country may be retained for family planning activities within that country'.⁶⁹

Alice was convinced not only that New Zealand should become a donor country but also that the NZFPA had a responsibility to be involved in this way. Drafting a letter to branch committees, she wrote,

> I have resolutely ... refused to consider asking IPPF for [further] funds for our NZFPA. My conscience would not allow me to compete with countries like the Phillipines [*sic*] where a whole family must live on $100 per year & failure to implement ... programmes for population control means stark malnutrition if not starvation.⁷⁰

Plans were initiated to extend NZFPA activities into fund-raising for the international body. On 6 April 1971 the Standing Committee decided to set up a subcommittee to 'look at the whole situation', and branches were requested to consider introducing a special membership with limited privileges and a reduced subscription for clinic patients (who usually did not join the association), so that NZFPA statistics would more truly reflect its 'activities and significance' in the community.[71] By this time Alice had another string to her bow: she had joined the conservation lobby and was adding ecology to her argument.

The emotive content of the ecology debate over the early 1970s is difficult to recapture but something of its flavour remains in the press reception given to an article published at the beginning of 1972 and supported by 33 British scientists and ecologists. Described as a 'blueprint for survival', the article suggested that a 'national doom-watch movement' should be set up to prevent the self-destruction of mankind and was reported in the usually staid *Herald* under the headline, 'Doom Warning by 33 Top U.K. Scientists'. If the world continued on its present path, it was argued, it would end in a succession of famines, epidemics, social crises and wars. To avoid this fate, governments must acknowledge the problem and 'declare their commitment to ending population growth', couples should not have more than two children, contraception and sterilisation should be free and abortion available on demand.[72] Running concurrently were articles with such titles as 'Stop the World – I Want to Get Off', featuring the latest news (all of it bad) from groups, including the Club of Rome and the Zero Population Growth Society, supported by the new forecasting tool, computer projections.[73] Headlines like 'Birth Control "only solution"',[74] and 'Birth Control Vital to World Survival'[75] at least offered the comfort of a practical response that was not beyond individuals. For established champions, like Alice, this was simply a logical extension of family planning. If birth control could benefit nuclear families and Western society, why should it not save the world?

In January 1971, the *Herald* ran leading articles about the 'two great dangers of the late twentieth century – shortage of food and irreversible pollution of the environment' and suggested two essential responses: increased food production and slowing of population growth. Alice responded with a letter to the editor which argued that New Zealand was doing neither. By subsidising secondary industry and leaving the primary producer to 'cope alone with rising costs and diminishing returns', the government was doing its best to reduce food production. By failing to officially recognise the need for birth control education at home or abroad, it was supporting increased population. If New Zealanders were to continue enjoying their high standard of living with a clear conscience they must keep down the costs of food production and give full support to programmes for population control everywhere.[76] By the end of the year, the conservation and population 'problems' had become so conflated in Alice's mind that she believed these were all the NZFPA's concern. 'Anti pollution, conservation, family planning, all these are striving for the same goal, and for preservation of the quality of life. Let us unite and help each other,' she announced in *Choice* in November 1971.[77]

Several facets of the conservation movement had a natural appeal for Alice, beyond her commitment to family planning. She had always been fond of outdoor life, attracted by the beauty of New Zealand's beaches, bush and mountains. Her values tended towards simplicity rather than ostentation. Naturally frugal, she was fond of setting limits on her spending and thought that others should do the same. She believed in present prudence to secure future benefit. Her view of society was essentially that of inter-linked individuals, where effects for good or evil on one resounded throughout the whole. These views made her receptive to the aims and strategies of the conservation lobby, while its links with population concerns and demonstrations of the high rate of resource consumption by developed nations gave credence to arguments that all countries should limit their population in the common good. In September 1972 Alice warned,

> Unwanted children in New Zealand are a much greater tragedy than those in India. It is the people of New Zealand who are using up the world's resources. The ocean and the atmosphere don't belong just to us. Our pollution is the pollution of the world.[78]

The same impetus lay behind her interest in an NCW sub-committee on immigration, a new cause that confused those to whom she had been preaching the virtues of a low birth rate. But, for Alice, immigration seemed a practical way for New Zealanders to demonstrate a real commitment to the international cause. To offer 500 Pakistani refugee families a permanent home in New Zealand, rather than to send medical aid to them in India, would indicate 'that we really wish to share with others the good things that we have, space to live and freedom to worship'.[79] In August 1971, *Choice* had carried an article on population growth and human environment that stated,

> The time has come for a full and open discussion of population growth in advanced societies and its environmental impact. Equally important, IPPF believes that the adoption of the "stable population goal" by the more developed countries will, to some extent "desensitize" the population and family planning programmes, by governments and by the international agencies involved, with consequent benefit to the global environment as a whole. For the environmental problems which now arise in advanced industrial economies, through the combination of population growth with affluence and technology, will certainly be repeated in the developing world as they attain ever-increasing standards of living, unless appropriate action is taken.[80]

As far as Alice was concerned, these arguments confirmed the need for the NZFPA to make a stronger commitment to the international scene at home. The same month she suggested that the Standing Committee should 'set out to assume leadership in this field in New Zealand'.[81] Raising money for the IPPF was a logical part of this scenario.

This was a significant misjudgment on Alice's part, going well beyond the inclinations of the majority of the NZFPA membership. Moreover, the New Zealand government was now becoming actively involved and, almost concurrently, announced a conribution of $25,000 towards 'population control activities'. Of this $18,750 was to go to the recently established United Nations Fund for Population Activities and $6,250 to the IPPF.[82] NZFPA's Wellington and Hutt Valley branches had already reacted discouragingly to Alice's proposal that they become fund-raisers for the IPPF, advising that they did not wish to be involved in any such scheme.[83] In October, South Island seminar delegates were also reported to be 'uneasy', and felt that they did not 'understand the implications sufficiently to be able to make a decision for or against it'.[84] At a special meeting held at Denestone on Thursday 25 May 1972, attended by the full Standing Committee and Peggy Zeisler, the recently appointed administrative secretary, who had a background in international relief organisations,[85] it was made clear that, although branches believed they had some ultimate responsibility to contribute to IPPF funds, they felt they had enough on their hands filling local needs.[86] By this time, even Alice was beginning to feel daunted. Nevertheless, she continued to push the fund-raising barrow. In her president's report for 1972 she suggested that, since local committees were fully committed, IPPF fund-raising 'must mean recruitment of a new group of workers, people with different skills and interests from those required to organise educational programmes and clinical services'. The 'moral support' of branch committees would be of 'inestimable value to fundraising teams'.[87]

Population issues and ecological concerns would remain to the forefront of Alice's mind. In September 1973 she was featured in a newspaper article entitled 'Every day a battered baby or neglected children'. Cases of extreme family distress were cited as examples of the 'population explosion' that Alice regularly came across in the course of her work. The NZFPA, the article continued, believed that the knowledge of planned parenthood was a fundamental human right and that 'a balance between world population and the world's natural resources and productivity is a necessary condition of human happiness, prosperity and peace'. Dr Bush could 'reel off one heart-rending case-history after another' to bring 'such lofty, global ideals down to local and human terms'.[88] But by clinging to her beliefs, Alice had placed herself at odds with many NZFPA members, though she continued to sustain a leading role within the association. This was also now her position within the changing worlds of women and of medicine.

CHAPTER 11

New Feminism
and New Medicine

> *I have no doubt that you wish to know where I stand on
> Women's Lib. Having been able to take it for granted that
> I would be able to take up a profession just because I
> wanted to and having a husband who could meet with
> good humour the jibes of his friends who suggested that
> because his wife didn't spend all her time looking after his
> needs he was underprivileged, I am tempted to say there
> is no need for a women's liberation movement but my
> experience is quite the opposite and I think that in
> general the ordinary woman today has fewer privileges
> and is more dependent on her husband than was her
> social equal of fifty years ago.*[1]

Women's rights had not played a prominent role in national affairs since 19th-century feminist groups had gained the vote. That movement, nurtured by liberal sentiments of personal equality and the social morality of the temperance cause, had argued that women had special qualities, which were essential in the public sphere to correct the evils of a 'man's world'. Alice can be seen as one of its finest fruits, a talented woman who had succeeded in a predominantly male profession and taken the benefits of that experience to the wider community, concerning herself with the problems of women and children. Now a new feminism was emerging from within the civil rights movement in the United States, the New Left, the youth counter-culture and the sexual revolution. It challenged existing social and political structures and called for the creation of alternatives that would allow for personal fulfilment, regardless of gender. 'Women's Liberation' was born. It found a ready constituency where women were critically examining their domestically centred lives and finding them lacking.

It did not take long for this new wave of feminism to reach New Zealand. 'Feminine' qualities were now seen as social constructs that denied women the chance to compete on equal terms with men because of the constrictions of 'ladylike' attitudes and behaviour. Church and state were held to account for institutionalising the notion of female subordination, which upheld social and economic policies discriminatory to women's self-fulfilment as individuals. The nuclear family came to be regarded as an oppressive structure for women because its functional success depended on the restriction of their individual ambitions and the subjection of their interests to the greater family good. Bowlby's theories of maternal deprivation became the *bête noire* of a movement that was calling for childcare centres for working mothers. Revelations of the medical profession's historical 'scientific' support for limitations on wider educational or employment opportunities for women, and their dominion over access to contraception and abortion, defined their role as oppressors. The socialist and civil rights origins of the new feminism raised issues of colonialism and racism, which brought into contention the motives of population movements exported into Third World countries. Questions began to be asked about the 'big business' aspects of new contraceptive techniques and the health problems associated with their use. These were all areas in which Alice was conspicuously involved, but though she and radical feminists both wanted advancement for women their differing strategies could only lead them into conflict. The new feminism was to prove a problem on several levels, not only for Alice but for the women's organisations with which she worked.

Even her professional and social achievements as a doctor, which had previously confirmed Alice's feminist status, now became suspect. Women doctors were seen as having internalised the values of their profession to the extent that they had become equal partners with male doctors in the oppression of their sex. Because radical feminists could find no answer to their concerns in women doctors, they attempted to reject the profession altogether, reverting to past healthcare practices such as midwifery and herbal remedies, which had traditionally been carried out by lay women. They set up alternative health centres with an emphasis on self-help, low cost and democratised structures, while a wave of revisionist literature provided a theoretical base for this and other developments of the new feminism. On the other hand, medical women could not remain aloof from radical feminism, because it was affecting every level of society, even within their own profession. In 1969, when women made up only 10.9 per cent of doctors holding annual practising certificates in New Zealand,[2] a report on the second intake of students at the new Auckland Medical School revealed that 'rather surprisingly 30 per cent of the places were offered to women students'.[3] This trend undoubtedly reflected the increased personal ambitions of women inspired by the new feminist challenge.

Coincidentally, the profession began to be concerned with 'wastage', or the diminished return on training of a doctor who did not practise full time after graduation, a circumstance that came to be linked particularly to the careers of women doctors.[4] The implications of this development were sufficient to politicise medical women internationally. A series of studies by women members of the profession and social scientists aimed at defining the 'problem' statistically, identifying the factors that precluded women's fulltime professional participation, and suggesting possible solutions. The results of a survey of medical women, which appeared in the *NZMJ* in April 1973, indicated that the dual demands of motherhood and the increasingly rigid requirements of professional advancement were the major stumbling blocks to women doctors' progress.[5] An editorial in the same issue described this as 'ambition deflected into a different destiny, that of children .... There is no other intrinsic bar to the top.' The editor then did what the survey did not, and linked the medical women's problems with those of other women, arguing that this was 'part and parcel of the whole problem of the employment of women after marriage'. Since it was 'unthinkable in the present state of the social climate that the entry of women to medicine can be restricted and indeed may increase', ways had to be found to allow women to be more active in the profession. Maternity leave and sick leave covering children's illnesses were suggested as two possible moves.[6] In February 1974 the NZMWA recorded with some bitterness that the profession's news sheet, 'News and Views', and the report of the Central Education Committee to the Medical Council, had 'misinterpreted the survey' and appeared to be using it to limit entry of women medical students, although further correspondence saw this concern relieved.[7]

Previously, women doctors had accepted the need to fit into a man's world and into male professional structures. Now, for the first time, they began to challenge those priorities, but for the remainder of Alice's lifetime this protest amounted only to requests for minor modifications to the system. This was not only because women doctors tended to come from a class background that was not comfortable with revolutionary strategies, but also because of a statistical disadvantage. Unlike radicals in the wider movement, who could argue that because women composed more than half of the world's population they were entitled to an equal share of power, medical women formed a small minority, clustered in the lower reaches of professional hierarchies. Alice's own position was a perfect reflection of this basic fact. In 1961, when senior staff at Auckland Hospital presented a statement on behalf of a colleague who had been dismissed under strained circumstances, she was the only woman among 22 signatories.[8] There had been only a slight improvement in her situation over the decade, most notably the appointments of Alison Hunter and Keitha Farmer to the fulltime staff of Princess Mary in the early 1960s.[9] As late as 1971, Alice could still wonder if she would be welcome at a dinner of the Microbiological Society of New Zealand, after giving a paper at their conference, because of her sex.[10] Like her female colleagues, she expressed her desire for women's progress within the profession in terms of modest reforms, arguing towards the end of her life that,

> It is quite practicable for a mother to put her medical interests on one side for the years while the children are young and then to take them up again when their children have become more independent. It might be argued that ... a doctor who has been out of practice for five or ten years will have become out of date, but ... medical procedure is advancing so rapidly that even a doctor who continues in practice will soon become

out of date without continual refreshment at study courses and there is no lack of these in this country. Even in ten years one cannot forget the rigid discipline of thinking honestly, observing correctly and examining carefully which has been acquired by every successful graduate from a good medical school and the wish to learn about new advances and the enthusiasm to undertake the arduous study required is perhaps more likely to be found in a woman who is going back to medicine because she loves it, than in a man who couldn't leave it, even if he would.[11]

This was not a strategy to impress radical feminists, who were putting themselves on the line by challenging social restrictions in the most 'unladylike' way. Despite their obvious need for support, it was not until 1972 that medical women found a new feminist group with which they felt in tune: the National Organisation of Women (NOW). This movement in direction was an innovation for Alice too. Before the mid-1960s she had been associated with lay groups that had formed around concerns in which women were interested and most, if not all, of whose members were women. When she did become involved in purely female organisations such as the NCW and Zonta, her activities had been directed principally toward promoting her particular interests. In the hearings of the Royal Commission of Inquiry into Social Security during the early 1970s, for example, Alice was involved with the submissions of several participating groups, including her reformed professional organisation, the Medical Association of New Zealand (MANZ), the Paediatric Society of New Zealand and its Auckland branch, the NZFPA, the Family Guidance Centre (of which she was now Director), the Lady Fergusson Family Counselling Service (LFFCS) and Zonta. The NZFPA submissions, which were presented by Mavis Hurrey, Ruth Black and Ron Meggett, were naturally concerned with increased access to contraceptive services,[12] but references to the same need also turned up in the submissions of Zonta, the Health Department, the Auckland branch of the Paediatric Society and the NCW.[13] Alice appeared personally before the commission to jointly present the LFFCS submissions. She had been involved in setting up this service in response to the 'battered babies' crisis of the late 1960s and they were seeking subsidies and more extensive training for social workers to work with troubled families.[14] The Zonta submissions, which she also helped to present, reflected all her current concerns, from parental education to criticism of the amount of money being directed to kidney transplants.[15]

Since the new feminism focused on the need for women to take strength from each other, working together in non-hierarchical groups, Alice's tendency to 'use' women's organisations in this way can be seen as evidence of domination, an accusation given added credence by her undoubted strength of character and purpose. Such a judgment, nevertheless, suggests a degree of one-sided compliance that simply did not exist and discounts the fact that she was equally active in pushing her views through other bodies. The Auckland branch of the Medical Association also received a list of suggestions for their submissions to the commission, among them the inclusion of oral contraceptives in pharmaceutical benefits, and some were used.[16] Although Alice undoubtedly gained useful support and tended to act in a leadership role, not always officially, within women's organisations, their members were not blind to her special pleading and supported only those causes with which they agreed. The assessment of the NCW's Betty Holt, that Alice's participation in that organisation was mutually beneficial to both parties,[17] is nearer the mark, for she possessed several qualities rarely found in women at the time, and was valued for these. They included practical experience of the professional and political worlds, combined with a willingness to contribute at a hands-on level. For these reasons, Zontians were prepared to accept Alice's comparatively poor showing at meetings, even though regular attendance was normally a prerequisite to continued membership.[18] Her propensity to respond with provocative and succinct statements on social issues of the day also made her attractive to the media, and women journalists in particular found her a prepossessing, even inspiring, personality.[19] As a result, she featured regularly in the news, an invaluable asset, particularly for those women's organisations just establishing themselves.

Zonta was typical of the new feminist organisations with which Alice became involved, catering, as it did, for middle class professional women of a liberal and reforming frame of mind. She also accepted an invitation to become a vice-president of NOW,[20] although whether she was inspired in this move by the movement's founder, Betty Friedan, is doubtful. She had been sent a copy of Friedan's book, *The Feminine Mystique*, in late 1967,[21] but there is no evidence that she ever read it. But when, in August 1970, Alice was invited along, with several other local women, to give her opinion on a one-day, non-union, all-purpose strike organised by NOW in the United States to protest the low status of women in the community, her response was framed in contemporary, even radical, language. The state of women in New Zealand, she said, was 'quite plainly appalling'. They lived 'in a state of slavery unequalled in the annals of history'. Intelligent women were required to do the most menial work, having been educated to do no other. Women had been 'brain-washed' into thinking that education was unnecessary for them 'to be only wives and mothers'. Four times as many women as men entered mental hospitals because of the 'insufficient satisfaction of their lives'. Children had to be put first but this did not mean a career must be abandoned, although people had to learn to be realistic and accept that children cared for by others would obviously give them part of their love.[22]

This was not the only time that Alice used the 'slavery' concept. In May 1971 she referred to many large families as being 'slavery' for the mother.[23] Her most likely source for this analogy was not new, or even old, feminist tracts, but Fraser Macdonald, an Auckland psychiatrist and popular speaker who approached women's liberation as an aspect of mental health and often used the concept of women as 'slaves' or 'serfs'.[24] He and Alice had already found one common cause in the Appeal for Population Control,[25] and she was naturally in tune with his psychological tack. As a speaker in a series organised to celebrate Auckland City's centenary in July 1971, she made the link between 'suburban neurosis' and the inequities of everyday life for contemporary women. She also took some pride in pointing out that, as the only woman speaker, she was 'a demonstration that even a woman can speak with the authority which is properly bestowed upon those who have sought and obtained first class scientific qualifications', and wore her academic robes to prove it.[26] All the same, her topic was 'The Family', which she now defined as a variable cultural construct, not always achievable in the ideal sense but still 'essential . . . for the development of humanity'.[27] For radical feminists such sentiments could only confirm that Alice, like her entire generation of women doctors, was too concerned with sustaining women in their familial role, however she might now intellectually define the family. Her strong identification with child-raising groups that had emphasised the importance of parent-child relations seemed only to augment this conclusion. Analysis by woman's rights campaigners during the 1970s presented this phenomenon as a reign of 'experts' who created child-dependent mothers loath to let their children go because they had no identity other than their child-raising role. Such maternal possessiveness, it was argued, had formed an important component of youth rebellion. Radical feminists would have been astounded to discover that Alice, whom they perceived as one of those discredited 'experts', had articulated exactly the same argument when she had written in 1953 that for women to have no other interest in life than their children was 'too heavy a burden to ask any child to bear'.[29]

Women doctors felt rebuffed by such criticisms. They had seen themselves as championing women, not imposing a social role on them. This was the view put forward in 1969 by both Elizabeth Hughes and Alice, speaking at an NZMWA dinner, when they referred to their special task of taking 'the woman's point of view into the sphere of medicine, especially maintaining vigilance on matters affecting women and children and the welfare of the family'.[30] Alice had gone about this more provocatively than most. Her childcare theories and her support of a woman's right to sexual knowledge and birth control had been the public face of her concern, but the time and energy she had put into challenging the destructive family dynamics of many of her patients remained obscured by the demands of professional confidentiality. Abuse of power within the family, or any other social structure, had always been abhorrent to her liberal, anti-authoritarian nature. Her belief that women should have other roles in society was now becoming more widely shared but where it was not Alice could still rise to the occasion. In April 1970 she wrote a scathing letter to the press, criticising the president of the League of Mothers, who had been quoted as saying that 'a woman has nothing if she does not have a happy marriage and a happy home'. 'Being a wife and mother,' Alice responded, 'is only one way of using the talents bestowed upon us. Those who serve the community without a marriage, or in spite of an unhappy one, are among our most valued citizens, and certainly have a great deal.'[31] Her attitudes in this respect were markedly different from those of men doctors, even when they were her contemporaries and, like her, involved in paediatrics. Neil Begg, in the 1974 edition of his book, *The New Zealand Family*, saw the role of wife and mother as 'the most important and most rewarding task a woman can have, even though it be both difficult and challenging . . . . Any other task is of less importance', although after the age of 40 a woman might 'take a useful place in a profession, commerce or industry'.[32]

Alice shared Begg's belief in the importance of women's familial role but was more forthcoming about the tedium and lack of recognition that accompanied it. In 1961 she reflected on the

> sacrifices which a good working class mother does make which are taken for granted by society. She is cooped up in a small house with children . . . endless washing, meals and housework and just no fun at all . . . broken nights, children who don't want to eat, and all too often a husband who criticizes because the whole house does not revolve around him.[33]

Because her perception of women's health covered a much wider spectrum than that of most of her professional peers, Alice's ideas of a woman's right to a life beyond the home went beyond doing good works or pursuing a career. In her 1971 centenary lecture she criticised the assumption that 'women are less than human, that they have no need for the type of pleasure and companionship which is taken for granted by practically every man as his proper inalienable right'. To illustrate this attitude, she related the tale of a patient whose husband had complained that she had gone to an expensive restaurant for lunch with a friend. Further questioning revealed that this had happened only once. On the other hand, he told Alice 'with patent virtue', he went to the pub with his mates 'only on Fridays and Saturdays'.[34] At a symposium in May 1973 she specifically criticised the limited vision of many general practitioners, pointing out that a worrying mother did not visit the doctor 'just for fun', and proposing the adoption of a broader perspective than that provided by purely clinical parameters. 'Puerperal depression,' she suggested, 'may be due to oral contraceptives, an inattentive husband, or indeed an openly hostile one, or deep disappointment that having a baby is not as satisfying an experience as the mother had been led to believe.' Doctors who could not put aside an hour to investigate a crying baby should refer these cases to someone who could. Mothers deserved more than platitudes to deal with their problems and their experience with their children should be respected.[35] This was the sort of backing that many women needed and seldom received. Alice's sympathetic understanding of their lot earned her a loyal following.

Alice had also become more sensitive, and therefore more outspoken, about the extent to which notions of class and race could influence social debate. In one of the last acts of her life, contributing to the Zonta submissions for the revised Children and Young Persons Act (1974), she argued that the proposed president of a Family Court should be 'above the prejudices of any particular social class'.[36] In an earlier paper to the Medico-Legal Society on the 'battered baby', she included psychological or emotional abuse in her definition and took issue with the impression that, in New Zealand, this was a lower class or 'Polynesian problem'. Such assumptions, she suggested, were 'more of a reflection on our attitude to Maori and European mothers than of the true insidence [sic] of those who maltreat their children'. A punitive attitude towards offending parents simply made them 'the scapegoats of a society that neither knows nor cares what happens to a large number of its children ... The problem will not be solved by punishing someone who is just one link in the chain of social inadequacy that leads to the battering of babies.'[37] For her, the best solution remained a combination of support and education for parents, a strategy that she pursued in a variety of ways.

In 1973 she suggested that a mother implicated in child abuse should be 'encouraged to go out to work to build a better image of herself' while relatives or friends approved by the Department of Social Welfare looked after the child.[38] On a wider scale she became involved in the establishment of the LFFCS, which favoured the provision of counselling and family support services by strengthening a lay agency that had worked in the field since the end of the 19th century, the Society for the Protection of Home and Family.[39] Other medical professionals had their doubts about this ultimately short-lived scheme. When Alice approached Peter Lewis, recently appointed senior lecturer in child psychiatry at Otago Medical School, a man she regarded as a potential leader in his field and to whom she had given personal encouragement, he criticised the involvement of 'amateurs'.[40] Nevertheless, Alice continued to support the LFFCS, referring more than half of the organisation's 17 clients in the 1968–69 year.[41]

Despite modifications in her outlook, and her continuing tendency to step outside accepted boundaries, Alice remained conservative in her preference for evolutionary rather than revolutionary change, with the reformation of individuals, not structures, as its primary engine. And her position was increasingly a matter of public record in a social and economic climate where shifts were occurring with a rapidity that had caught everybody by surprise and where her opinions were frequently sought. Media exposure at this level was as likely to work against Alice as for her. Pithy, off-the-cuff remarks did not always fare well in print. In 1972, *Thursday*, a new magazine especially designed for, and popular with, young women, reported that Alice, as leading speaker at a Mothers' Day afternoon tea organised by NOW, had voiced the opinion that, among other things, she was against 'casual breeders. I don't think they're very good for society.'[42] This might have made entertaining copy but it was undoubtedly offensive and offputting to many. To radical feminists such a remark would have confirmed Alice as just another old-fashioned controlling doctor. Ironically, it was around this time that Alice reached the pinnacle of her profession. In 1970, on her second nomination,[43] she became a fellow of the Royal College of Physicians.[44] Of the 139 fellows elected at the same time, only nine were women, only five had a primary New Zealand qualification, and only Alice had practised all her life in that country.[45] In the eyes of older feminists this was the peak of her achievements, the one for which she was honoured in a 1975 pageant organised by the NCW to mark International Women's Year; it recorded the post-suffrage progress of women in New Zealand as a series of significant milestones.[46] For radicals, Alice's very success in her profession marked her as captured by it.

This viewpoint was not shared by many of those most influential within the medical world. Despite her worldly success as a doctor, several aspects of Alice's mature medical practice and personality isolated her within her profession. That she was a woman was only one factor, though her persistence and determination to voice her opinions must have been particularly grating in a profession where, even in the 1990s, mature women practitioners recalling their own experiences seemed concerned not to 'express too strongly verbally any dissatisfaction with their male colleagues'.[47] Alice's constant championing of the inclusion of family planning within health structures still had the power to irritate, and her special interest in allergies was only just beginning to be shared. It was too easy to classify her as 'Allergy Alice', who took babies off milk and put their mothers on the Pill, a limited and even cranky practitioner. That she was, in many ways, out of step cannot be denied. Unlike most of her peers, whose pursuit of specialisation had narrowed their range of interests, Alice's perspective on health care had broadened, increasing her commitment to social responsibility and action. Although she had her admirers, her priorities, and the strategies she used to pursue them, were often not widely shared or applauded. Her differences with the medical mainstream would be highlighted from the late 1960s as New Zealand entered a period of economic stagnation and inflation, forcing the first major re-evaluation of the welfare state in over 30 years. The setting up of a royal commission was its public face. Calls for economies within hospital structures could only exacerbate funding rivalry between interest groups.[48]

Within hospital circles it was paediatrics, consistently relegated to a subordinate position in the competition for resources, which was most likely to lead Alice into conflict. Despite a veritable building boom by the board over the 1960s, the prospects of a modern children's hospital in Auckland had receded. In 1963, after overseas leave, Ronald Caughey submitted a report, part of which re-emphasised the need for a single comprehensive paediatric hospital in Auckland and for the first time a completely new, purpose-built unit was mooted. The matter was discussed at a July meeting, chaired by Alice, between Wilton Henley, the board's superintendent-in-chief, and the paediatricians, including Sammy Ludbrook. They had to accept the board's argument that existing commitments made the completion of a new building unlikely before 1981, but used the opportunity to strengthen their old proposal, that the combination of Princess Mary,' brought up to full efficiency', and the annexation of the Infectious Diseases block could provide 250 conveniently situated paediatric inpatient beds long before the proposed new 300-bed hospital would be ready.[49] Alice augmented the argument in a letter to the chairman of the board's Hospitals Committee, stressing that these developments were essential, not just to raise local and national standards of child health care 'above the present mediocrity which is the best that can be said for it', but also to establish a paediatric teaching unit for doctors and nurses.[50] The setting up of such a unit had been approved by the board in 1955 but never acted upon.[51] With a medical school due to open in Auckland within the next few years, the need was now urgent.

By 1966 the unit had still not been established, but Alice and the other paediatricians appear to have assumed that, though developments were tardy, the board shared their ultimate aim of centralisation and this provided the dominant theme of a blueprint for the city's future paediatric services which the board encouraged them to produce over this period. In May 1966, before the report was completed, the board circulated its own proposals for future planning.[52] It was only then that the paediatricians became aware that a policy of decentralisation, with a cap of 150 beds on the Auckland site and no prospect of a teaching unit until at least 1972, had been in place since September 1963, the result of a meeting between Henley and Health Department officials at that time.[53] They prepared to argue the case within board and Health Department structures, but Alice had some additional measures in mind. She immediately placed before Princess Mary staff proposals for the establishment of a research project on malnutrition in children, the admission of more neonatal patients to Princess Mary and the allocation of beds there to paediatricians employed by the board but not allocated hospital beds of their own. She was quite clear about the strategic implications of these suggestions.

> ... the possibility of establishing one first class children's hospital in Auckland will be gone for ever if units for the care of sick children become established in the meantime in satellite sites. I believe that at the moment the danger that such units may be established in the near future is very real and I think it would be averted if some means were found whereby paediatricians employed by the Hospital Board but without general paediatric beds might be given an opportunity to care for their own children in the Princess Mary Hospital.[54]

Moves of this kind, looking after sectional interests within hospital circles, constituted acceptable practice and were generally tolerated, if not universally supported, by other staff. But Alice then overstepped the mark. In July she gave an address about the lack of a centralised children's hospital to an open meeting organised by Parents' Centres.[55] As was customary, a report of the meeting was sent to the media and appeared in the *Herald* under the headline 'Big Hospital Needed for Children'. The newspaper sought a response from the chairman of the Hospital Board, T.H.C. Caughey, who, obviously caught on the back foot, felt unable to give one.[56] Alice, unfazed, promptly sent off a letter to Caughey, offering him 'an unofficial look at letters and recommendations from the Paediatric Staff' so that he might be fully informed before he made his 'statement about the possibility of a Children's Hospital in Auckland'.[57] She received a diplomatically worded response to the effect that no statement would be made in the near future,[58] but by this time the publicity had led to such agitation among the board's medical fraternity that Alice had to circulate a conciliatory, private, communication of her own, partly because the press reports had referred to her only as 'a leading paediatrician'.[59] Henley, who had also felt it necessary to dampen down reaction with an internal circular, privately cautioned Alice that 'any extension of the argument in the press might prejudice your later approach to the Board'.[60]

It must have been clear that to take the children's hospital debate outside board structures would not endear her to her colleagues but, even after Henley's cautionary note, Alice attempted to do it again. She had recently become a Zontian and, following the *Herald* article, the club wrote to the medical superintendent of Auckland Hospital offering help with 'the children's hospital'.[61] The offer was politely rejected 'at present' by the August meeting of Princess Mary staff,[62] but apparently not by Alice. At the December staff meeting she produced a reply to the club which was read to those present, who now agreed that it should be sent through the medical superintendent's office.[63] At the same time, she privately forwarded to the club's secretary a 'personal supplement' of suggestions, posited on the belief that Zontians 'are a group of women who, by virtue of their intelligence, training and positions of responsibility could weild [*sic*] considerable power in moulding public opinion and spreading new ideas'. There followed an argument along the lines that there was no children's hospital in Auckland, or even in New Zealand, and that even 'our own most experienced hospital administrators', who lacked modern paediatric experience, had consistently followed a policy of decentralisation, ignoring the paediatricians' advice. She then suggested that Zontians could assist in establishing an association, 'The Friends of the Children's Hospital', which could mould opinion and educate the public about the need for such an institution.[64] The eventual fate of this proposal is unknown, but no such group seems to have been formed.

By 1970, continued frustration had lent Alice's approach an even more unwise and cutting edge. In a letter to Wilton Henley in January of that year she complained, 'I realise that the building of a Children's Hospital is a long way away but I am disturbed to learn that apparently it has not yet even been considered by the Board. It is obvious that Paediatricians are inept at power politics.' Accusations of 'second and third rate treatment' and 'a continued wastage with babies dying or becoming permanently handicapped from illness[es] which are preventable and curable' followed.[65] Henley, an urbane man, dispatched a reproachful reply, regretting the emotional tone and factual inconsistencies in her letter and suggesting that more would be gained if she put specific proposals to the Medical Superintendent and the Hospital Medical Committee.[66] Now that Alice had been put in her place as an emotional and unscientific medical woman, it was, perhaps, just as well that, in October 1970, the Paediatric Society took up promotion of a children's hospital as a national enterprise.[67] At the same time, a campaign to raise funds for a research chair in child health at the Auckland Medical School, backed by Rotary through the influence of Ronald Caughey, advanced the project locally in a more acceptable way.[68]

By this time, paediatrics was beginning to receive the academic recognition Alice had always regarded as its due, but that very achievement distanced her from the central role she had played in earlier years. Although she recognised the importance of research, Alice's working life had been taken up primarily with patient care. As a result, by the late 1960s she had published very little in medical journals, and neither of her scientific papers in the *NZMJ*, 'An Evaluation of Methacycline Hydrochloride (6 Methylene Oxytetracycline)' in April 1967, and 'Precipitating Antibodies in Asthma: A Preliminary Communication' (with D.J. Bryant) in July 1970, made an impact. By the time the establishment of chairs in paediatrics in Otago (1967) and Auckland (1970) offered opportunities to take up an academic career, Alice's attention was directed elsewhere. Her appointment as a part-time clinical teacher at the Auckland Medical School in 1971 was simply an extension of her hospital appointment. Staff at National Women's, where the postgraduate chair of obstetrics and gynaecology had long provided the university links necessary for a sustained research programme, fitted more easily into this new professional climate. When the Paediatric Society's executive returned to the city in the early 1970s, it was based at National Women's. It consisted of a new generation whose ideas seem often to have been out of tune with Alice's own, so that she remained an interested, sometimes contentious, member but no longer a driving force.

At the same time Alice actively supported these new academic and research opportunities for others. Her suggested project on malnutrition in children eased Dr Morag Hardy's entry into paediatric practice after taking time out to have a family, and Alice was a member of the panel that selected R.B. (Bob) Elliott, an Australian paediatrician with a background in teaching and postgraduate research, as foundation professor of paediatrics at the Auckland Medical School in January 1970. When the new professor arrived to find no ward space set aside for his personal use, Alice offered him her own.[69] This was a generous professional act that required the co-operation of her colleague, Alison Hunter, who transferred to another team. There may also have been a more personal cost: Alison Hunter believed Alice felt guilty when she didn't have a ward but continued to receive her usual salary.[70] Alice was prepared to go to such remarkable lengths because Elliott's appointment not only made research a viable activity at Princess Mary but also gave added credibility to the establishment of a children's hospital. She was less inclined to support other research activities that she believed were taking medicine in quite the wrong direction. We can be sure, from notes she made while considering Zonta's submissions to the Royal Commission on Social Security, just what she thought was the 'right' direction. Her views were shaped by her own ideas about medical and social need, economic prudence and the pursuit of a 'happy medium' between provision of free services and the erection of financial barriers. She did not think it fair, for instance, that when a patient was nursed at home, the family bore the full costs, but inpatient care at a public hospital came free. To achieve the ends she favoured, priorities would have to be reordered. Spending on preventive health programmes should be increased, with all healthcare personnel expected to participate in this area, providing 'proven preventive health measures' free to all. Curative services should continue with a 'fee for service' of 25 per cent of the total cost, and some hospital services paid for, subject to an almoner's report and the possible arrangement of time payment.[71] She pursued the same argument in the press, asserting that, over the previous 15 years, government spending on hospitals had increased by 44 per cent, but expenditure on preventive health had decreased by 8 per cent.[72] Even if her notion of preventive medicine had not included family planning services, this prescription was bound to place her at odds with many in her own profession, which had been developing in exciting new, but expensive, directions.

In June 1965, Auckland Hospital had stepped into the limelight with a successful kidney transplant between identical twins, the culmination of over a year's work in Medical and Surgical Units specially set up, as a Paediatric Unit had not been, to foster research and prepare for the establishment of the new medical school. Organ transplantation was one area of medical spending that nobody was keen to restrict. A meeting of the Combined Staff of Auckland Hospital approved the establishment of a renal homotransplantation service centred on the unit, and supported plans for further development.[73] Alice found this decision hard to take. When there was direct competition for resources, paediatrics did not fare well. At a meeting on 1 August 1966, Princess Mary staff discussed the news that a ward in the Infectious Diseases Block, which they had hoped to take over, was to become an outpatient clinic for renal dialysis. The alternative use they had in mind, to house cases of gastroenteritis and other intestinal infections, hardly had the same ring to it.[74]

Alice argued that the medical world's emerging interest in, and concentration on, organ transplantation was overriding more basic medical needs. Over these years, the concept of improving the 'quality of life' became the constant subtext to her activities. Family planners had always favoured this approach and Alice's concern with the preventive aspects of paediatrics and the sustenance of mental health services was similarly focused. Maintaining a quality of life was even more obvious in the treatment of allergies and she feared that concentration on this new field would push allergy, with which it shared an immunological basis, even further to the margins of medical education and practice. This belief was intensified after she spent three months at the beginning of 1968 at the Hospital for Sick Children in Toronto, where she worked with Dr Cecil Collins-Williams, a noted allergist.[75] Alice came away from the North American experience critical of two particular developments. The first was that the treatment of allergy had become 'distorted by the financial aspect and the extremely lucrative practice than can be based on a system of skin testing and injections for desensitisation'.[76] The second was the priority being given to organ transplantation. She recalled how,

> On more than one occasion I expressed to clinicians my envy of the resources which they must have available to them as a result of their proximity to institutes in which all sorts of sophisticated immunological techniques were practised, only to be told that the institution was

devoted to the service of a transplant programme and its resources were not available for the diagnosis or management of curable disease. I don't think that New Zealand can afford this type of medicine. I don't think the United States can either, but it is unlikely that I can do anything much about this.[77]

Alice clearly thought she could do something about the New Zealand situation. She returned home primed for action, and very probably some people were soon wishing she had stayed away. In August, a special edition of the *NZMJ*, marking the 50th anniversary of the opening of the original Princess Mary Hospital, included an article that Alice had written while in North America. In it she complained that, though medical students were 'now learning about the immunology which pertains to tissue grafting', they continued to 'regard with suspicion that particular immunological reaction which will account for minor or major symptoms in a large proportion of their patients and will require specific therapy'.[78] Later in the year she stood unsuccessfully as an Independent candidate for the Hospital Board on a platform of reducing the need for hospital beds (particularly for children) by establishing alternative services and suggesting that she 'had something to contribute towards the wise management of hospital affairs'.[79] In December, at the annual general meeting of the Medical Women's Association, she questioned whether large amounts should be spent on grafting organs while other fields suffered from funding deficits.[80] When she heard, in January 1969, that the Medical Research Foundation had made a grant to help the training of a doctor in immunology to assist in tissue grafting, Alice wrote to the head of the programme, Derek North, the recently appointed professor of medicine at the Auckland Medical School, urging that the training should be broadly based so that the immunologist

> will be able to assist in the diagnosis and treatment of common diseases as well as contribute to the management of patients requiring the transplantation of organs because their own have been destroyed.
>
> I'm sure that transplantation is a very fascinating pursuit for the physicians and surgeons engaged in it, but I believe that you would agree that from the patient's point of view, life is much more comfortable with their own functioning organs. Most of the disorders that progress to the destruction of the kidneys have immunological disturbance as their basic

pathology ... the students who will be your main responsibility in the near future will be going into practice to care for patients in the earliest stages of pathology and almost certainly responsive to treatment based on sound immunological principles.[81]

Alice's very personal campaign marked her out to the emerging leaders of her profession as a woman out of step with progress and tied to the past. Perhaps more unhappily, this was also becoming the case in her social role.

CHAPTER 12

Reproductive Politics

> *When an unwanted pregnancy threatens the welfare of a family or the cherished plans of a woman past the time of being prepared to devote herself to motherhood the conceptus is not a child in any respect, it is not a loved object, its destruction is a gesture of self defence as surely as the actions of a member of the armed forces, only the threat is individual rather than communal; the decision is an individual responsibility.*[1]

Alice was used to taking a stand on contentious issues in her public life. Now she was outflanked, not only by radical feminism but also by sexual libertarianism. Although she welcomed the discussion and debate that the new age promoted, and was willing to enter into it, she could not countenance what she saw as the abdication of personal responsibility to respect the rights of others, which accompanied the extremes of the sexual revolution. In June 1970, she congratulated the Students' Association of the University of Canterbury on their production of a 'Living with Sex' booklet, which she considered 'a significant contribution to the dispelling of ignorance and prejudice in this most important part of human feeling and behaviour'. While she agreed that 'each person must work out for themselves what will be satisfying and acceptable behaviour', she argued that this process should include not only recognition of 'the pain which their actions may inflict on another person' but also an examination of 'their own inheritance of behavioural drives'. For some, she suggested, frustration might be a 'biologically more normal and human' option until they wished for a deep emotional involvement.[2]

Although aware that her approach was unlikely to appeal to those intoxicated by the heady atmosphere of the 1960s Alice continued to propound it, particularly where she believed accuracy was being sacrificed to enthusiasm. This meant that any proposal to co-opt her into an alliance with sexual libertarianism soon collapsed. In 1972, after reading *The Little Red Schoolbook*, a publication aimed at young readers which raised the hackles of more conservative members of the public, Alice wrote to the editors, telling them she thought the concept generally a good one. But she had specific concerns with the text, including its vagueness about the age of consent and the chances of young people obtaining an abortion, which she considered would be dubious, 'however hard they try'. She also pointed out that doctors were legally prohibited from providing contraceptives to those under 16, and objected to the fact that abstention from casual sexual relations was not offered as an option. On the other hand, contraception was presented as 'easy and free from problems', which her own experience had revealed was not so. Moreover, in her opinion, the book presented an unnecessarily negative view of career opportunities for girls and, though she agreed that 'teachers should not call children stupid' and that environment was connected with 'expression of intelligence', she could not go along with the assertion that 'all kids start life with the same potential'.[3] Her letter resulted in a request from the publisher, Alister Taylor, that she act as an adviser for a forthcoming book designed 'to meet the needs in the sex education field in New Zealand'.[4] After initially agreeing to lend her name to the enterprise, Alice found her views to be so much at odds with the text that she extricated herself from the venture almost immediately.[5] An invitation to contribute to a proposed publication to be called 'Sexism, Sexuality and the Future of Marriage in New Zealand', edited by Alan Webster of Massey University, also foundered.[6]

Alice was equally uncomfortable with what had become the central plank of radical feminism: free access to abortion. This, she argued, was an issue which could divide the women's movement, undermining other possible advances. In June 1972, when reports of disrupted meetings of NOW reached her ears, she wrote to the secretary, Deirdre Milne:

> I consider that if the aims of the National Organisation of Women are to be persued [sic], they must be given priority over any side issues which would weaken the structure of the Association.
>
> I think it is improper for this Association to have an official policy on abortion. Whatever one's feelings about the present law, it is probable they are sincerely held and an official policy on this issue must weaken the organisation by reducing its membership.[7]

There was rather more to it than that. The abortion debate was to prove difficult for most people. Only those with an unquestioning religious or moral standpoint saw it as a black and white issue with one possible outcome. In facing up to the controversy that developed over the late 1960s and early 1970s, Alice was forced to review her entire experience. During her working life, termination of pregnancy could be performed legally only when medical practitioners decided it was necessary 'to protect the life of the mother'. These, referred to as 'therapeutic' abortions, were generally accepted by all but devout Roman Catholics. During the late 1930s the *Rex* v. *Bourne* judgment in Britain had extended the criteria to include psychological as well as physical grounds, although the wording of the law remained unchanged. Doctors who had a 'sympathetic' reputation could be certain that, from time to time, they would be asked to recommend, or perform, the procedure. Alice had found herself in this situation as early as May 1940, when a patient who thought she might be pregnant asked Alice 'to do something about it'. Although she confessed to 'a tremendous amount of sympathy' for the woman and wished she could 'give some real assistance instead of just a lot of advice', Alice was quite certain that, in this case, the procedure was legally out of the question.[8]

She had confided the experience to Faulkner, who was in his radical phase and took her to task. 'To the winds with such taboos,' he had written. 'In certain cases the principle is admitted. Why not in that case when to not have the child would have eased that woman's life? Sympathy is not enough.'[9] This little outburst brought out all Alice's shiny new professional resolve, so she continued the debate, even though the woman proved not to be pregnant.

> The principle is admitted only in cases in which the pregnancy is considered to be prejudicial to the health of the mother. In this case there was no real reason why she shouldn't have gone thro' with it except that it would have been very inconvenient .... an unborn child has as much right to live as anyone. There is also another side to the question, do you think that there is any call upon me to risk my livelihood, & take the chance of going to prison for a woman just because she wants to shirk a normal duty.[10]

Never one to back away from a good argument, Faulkner replied

> 'An unborn child has as much right to live as anyone'. O.K? Then why not adopt the R.C. principle & not even make an exception in the case where the mother might die. After all, it is one or the other sometimes. I think that if such exceptions are admitted, then the principle is established for further cases.[11]

Alice remained unmoved. By 1943, her desire to do something positive was being fulfilled by her involvement with the NZFPA, which regarded contraception as the way to reduce the rate of induced abortions, for married women anyway.

Alice's attitudes to abortion were not shaped wholly by her professional allegiance. In 1944 she had written an article for the Auckland University student paper *Craccum*.[12] Entitled, 'Abortion – What of it?', it was attributed to 'an Auckland Woman Doctor'.[13] Here Alice took the view that the issue of abortion was no exception to the rule that there were two sides to every question. But where she had earlier seen these as mother versus unborn child, she now examined more closely the complexities of the woman's experience, attempting to transform her from 'a mere entity into an individual human being' and making an effort 'to try to understand her problems'. From this perspective, she could sympathise with the overburdened housewife who had more children than she could manage, or the ill-informed young girl, but not the working wife who refused to bear children 'lest they should endanger' her career, or the 'young woman . . . well-schooled in the ways of life who had acted recklessly and irresponsibly'. Discreetly avoiding any mention of contraception, Alice listed some 'social improvements which would at least diminish the magnitude of this menace to the lives of the mothers in our community', including adequate housing, family allowances and subsidised domestic help for married women. Young girls should receive 'a proper education in all matters pertaining to sex, including an explanation of the power of the sex instinct and its proper control', while it should be emphasised to young men and women alike 'that all privilege is accompanied by responsibility, that for most of us life is long and includes no isolated instances. Every action, however insignificant, has its effect on the whole of life and as we sow, so shall we also reap.'

Her attitudes were entirely in tune with those held by family planners and in September 1944 a synthesis of the article was attached to a piece about the NZFPA in the *New Zealand Woman's Weekly*.[14] By then Faulkner had done an about face and was concerning himself, as was much of New Zealand officialdom, with the apparently low New Zealand birth rate. In May 1944 he had written to Alice, 'It's time this question of abortion was looked into and the police given a bit more assistance.' 'How views change with time,' he reflected, after Alice's death.[15] Over the postwar years Alice continued to be consulted occasionally by women wanting abortions. Some appeals she supported on the grounds of impairment of mental or physical health, but not all.[16] These were decisions made in consultation with only one other medical practitioner and the patient, but by the late 1960s legal abortion had become an ongoing public issue. Britain, and several American states had reformed, or were reforming, their abortion laws. Established guidelines were challenged, and opinions and outcomes were influenced by professional viewpoints, interest group commitments, moral, religious or philosophical inclinations and gender. Often these various standpoints were at war, not only in public but within individuals. This was the case with Alice. She was a woman doctor and a liberal feminist, dedicated to the interests of both mother and child, a reformer who believed in the necessity of evolutionary change. She was also dominion president of the NZFPA.

Family planners had always needed to be particularly careful to distance their services from abortion. They had avoided use of the term 'birth control' for this reason. In 1938, Jean Dawson, a founder of the NZFPA, had been warned by a British colleague,

> The R.C.s speak of abortion as a method of "birth control" and I am sorry to say some of our own friends do the same. I quite agree that

"birth control" is an ambiguous term, and I have often wished that it had never been invented; but at the time when M.S. [Margaret Sanger] coined it, to speak openly of "contraception" would have been impossible.[17]

Confusion was still surfacing in the 1960s. Following press reports of the NZFPA's 1964 conference, a correspondent to Wellington's *Evening Post*, who described herself as 'a Catholic, a Maori, and one of a family of 10', warned readers

None of us I am sure can understand the philosophy of these perverted "planners" who advocate a form of genocide – for you must know that family planning does not cease at preventing conception but that it includes the establishment of abortion clinics, if necessary on a national scale.[18]

Links could also be discerned through the NZFPA's connections with the IPPF, which favoured liberalised laws on the grounds of 'reducing or abolishing clandestine, back-street procedures, with their legacy of morbidity and even death. If abortion is to be performed at all it had better be done by competent gynaecologists in properly equipped hospitals.'[19] So the NZFPA had to tread a careful line, distancing itself from any pro-abortion implications, while using the debate to extend contraceptive services. In June 1969 Alice, as NZFPA president, expressed her personal opinions in a letter to Mrs M. Pearson of IPPF in London.

I don't think that abortion law reform will happen in New Zealand in the next few years. It has been discussed at the Medical Association Meeting but in general the comment was extremely unfavourable. New Zealanders are a very conservative group. They are only just beginning to accept family planning. I think we will have to give them a breathing space before they think of abortion. From our own point of view we would rather push sterilization and get social acceptance of this particularly in men. Nobody knows how many legal abortions are performed in this country but from the extremely high illegitimacy rate, I suspect that the number is fairly small. There is a certain amount of regular traffic from New Zealand to Sydney. While the law remains what it is, I am careful not to know how one may obtain an abortion in this country.[20]

The trouble was that, as a doctor and as a progressive liberal, Alice had come to believe that law reform was necessary. Her stand was initially based on her continuing aim to improve the physical and mental health of individuals and families and was bolstered by the development of the amniocentesis technique and advances in the study of genetics, which allowed some inherited diseases or disabilities to be detected before birth. Used with 'moderation and judgment', she argued, such new procedures 'could be as big a blessing to parents as the techniques that now allow infertile women to have children'.[21] In September 1969, in the Christchurch *Press*, she publicly advocated change, arguing that existing 'considerations for the physical and mental health of the mother' should be written in law and 'not left to doctors to interpret', while the diagnosis of a 'defective foetus' should be accepted as grounds for abortion because of the destructive effect caring for a handicapped child could have on the rest of the family. Alice was also concerned that 'there was one operation of the abortion law for the rich and another for the poor'. Abortions could be performed privately with very little delay, but this was not always the case for those who depended on public hospital services. She did not believe in automatic abortion in cases of rape because 'this is destruction of a potentially useful life', but added that the child would be better adopted, since the mother 'will probably hate it'. Never one to lose an opportunity, she asserted that the most effective method of preventing abortions was by the 'prevention of conception through family planning'.[22] The article drew at least one castigating personal response.[23] It may also have been a factor in the NZFPA Standing Committee's warning in November that, as a

> number of medical people have been asked their opinions by mass communications media, ... IT IS IMPORTANT THAT THIS ASSOCIATION HAS NO OFFICIAL POLICY ON ABORTION AND ANYONE MAKING A STATEMENT DOES SO ON HER OWN PERSONAL CONVICTIONS AND NOT ON BEHALF OF THE NEW ZEALAND FAMILY PLANNING ASSOCIATION.[24]

This clearly included Alice, identified in the *Press* article both as a paediatrician and dominion president of the NZFPA. Lay members of the association, too, needed to examine their situations at this time: Isabel Stanton, who was active on behalf of the Abortion Law Reform Association of New Zealand (ALRANZ), resigned from the presidency of the Auckland branch of the NZFPA at the end of the year.[25]

By 1970 the demand for abortion as a woman's right was gaining ground and Alice, both as president of the NZFPA and as an individual, was repeatedly asked for her opinion. Clearly, it was going to be increasingly difficult for organisations interested in reproductive matters not to have one. On 10 September 1970, the AKMWA held a special meeting to discuss the issue and decided almost unanimously to support the legal extension of grounds to include the mother's health as well as her life, with the added recommendation that 'substantial risk' of the birth of a seriously handicapped child should also be included.[26] Alice now had an official group policy with which she could align herself, while explicitly absolving the NZFPA, and she did this 11 days later when she took part in the second of three discussions held at Auckland University in the lead-up to a student referendum on abortion. She also took the opportunity to make it clear that she was 'firmly entrenched' against abortion on demand, which she defined as using 'sociological and economic circumstances' as grounds.[27] The following weekend, the NZFPA held its conference. Following discussion by a subcommittee consisting of three doctors (but not Alice) and one lay person, the association also supported reform on the same lines, after first emphasising that abortion could 'never be an alternative to satisfactory contraception'.[28] But by the end of 1971, when she was approached by Dr Carol Shand, the wife of Erich Geiringer, to share her opinions with a small group of reform-minded doctors, Alice emphasised that she now did not think this went far enough.

To get the ball rolling, Shand had suggested radical reform: doing away with abortion statutes altogether. Termination of pregnancy would then be controlled by existing laws that protected the individual against assault and would require the medical profession to observe good faith and professional skill, undertaking only medical procedures genuinely felt to be in the interests of patients.[29] Alice could not agree; she felt that there must be a law. It should not only define grounds but include 'control over places and prices', to guard against 'the performance of terminations of pregnancies for profit', and 'give the woman rights as well as protect the doctor', something which Shand may have felt her position covered, but which Alice did not. Alice had a specific circumstance in mind, however, when she spoke of a woman's rights; requests for abortions by mothers in cases where there was 'reasonable doubt' about 'the normality of the foetus'.[30] Her opinions therefore placed her somewhere between most doctors, primarily concerned to protect their own legal position, and radical feminists, who believed that women should be able to obtain an abortion as of right.

In the meantime an organised anti-abortion lobby, the Society for the Protection of the Unborn Child (SPUC), had been developed from an initiative by Auckland obstetrician and Roman Catholic, Dr Pat Dunn.[31] Increasingly prominent in this movement was Dr, later Sir William, Liley, whose own pioneering work in the study and treatment of the foetus had confirmed for him the belief that 'life begins at conception and ends at death'.[32] This was also the view of the Roman Catholic church and was presented by Dunn as confirmation of 'the foetus as a patient' in the October 1968 edition of the *NZMJ*. Concentration on the rights of the foetus extended the moral authority of SPUC supporters, at least in their own eyes, over every pregnant woman in the country, whether or not she sympathised with their views. The authoritarianism of the anti-abortion lobby undoubtedly intensified Alice's pro-reform stance, pushing her further than she might originally have gone as she saw the rising public profile of SPUC increase problems for all women trying to get abortions. Her antipathy was considerably increased when it became clear that this pressure group was not inclined to see contraception as an answer to the problem. William Liley addressed SPUC rallies and was quoted in the papers as saying there was not 'a cracker of evidence' to show that contraception obviated the need for abortion.[33] In 1966, Alice and Liley had shared a mutual interest in supporting Geiringer's APC.[34] By the end of 1970, Liley's tactics were irritating Alice to such an extent that, when his name came up for an honorary life membership of the Paediatric Society, she formally objected because of his activities 'for the rights of the unborn child versus the welfare of the family as a whole'.[35] This was not how the society's executive saw it. 'Honouring a person does not, after all', the secretary replied, 'mean that the body concerned (whether it is the Paediatric Society of New Zealand or the Royal College of Physicians of London) [Alice had been elected a fellow shortly before] necessarily endorses all his or her views.'[36]

The best evidence of the personal turmoil that the abortion debate aroused in Alice lies in a four-page cyclostyled typescript, 'Abortion: A Personal View', which she wrote over this period and which was released in August 1971 by ALRANZ, now a national society with Isabel Stanton as president.[37] The text argued for legal reform on the grounds of 'quality of life' from the perspective of 'a Christian, a doctor and a mother'. Alice discussed various viewpoints, from the analogy of supporting abortion or war as mutually hard choices, to the desirability of providing terminations for women with diagnosed, even suspected, foetal abnormality. Yet there was something atypical about the document. It was not simply the contentious nature of the issue. Alice had always had the courage of her convictions, and it was impossible to enter this debate and be otherwise. Rather, it was the construction of the text. Essentially, she produced a counter-argument to the anti-abortion lobby's focus on the evils of abortion by concerning herself with the evils that she believed could result from the inability to obtain a termination. This emphasis on the negative resulted in a pessimistic tone and an often emotional argument, which contrasted with Alice's usual concise, cogent and ultimately optimistic reasoning. Uncharacteristically, she also ventured into profitless areas, at times expressing herself in terms that provided ammunition her opponents.

Here, Alice's belief in the links between the childhood experience and later social adjustment took on a dark determinism. There were people, she claimed, 'whose early life has been such that they reach adult life incapable of responding to anything good'. They were 'cruel, tyrannical and completely egotistical' and society could do nothing with them. Similarly, touching on the physical and emotional aspects of 'battered baby' syndrome, Alice drew a much bleaker picture than the one she had offered not so long before, describing parents

> ... whose emotions can never be really involved with another person either old or young and even the cry of the infant arouses not maternal love but punitive aggressiveness, their babies are beaten and battered from the early months. Less dramatic but far more common than the truly battering mother is the one who can never forgive a child for coming, unwanted.... Seen by his mother as an enemy this child is likely to swell the ranks of those who occupy our gaols or mental hospitals; indeed often alternating between the two.[38]

And these were not people for whom contraception could provide a solution. To insist that it should have been practised was 'to ignore the way the world was made as surely as did the courtiers of King

Canute. A couple of bottles of beer will make any risk seem infinitesimal.' Even the use of religion as an authority for her position, so often Alice's ally in the past, took on a harder line when combined with her analogous use of participation in a war. 'If ever there could be a "Holy War",' she asserted, 'for the preservation of good and the prevention of evil, selective termination of pregnancy would qualify to be so called.' This, and her expressed belief that the pregnancy of a mother suffering from Down's syndrome, who had a 50/50 chance of producing a similarly affected child, would best have been prevented by 'timely sterilisation', had dangerously eugenic connotations.

Alice's conclusion was also unwise, a gift to those who wished to make a direct connection between abortion and contraception: 'To summarise, early terminations [sic] of pregnancy is not killing a child. It is preventing a child. A child is a human being in its own right with a separate existence of its own . . .'.[39] Revisiting the 'quality of life' and the priority of the rights of the born over the unborn child, she referred to Roman Catholic beliefs in a slighting way that contrasted with the measured tone of her 1968 response to *Humanae Vitae*.

> The foetus can do no wrong. In some people's philosophy, it is ensured eternal life if it dies, but the born unwanted child is a stumbling block to us all, it has human needs but no human satisfactions. If we are concerned with the preservation of the life of the unborn, let us first be concerned that what we can ensure for it is a human life not just an animal existence with no knowledge of the Grace of God.[40]

Alice also left no doubt that she was presenting the choice to have an abortion as 'a woman's right', not just to preserve her own health but also for reasons other than the possible birth of a handicapped child.

> When an unwanted pregnancy threatens the welfare of a family or the cherished plans of a woman past the time of being prepared to devote herself to motherhood the conceptus is not a child in any respect, it is not a loved object, its destruction is a gesture of self defence as surely as the actions of the armed forces, only the threat is individual rather than communal; the decision is an individual responsibility.[41]

Since economic or social issues cannot be excluded from undefined threats to family welfare or 'the cherished plans of a woman past the time of being prepared to devote herself to motherhood', this was effectively, and by Alice's own previous definition, an argument for abortion on demand. She may have given authority to her argument with her long-held liberal credo of 'individual responsibility', but it was her opposition to the tactics and arguments of SPUC that had ultimately led her to this position.

Alice allowed this document to be circulated in the full knowledge that it would be critically received. At some time before June 1970 she had sent a copy to the Anglican Bishop of Auckland, Eric Gowing. The bishop responded very politely, but from his own perspective of 'belief in the sanctity of human life', which for him included irrevocable opposition to war, capital punishment and 'the killing of human life when that life is in the womb rather than in the world outside'. He was 'very doubtful about your argument with regard to the elimination of those who are going to be misfits in society "incapable of anything good"'. How could this be predicted, he asked? Mothers who did not want their babies 'should be given all the spiritual, psychological, medical and social help that society can offer', and if their attitude to the child continued it should be 'cared for by society'. He agreed that the quality of life was more important than its quantity, but suggested that this was a matter for community education. He could not agree that 'early termination of pregnancy is not killing a child – it is preventing a child'. He was sure she would not say that the 'elimination' of a child who may be mentally retarded was '"not killing a child" – it is preventing a man or woman. Such an argument would not make sense.'[42] Despite this response, Alice apparently saw no reason to revise these points.

Relating the extremities of Alice's text to the equally emotional and extreme views she was opposing does not seem to fully explain 'Abortion: A Personal View'. She was no stranger to fiery debate. One of her principal strengths had been her ability to maintain logical argument, strategic astuteness and a certain amount of grace and flair. During the early 1970s she often seems to have had trouble achieving this admittedly delicate balance. Her confrontation with Wilton Henley over the lack of progress on a children's hospital and her challenge to William Liley's life membership of the Paediatric Society were both uncharacteristically awkward. Although she was still a comparatively young woman, the answer may well have lain in a failing constitution. Many colleagues felt that Alice was pushing herself too hard, spreading herself too thinly. Her diaries and Faulkner's recollections testify to a life proceeding at full pace, even on holiday and especially during overseas trips. When asked, in May 1971, for her hobbies, she proffered the Play Centres Association, Parents' Centres and her vice-presidency of the Speech Therapy Association, an involvement that had grown out of her interest in emotional health and education. That these should have been considered recreational pastimes must have struck even Alice as bizarre, since she immediately added, 'I suppose I'm culturally retarded . . . but there is so much to keep up with in medicine these days, and so much that needs doing that I don't seem to have time for anything else.'[43]

Perhaps not, but this lifestyle was taking its toll. In a photograph taken at the 1972 NCW conference in Nelson, Alice looks drawn and strained. Still, she kept up the pace and her equanimity, so often her ally in the past, had not entirely deserted her. At the time, the more charitable of her acquaintances put any lapses down to the menopause;[44] only in hindsight would they take on any greater significance. Just a month after her 'Personal View' appeared, Alice was once more using the abortion issue constructively to further the interests of the NZFPA.[45] The same preference for contraception over abortion emerged from the first Health Department seminar on family planning held at National Women's Hospital in November 1971,[46] and from a survey conducted by the New Zealand Council of the Royal College of Obstetricians and Gynaecologists.[47] This should have been the heyday of the NZFPA, but the turbulence of the abortion debate was giving old foes new vigour.

The Roman Catholic church continued its campaign against 'artificial' contraception with plans for 'appropriate general education programmes', opening its own '"Natural" Family Limitation Advisory clinics' and giving practical and moral support to research into acceptable techniques. Parish councils were urged to be active in the anti-abortion struggle and to oppose sterilisation as a form of contraception. All parishes were recommended to join SPUC and publicise its work.[48] In January 1972 Pat Dunn wrote a pronatalist piece entitled 'Is Population Pollution or Progress?', which was published in the local press. The article came down heavily on the side of people as 'progress, ideas, vitality, stimulus, hands to work with'. Those who were against population increase were 'pessimists and xenophobes'.⁴⁹ Alice responded by pointing out that she and Dunn were looking at the issue from perspectives attributable to more than just their religious views.

> ... a child needs more than food and clothing and fresh air. When I see 20-year-old parents trying to cope with a family of five, mothers taking to tranquillizers as a refuge from their three in three years, fathers continuing to prefer alcohol, babies with fractured skulls and limbs inflicted by parents who, themselves, grew up without affection, then I am forced to the conclusion that increased finance for families is no adequate solution. "The more the merrier" may be a good slogan for obstetricians, but to those who care for children, planning seems better.⁵⁰

Alice might have added that, for men, birth control still tended to be a national issue, for women a personal one. Male Maori and Pacific Island leaders addressing the 1971 family planning course at National Women's Hospital had claimed that their women wanted nothing to do with it, opinions that were hotly denied by leading members of the MWWL,⁵¹ and that seem doubtful in the face of a Maori birth rate which would halve between 1963 and 1977.⁵² Alice interpreted this debate as a difference between leaders and led.

> The Polynesian leaders who addressed the Health Department seminar on their attitudes to family planning may perhaps be forgiven for their lack of knowledge of the attitudes of the majority of their womenkind. It is not fashionable for leaders of racial groups, political groups, or apparently of trade unions, to study the attitudes of the lower echelons, they think they know what is good for them.⁵³

The new feminism was to indict Alice on the same charge in regard to her own activities as leader of the NZFPA.

Alice was used to fending off criticism of NZFPA activities from outside sources, but over the 1960s she had enjoyed unchallenged leadership within the organisation. During that decade the association had moved from a struggling, marginalised group, to a state-funded chain of clinics, boasting vice-regal patronage and offering professional services and the latest contraceptive techniques. For older family planners, this was the dream of access to 'scientific and reliable contraception' realised. By the end of the 1960s, however, the association's membership had changed significantly.

After the 1968 conference *Choice* noted that a new generation was making an impression.

> The delegates old in experience listened to and welcomed the opinions of the newer members of our groups. It was refreshing to see and hear so many younger delegates. This sense of full participation helped the discussions to be conducted in a good atmosphere and lead [*sic*] people to accept majority decisions they did not really like. A number of decisions were carried by a narrow vote but I for one never heard an upstairs out of meeting complaint from those who voted against these decisions.[54]

There were several aspects of the NZFPA in the early 1970s that new members, especially more radical ones, could find wanting. They were less inclined to make the same comfortable connection between contraception, woman's rights and family health. When women were increasingly identifying their right to control their own bodies, there was resentment of the central role of the association's doctors, who undoubtedly acted as the gatekeepers to contraceptive accessibility for single women, and complaints about the 'embarrassing and probing questioning and moralising' which, it was alleged, preceded any distribution of the Pill at clinics, even for married women.[55] The NZFPA's refusal to officially support free access to abortion and the association's recent inclusion within state health structures provided further evidence that this was a woman's organisation subverted by 'male' values and exposed to political and medical power.

Under such analysis, Alice could easily be identified as the chief mediator of that subversion.[56] The evidence was overwhelming. It was only after she had become president that the association had managed to expand its clinic services after reaching an accommodation with the NZBMA – and from that point what had been a lay women's group became an organisation dominated by doctors. Alice had also masterminded negotiations with the Health Department and publicly supported developments in contraceptive techniques in areas where women's welfare was now being seen as overridden by profiteering drug companies. Moreover, under her leadership the NZFPA had increasingly accepted money from these companies and had begun participating in clinical trials. As a doctor, Alice was used to moving in a world where drug companies, keen to promote their products, gave travel grants, assisted with the costs of clinical meetings and financed research.[57] She could not see why financially strapped and worthy lay bodies, not just the NZFPA, should not accept some of these benefits as well and had no hesitation in going out of her way to arrange these. In March 1971, taking advantage of a pharmaceutical representative's visit to her rooms, she was instrumental in arranging for his company to cover the costs of an Auckland doctor's attendance at a national executive meeting of the Asthma Society in Taupo.[58]

In the case of contraceptive clinical trials, economics was not Alice's primary motive. She believed they were essential to evaluate safety standards,[59] and that NZFPA branches had a particular role to play because they held records of satisfied users which would counterbalance the unsatisfactory case histories usually recorded in medical literature.[60] There was, though, a natural confluence between financed trials and a well-intentioned desire to take family planning to those 'most in need'. The 1963 clinic held in a South Auckland school, and aimed at attracting women from lower socio-economic and cultural groups who had not previously patronised the NZFPA, had been 'a small part of the trial on the sequential method of oral contraception' being carried out at National Women's Hospital by Dr G.C. Liggins.[61] The ethics of such exercises were not lost on Alice or NZFPA organisers. She insisted on informed consent, that it should be 'made very clear' to patients that they were participating in trials where 'the pills used have not had a full acceptance in the same way of [sic] those that are specially available',[62] and the Standing Committee spent several meetings agonising over the implications of receiving money and supplies from drug companies, and how this should be balanced against the interests of clients, the additional work generated for clinic staff and the chance to extend their services.[63] By the late 1960s, poor patients were not seen as good trial participants since they tended to be 'frequent defaulters and not easy to follow up because of the way they move around from one place to another', and at least one trial based on an NZFPA control group acknowledged that the sample was skewed because it contained 'a significantly lower proportion' of the lower socio-economic group than that 'present in the clinic population'.[64] But, in the early 1970s, any such exercise could only arouse disquiet in minds becoming increasingly aware of the politics, and big business aspects, of reproductive technology.

Radical feminists could also find plenty to criticise in Alice's persistent efforts to involve the NZFPA in the international population movement and to take contraception to Maori and Pacific Islanders,[65] particularly when she resorted to the language of the old evolutionary model. Uneasiness could only increase when, as in January 1972, she publicly suggested that New Zealand should 'follow the example of the World Bank' and make financial aid to the Cook Islands dependent on their adopting 'a realistic attitude to their population explosion'.[66] The professionalisation of the association, which Alice saw as a necessary corollary to expansion of services following Health Department involvement, became another bone of contention. In December 1970, during preliminary talks concerning the setting up of a 'top level academic' National Medical Committee, Alice urged that the 'new committee would appreciate the importance of co-operation between medical and non-medical members of the association'.[67] But lay workers were already feeling marginalised. There were clear indications of unrest along these lines as early as 1968,[68] and over the next year Alice received at least two personal approaches from members concerned about differences with their clinic doctors.[69] She tried to smooth things over publicly and behind the scenes, but the rumblings continued.[70] By 1972, when Alice paid tribute to lay workers' achievements over the preceeding years and expressed the hope that, as expansion proceeded and a wider range of professionals needed to be employed, they would not 'make the mistake of thinking that this is a takeover',[71] it was clear that her efforts had not been enough.

Alice had always been too conservative in her ends for radicals and too radical in her means for conservatives. Upsetting both groups at the same time could create a significant opposition. An influx of a new, radically informed, membership, together with established members uneasy about ambitious plans for involvement with the international population cause, and a general wider mood for change was sufficient to alter the balance of power within NZFPA. At the 1972 conference, the second to be held in Auckland, voting for national office saw the election of an almost completely new Standing Committee, and Glenys Lowe lost the editorship of *Choice*. A remit was passed limiting all dominion executive officers to a term of four consecutive years, after which they must stand down for at least a year.[72] Alice had now occupied the presidency for 12 years and, though she was returned unopposed, she was clearly on notice. Glenys Lowe maintained her equilibrium in her last editorial in *Choice*, interpreting this turn of events in terms of natural progress,

> The last two years have seen growth within the NZFPA – growth unprecedented at any other juncture in the history of the Association. But growth means expansion, and expansion needs continuous evaluation of resources. The dead wood must be removed from the tree and new buds be grafted in its place.[73]

It was the end of an era in the NZFPA, an era that had been moulded by the introduction to New Zealand women of new ideas about sexuality, mental health and reproduction. From the 1940s to the 1960s, they had increasingly responded to opportunities offered to control their fertility and better understand their bodies and their lives. For many it had resulted in widening personal horizons and more confidence and autonomy in personal decision-making. For some, educational and leadership opportunities within the association, or within related organisations, had led to lives of a new, undreamt of breadth. All this was centred on enriching life for women within an improved family life, and as such it was in tune, if not always in tandem, with the general political climate of the time. Now, a generation later, the children of these women, with different needs and experiences, were reaching further still. Although it did not necessarily seem so from the perspective of the early 1970s, it was the hard-won advances of the previous 30 years that bridged the gap between late-19th-century and mid-20th-century feminism. In this sense, Alice's notions of evolutionary social change had been validated, but the reasons behind her own fall from grace were more personal.

Alice's hallmark had always been to aim higher than her peers and pursue those aims with extraordinary tenacity. This tendency was seldom a problem when she was acting as an individual. It had worked to her advantage professionally, and when, as president of the NZFPA, she had taken the association where its members wished it to go. The trouble began only when this unity of purpose was eroded, but it was not within Alice's nature to see a need and turn away. She was used to voicing alternative viewpoints and, in full flight, cut a formidable figure, perhaps more so in the crowded last years of her life, when erratic behaviour occasionally impinged on her self-control. Even Faulkner, who saw her as essentially kind, gentle, always a lady, had to admit that the strength of her convictions was powerful indeed. She was, he remembered, 'inclined to expect people to agree with her because in her mind she was quite sure she was right' and would not be 'fobbed off' unless she could be convinced that she was wrong.[74] The equivocal opinions expressed by family planners after her death show that this determination was not only her great virtue but also her Achilles' heel. While Alice was admired for her strength of purpose, her leadership, her humanitarianism, the acceptable image she had created for the association and its work, she was criticised for her 'directing' influence.[75] It was the ultimate irony that Alice, who had opposed authoritarianism all her adult life, would herself be branded in just this way.

Alice continued to pursue her ideals after the 1972 elections, but the challenges were now coming more rapidly. During the early months of 1973, after the appearance of a letter from Mary Littlewood in *Choice*, differences surrounding NZFPA involvement in the international population movement were aired openly.[76] Dispute hinged on the nice distinction that family planners had always made between 'family planning' as 'family spacing' and 'population control' as 'family limitation'. How could family planners reconcile these two philosophies, especially when they drew parallels between the world situation and that at home? For Mary Littlewood, the danger was that NZFPA personnel might be seen as 'judges of morality – which we would do if the moral issues of family size and population control become our business'. One voice was strangely silent in this debate.[77] On the morning of 26 May Alice had suffered a coronary during her ward round at Princess Mary.

CHAPTER 13

The Quality of Life

> *There is a real need for concern about the quality of life rather than the quantity of it . . .*[1]

In 1973 Alice was in her late 50s, Faulkner his early 60s. Their personal life was settled, even serene. In 1969 Alice had decided to work from home, and she had a suite of professional rooms installed at Denestone, part of which she sub-let.[2] Faulkner, who had been semi-retired since their return from Canada in 1968, now had more time to help with the practice accounts, deal with patient telephone calls and even, in his inimitable way, occasionally act as 'nurse' in the rooms.[3] There had been other changes. Since 1959, three quarter-acre sections had been sold off so that the house stood in very much reduced grounds. There were also fewer people around. Alice now had only weekly household help. Peter was attending university in Palmerston North and after July 1972 when Christine, recently graduated in law, left for a working holiday in London, neither of the children was living at home. There were no more gatherings at Deep Creek. It had been sold to the local council in 1969 to form part of what is presently the beach reserve at Torbay. Instead, Alice and Faulkner spent their holidays travelling around New Zealand and he would often accompany her when she had speaking engagements or conferences out of town. In July 1970 they went abroad for two months, visiting Hawaii, Canada, Britain, Brussels, Germany,

Israel (where Alice attended a conference on child psychiatry), India and Australia.

Only one major cloud darkened their personal horizon over this last decade. In mid-July 1966 Faulkner became seriously ill as the result of a leaking abdominal aorta. This was successfully replaced, but he was unable to return to work until 5 September,[4] and the episode worried Alice. Her own health had been good all her life, apart from the development of a hiatus hernia during her pregnancy in 1949 (which she had presented as a 'case' to the Clinical Society that year)[5] and an episode of thyrotoxicosis in 1960. Although her hair had greyed prematurely, Alice was still a vital figure, slimmer than she had been as a teenager and seldom seen in repose. When she talked, her hands moved incessantly to emphasise her words, while the glasses that she now wore seemed at times to be struggling to stay on as she rushed here and there to fulfil her busy schedule. True, she sometimes looked strained, but her stride was as purposeful as ever. When she refused speaking engagements and resisted new ventures,[6] she offered as an excuse only the pressure of existing commitments, not failing health. If something that really interested her came along, the old sense of 'keenness' could not be suppressed. In 1970 she arranged the inaugural meeting of the Auckland branch of the Asthma Society at Denestone, but cautioned that her own contribution would be confined to 'moral support' and perhaps the occasional talk.[7] An interim committee had hardly been established, however, when its secretary, Mary Taylor, a mainstay of the society over following years, received a letter from Alice containing a list of suggestions which the committee was 'entirely free to accept . . . or reject as they choose'. These included organising a meeting around the theme of the house dust mite, a recent development in asthma research being pursued by Brian Cornere at Green Lane Hospital. Cornere could speak, microscopes for viewing living mites could be placed around the room, practical ways to reduce mite counts could be suggested, and skin tests with mite extract at $1 a time could be offered as a fund-raiser. She also proposed the new professor of psychiatry at the Auckland Medical School, John Werry, physiotherapists and dietitians as other prospective speakers. Members could exchange recipes and combine with other societies 'to have things on display at the Easter Show'. A copy of the Australian *Asthma Welfarer* was enclosed for ideas on additional activities.[8] This 'moral support' continued until her death.

Because of Alice's energetic approach to life, most people were shocked when she suffered her first coronary in May 1973. It was only then that they recalled a recent loss of weight, her occasionally erratic behaviour and the fact that she did look older. After Alice's death, Faulkner came to the conclusion that she had been unwell for some time but that he had 'missed' it.[9] His suspicions increased when he discovered amongst her papers a 1971 *British Medical Journal* article on the treatment of crescendo angina in a 40-year-old man and a 60-year-old woman with thyroid disease.[10] A similar significance might also be attached to Alice's decision between January and June 1970 not to proceed with an application to join a staff superannuation scheme,[11] and her remark in 1972, when writing to a close friend living overseas, 'I haven't had a free night during the week for a long time and I am not as young as I once was'.[12] Speculation is all we have to go on because Alice had never been in the habit of discussing, or even drawing attention to, her health and felt that minor discomfort was something one should not 'lie down to'.[13] Even when she experienced cardiac distress during her Saturday morning ward round at Princess Mary, she dismissed the pain as her old hiatus hernia playing up and asked for bicarbonate of soda to relieve it.[14]

Instead she was admitted to the hospital's coronary care unit for three days and discharged with orders to rest at home for six weeks. Chafing at the restrictions of convalescence, she was soon preparing submissions to the Statutes Revision Committee on contraception for minors,[15] sending off suggestions to improve an information booklet for the parents of children with adreno-genital syndrome,[16] and organising the testing of lambskin rugs for house dust mites.[17] Solicitous enquiries about her health were rebuffed.[18] Towards the end of June she contemplated her return to work. She had been advised to lighten her clinical load and so resigned from her appointment at the Green Lane Allergy Clinic.[19] Considering she was still working at Princess Mary, Karitane, the Child Health Clinic and in her private practice, this was something of a token gesture, and Alice's attitude to work seems to have changed hardly at all. Although she now had fewer paediatric beds at Princess Mary, the Medical Superintendent of Auckland Hospital reported at the end of 1973,

> Dr Bush used this period to very great advantage in developing out-patient services related to her in-patient bed usage and the workload has

been very heavy. Although she had only 14 beds, her patient turnover was greater than with other teams.[20]

Her commitment to the NZFPA and other organisations and interests continued. At the same time, she was apparently prepared for death, telling her practice nurse Betty Neal in July 1973, 'I won't make old bones, an ECG [electrocardiogram] doesn't lie.'[21] It was a reaction that reflected her attitude to life itself.

By her final year, Alice's commitment to the practice of religion had become openly perfunctory,[22] though the moral imperatives of Christianity remained important to her worldly activities and she had always been happy to contribute to church discussions on family life.[23] She did not believe in religious orthodoxies such as a 'hereafter or continuing existence'.[24] The extent to which the pursuit of mental health had provided an alternative for her was made explicit in Alice's 1971 centenary lecture, when she suggested that 'the creation of heaven on earth is a realistic goal that we must strive for with faith ... not praying for a miracle, but by working for success in mental health as we have worked for success in physical health'.[25] The philosophy that it was life itself, or the way in which it was lived, which provided true immortality and peace of mind not only lay behind many of her public stands but also released Alice from the dominion of death as surely as any religious faith. In her 'personal view' of abortion, she had written 'the quality of life is more important than the quantity of it. I believe that under certain conditions life is worse than death. I hope I die before I lose the power of thought and action which makes me the person I am.'[26] In October 1971 she had criticised persistent medical intervention in the *NZMJ*, citing cases involving both young and old 'where nature unhindered would have brought only blessed peace'.[27] In a subsequent interview in the weekly paper the *8 O'Clock*, she argued that the doctor's role was 'to preserve life – not existence'. Her added opinion that, at a practical level, prolonging life for extended periods was usually costly in terms of emotion and of money that could be better spent on community health and preventive medicine, raised the flammable potential of these assertions by several degrees and ignition was assured when the headline on the article read, 'Mercy Killing? I Say Yes'.[28] This was not what Alice had said at all, and a flurry of communications ensued to contain the damage to her personal and professional reputation.²⁹ The incident was typical of Alice: a commitment to speak out on what seemed to her the most important issues, no matter how controversial, dealing with the consequences as they came. In 1940 she had written, 'I just want to feel at the end that living had been worth while, that there have been no talents wasted, & no time misspent'.³⁰ Thirty-three years later, a sense of time running out did not signal a retreat for her; rather, it focused her attitudes and energies.

Members of her own profession were among those who would be publicly subjected to the sharp edge of Alice's tongue during 1973. General practitioners were now feeling disadvantaged by the NZFPA's Health Department connections and government grants, and its occasional provision of free contraceptives.³¹ The fact that the country again had a Labour government and that there was a shortage of doctors, which family planners could cite as grounds for extending their clinic services,³² did not help the doctors' case. In February 1973 the Minister of Health, R.J. Tizard, was quoted in *Choice* as having 'strong reservations' about objections from the New Zealand Council of General Practitioners regarding continued expansion of family planning clinics.³³ Alice put it more bluntly. In a lengthy article in the *Herald* the following month, she was quoted as saying, 'Believe me, no family planning clinic would survive if doctors gave the help they ought to give. A lot of doctors have failed to realise that women get fed up waiting two and a half hours in a doctor's rooms only to have a prescription thrust at them.' She went on to argue that general practitioners' concerns were self-serving. 'In effect the doctors are saying: "What we can't give you, you can't have" ... and the patients are no longer prepared to go along with this and be anybody's property.' Women in particular, she said, had been educated to appreciate the value of preventive medicine, 'while doctors tended to have a "dog-in-the-manger attitude toward it"'. The article also included a discourse by Alice on the changing attitudes of women towards their own sexuality and the value of family planning clinics.³⁴

This outburst initiated a debate in the press between representatives of the medical profession and the NZFPA,³⁵ and an internal review of clinic doctors' procedures in their relations with patients' private practitioners and the right of self-referred patients to maintain their privacy.³⁶ The interesting feature of this debate is why, when some women went to family planning clinics, they should not want to tell their doctor. For Alice, it was clearly a reflection of poor doctor–patient relations. Speaking at a public meeting in South Auckland later in the year, she claimed that the attitude of many general practitioners remained off-putting, particularly when they were dealing with the 'less vocal parts of the community'. She explained that she had originally become involved with the NZFPA 'because she knew it was difficult for lay people to argue with doctors'.[37] But, the differences between the services offered by the medical profession and those Alice thought should be provided went deeper than this debate implies. For her, 'Family planning was a skilled, medical and psychological undertaking and counselling was an important part of the work'.[38] If doctors could not provide these services, they should refer patients to people who could. 'People get too much medicine and too little personal service,' she complained in late 1973, suggesting that many patients really needed a social worker rather than a doctor, and that, like physiotherapists, these should be subsidised by the government.[39]

Schools, too, in Alice's opinion, were still not meeting needs as they should. Over the early 1970s, the NZFPA had made particular efforts to reach young people with the organisation of an education subcommittee under the leadership of Bobbie Swinburn. Alice approved of this, but believed it was beyond any voluntary organisation to provide what was really needed. In April 1973, she wrote to Angela Jelicich-Ranford, the new editor of *Choice*, concerning 'kids who need counselling and guidance the most' and were not getting it.

> I think that teaching and counselling are both professional jobs and they should be done by people professionally trained and this type of problem will only be solved when there is a fully trained counsellor to every school and when all teachers in both primary and secondary schools are adequately trained in human biology and human relationships so that information about living and loving and having children is imparted gradually to children from the time they are admitted to primary schools . . . . In the schools there is a captive audience and the teachers are there.[40]

Later in the year, when an Education Department subcommittee released its report, *Human Development and Relationships in the School Curriculum*, containing a suggested programme for inclusion in the basic curriculum in primary and secondary schools, with teachers trained to accept this as part of their normal responsibilities, Alice was delighted. It was, she said, an 'appreciation that behaviour depends on freely made choices' and the provision of the knowledge on which to make them. This was 'more effective in encouraging responsible behaviour than any set of rules demanding blind obedience' and the most hopeful sign yet that 'educators truly appreciate the great privilege and responsibility of their profession'.[41]

Alice's commitment to the international population and ecological movements remained unshaken. In August 1973, she and Mavis Hurrey were elected to the IPPF council.[42] The same month, after taking part in a seminar, 'Population – is there a Problem?', organised by the Workers' Educational Association at Auckland University, Alice was reported to have 'reaffirmed her optimism that mankind could be saved by the curbing of population growth. She was so convinced . . . that she was prepared to devote all her leisure time towards helping to lower the birth rate.'[43] For her, optimism was never a substitute for activism, no matter how big the problem might seem. She could find no common ground with those who felt things would work out for themselves.[44] In this respect, Alice was in tune with a Labour government who pledged $200,000 to the United Nations Fund for Population Activities and to the IPPF, five times the previous contribution of $40,000. It was, said Prime Minister Norman Kirk, a 'fitting way to usher in World Population Year', as 1974 had been designated by the United Nations, and to make up for the 'quite inadequate assessment in the past of the development significance of population considerations'.[45] In September, Alice and Peggy Zeisler attended a meeting convened by Zero Population Growth Auckland and attended by representatives of Ecology Action (a university group), the Values Party, Abortion Law Reform and the United Nations. The meeting unanimously agreed 'to work together for an improved "quality of life" for all people' in World Population Year; the committee was to use the NZFPA's box number and meet at its dominion office.[46]

The international connections provided by the NZFPA's affiliation with the IPPF led to Alice spending several weeks out of New Zealand during 1973. In October she attended the 21st anniversary of the IPPF, marked by a world conference in Brighton to 'reassess the role of planned parenthood in this age of complicated socio-economic and environmental problems'.⁴⁷ A regional meeting in Kuala Lumpur followed in December. Earlier in the year she travelled to Europe to attend a conference organised by the International Project of the Association for Voluntary Sterilization, which was based in New York and described itself as a 'voluntary health agency' whose role was 'different but complementary' to that of the IPPF.⁴⁸ Alice was interested in surgical sterilisation as an alternative to long-term pill taking when parents had decided their family was complete,⁴⁹ and also supported its use by some sufferers of genetically determined disease.⁵⁰ By the early 1970s, vasectomy, surgical sterilisation for men, was gaining popularity. It was a much simpler procedure than tubal ligation of women, but for New Zealanders it was not available in a public hospital. This raised the issue of unequal access for those who could not afford private treatment, Alice's primary concern at the time.⁵¹ There were other reasons why the trip appealed to her. The conference was to be held in Geneva in March and her travel expenses would be paid. It was a heaven-sent opportunity to see Christine, who was still in London.

The conference itself took up very little of Alice's time. She arrived late because of flight delays and later discovered she had been invited merely 'on principle because they [the organisers] feel that NZers can get places where U.S. is not acceptable & [the] willingness to provide expertise is what they wanted from us'.⁵² Her only recorded activity was a suggestion at the final meeting on 1 March that 'several countries, including Australia, have training resources that they would be willing to share with other countries'.⁵³ The rest of her trip passed pleasantly. She and Christine, after living in style for a few days at a hotel, stayed with Les Clements and his family, now based in Geneva, before driving back to Boulogne by way of Lucerne, Basel, Strasburg, the Black Forest, Luxembourg, Rheims and Paris. 'I hope we'll be back one day to see things in greater detail,' she wrote to Faulkner, '. . . it has all been a wonderful experience & I'd love to share it with you.'⁵⁴

Unexpectedly, the Geneva conference led Alice back into the abortion debate. Les Clements was on the staff of the World Council of Churches' Office of Family Education, which had organised an 'Abortion Consultation' as a preparatory step in producing a report designed to help churches care for members who had to make such choices. Since Alice was in town and had some time on her hands, he invited her to attend.[55] Her contributions centred on her belief in the importance of the quality of life. She challenged the idea of biblical absolutism, argued that parents had 'a right to a healthy child' and could not agree that suffering brought people together. She spoke of the family as existing for the welfare of children, and of their need to be loved, but also suggested that one question to be considered should be, 'Does the church insist on the superiority of the male?'[56] It was the kind of lively, multi-faceted discussion that Alice enjoyed,[57] but back in New Zealand the topic was losing any pretence to be classed as considered debate. During Alice's absence, William Liley, now SPUC's first national president, had advanced his argument by telling the annual meeting in Auckland that a survey of 400 battered babies showed that nearly all of them were 'planned pregnancies'. 'Is family planning the answer,' he went on, 'or does it supply another and more lethal manifestation – a trend which no longer regards children as children but as possessions and chattels to be disposed of on a parent's whim?'[58] Division, emotion and activity were running wild, even within the reform lobby. Matters came to a head at a National Abortion Conference in Wellington during July 1973, when radical feminists formed the Women's National Abortion Action Campaign (WONAAC) to press for total repeal of the law, while ALRANZ continued with its more moderate campaign of reform.[59]

The NZFPA had its own particular problems. Techniques such as the 'morning after pill' and 'menstrual regulation' blurred the boundaries between contraception and abortion.[60] Accepting that the 'morning after pill' worked in the same way as an IUD, preventing implantation of an embryo, the NZFPA offered it as part of its service. In late 1973, Alice, speaking as president and mindful of the law forbidding the provision of contraception to minors, declared it to be available to any woman over 16 from NZFPA clinics, or 'if she is lucky' from the family doctor. She added that this was 'strictly an emergency method', not pleasant but 'better than an unwanted pregnancy'.[61] Alice's public involvement in the abortion law reform movement remained low-key, mainly because of her obligations to the NZFPA. Her subdued approach could nevertheless lend significant strength to the reform position. In August 1973, she spoke briefly at a meeting arranged by ALRANZ at Green Lane Hospital. Newspapers recorded her contribution as concerned with abortion for foetal abnormality, specifically in cases of women contracting German measles during pregnancy.⁶² 'It is fine that responsible doctors such as Professor Bonham and Dr Alice Bush are taking a lead in advocating change in the law on this question,' wrote a correspondent to the local paper. 'It seems that those opposing such a change fail to understand that the other side is not advocating wholesale abortions.'⁶³

Alice's public standing was similarly demonstrated in the same month when the Minister for Social Welfare, Norman King, invited comments on the problem of juvenile crime in New Zealand. She submitted a personal response containing an extensive list of shortcomings that she felt needed to be addressed before a solution might be found. King referred her letter to the Ministers of Education and Health, and each sent personal replies, including references to Alice's well-known concern for the welfare of children and families.⁶⁴ Her proposals not only illustrated Alice's continuing faith in family planning but also the breadth of related and equally important strategies that she believed should support its practice. They included research into the relationship between family size and delinquency, access to contraception for minors and free contraceptives on both economic and medical grounds in the interests of equality of opportunity and the promotion of family health. For the same reasons, the caseload of public health nurses in low socio-economic areas should be lightened, trained social workers should be placed in every health district and there should be professional counsellors and remedial reading teachers in all schools. For the minister's department to plead that extending services was impossible because of a lack of trained people in the foreseeable future seemed to her 'typical of the department which has defeated itself by its own attitudes'. People must be actively encouraged, even imported, to take on this important work, which could never be sustained by untrained volunteers. It remained, Alice argued, a matter of priorities. Delinquency was not being held 'in check because preventive medicine & mental health are rated as less important than curative medicine'.⁶⁵ Her health might be failing, but Alice's life was clearly not ending with a whimper.

She remained accessible to all the news media and appreciated the emerging power of the television screen, seeking publicity for her causes on the current affairs programme *Gallery*, supporting the idea of an educational series for parents on infant and child health, and appearing in interviews and discussions.⁶⁶ When British television personality David Frost made a whirlwind visit to Auckland in September 1973, Alice agreed to appear on a programme about marriage. We do not know what she envisaged, but it certainly was not being placed in a large audience that might feel free to participate – if anyone could get a word in. She sat silently through the hour of filming and, according to Faulkner, regarded the experience as a waste of time.[67] Her appearance was not without its moment of magic, however: she was seated beside country and western singer Rusty Greaves, the father of 14 children.[68] Had she been given the opportunity, the audience would no doubt have heard the argument she had put forward earlier that year, introducing a revised model of personal responsibility relative to the needs of the age. Marriage and family life was 'not the road to happiness for all people' but 'a true appreciation of the present population situation' could bring 'freedom from the social pressures that try to squeeze everyone into the same mould'. Now individuals 'need have no fear that the world will be poorer because they have chosen to opt out of the responsibilities of parenthood'; rather, their responsibility was to find a method of contraception that was 'possible and reliable for them'. By doing so, they could guard against the failures of parenting that occurred in all racial groups and classes. Such failures were 'not only against the interests of the community' but also involved 'heartbreaking [personal] frustration'. The new society's 'worst enemies' were careless creators of new life.[69]

The same month the NZFPA organised a Family Planning Week, the highlight of which was to be a 'happening' in Albert Park. This was to feature a rock band, loudspeakers, banners and 'soapbox oratory on the subject of responsible parenthood by popular speakers such as Dr Rex Hunton, Dr Alice Bush . . . young people from Youthline and students from the University School of Medicine'.[70] How would Alice, in her 60th year, cope with this? If earlier events were anything to go by, she was no fuddy-duddy. In 1970 she had managed to outlast her children at a showing of the film based on the rock festival Woodstock, though she found it 'more of an experience than an enjoyment'.[71] She had enjoyed the controversial stage show *Hair* in 1972,[72] but she was no child of the Age of Aquarius and was quietly experiencing recurring pains in her chest.[73] The same week was a full working one and she was scheduled to spend several hours on the Saturday and Sunday helping, as a Zontian, to make cut lunches for participants at the first United Women's Convention. On 6 October she was due to leave for the IPPF conference in London, taking extra time beforehand for a holiday with Christine in Mexico. Nevertheless, she was pleased to pull her weight. She was interviewed by a local journalist and addressed a meeting at the Arahanga Intermediate School in Mangere Central, as well as attending a Standing Committee meeting. Because of bad weather the happening was cancelled. The NZFPA consoled itself that the advertising, even the cancellation notices, had still publicised the cause,[74] but Alice, on her way home from preparing convention lunches, decided to drop in at the park. There she found two other NZFPA members who were handing out leaflets to a few stragglers and together they sat in the bandstand and held an informal discussion. It was typical of many small incidents throughout Alice's life which endeared her to individuals,[75] but it paled in comparison with the impact that the United Women's Convention, taking place just a few city blocks away, was making on a very much larger number of participants.

It is doubtful whether Alice actually saw or heard much of the convention since the Zontians who prepared lunches missed most of the proceedings,[76] but several organisations with which she was connected were represented, including the NZFPA, Parents' Centres, the NCW, ALRANZ and NOW.[77] One NZFPA supporter, probably Colleen King, put together a euphoric account of the experience.

> An intangible something happened at the Convention; it was as if the sisterhood of 80 years ago had been asleep – but suddenly stirred. . . . Such "togetherness" was all the more astonishing, when one takes account of the varied representation. . . . Yet sweeping through the crowd were feelings of pride, fellow feeling, sometimes indignation, and finally elation which revealed itself in the spontaneous arm-in-arm singing as the programme closed.[78]

The recommendations of the convention included the provision of 'free and freely available' contraceptives and advice to any age group by 'trained and sympathetic people'; education in schools on individual responsibility in social, personal and sexual relationships; support for abortion law reform so that termination of pregnancy should be the choice of the woman involved; legal sterilisation available to men and women who wanted it; and the mobilisation of media to encourage awareness of population problems.[79] This confirmed for family planners the crucial role that they had played in the pursuit of women's independence and fulfilment, and, for many, that involvement was inextricably linked with Alice. They felt the time had come when she should receive her due.

Rising feminist consciousness had highlighted the low level of official recognition of women's contribution to New Zealand society. Although seven medical women had appeared in the biennial honours lists, none had been given the equivalent of a knighthood.[80] Among NZFPA stalwarts, only Marie Griffin and Doris Nicholson had received any recognition, in both cases for their general services to the community. When, early in November, the *Herald* conducted a 'Name a Dame' poll, Alice attracted by far the largest number of nominations. She was praised for her 'outstanding qualities as both physician and humanitarian', her activities on behalf of mothers and children, her fearless outspokenness, her altruism, her role in the NZFPA and her outstanding medical career.[81] Towards the end of 1973, her name was submitted to the government for the real thing. There can be little doubt that Alice approved of such a move. She had retained many of her conservative social values, had accepted invitations to Government House over the course of her career and would not have allowed her name to proceed if she had not respected the system. Faulkner's recollections confirm that this was so.[82] Moreover, all those concerned would have seen the areas in which she had worked as deserving of this kind of recognition, but by the time her name was put forward it was too late for inclusion in the New Year's honours.[63]

Alice celebrated Christmas Day quietly at home, with Faulkner and Peter; Christine phoned from London. Earlier in the month, she had attended what was to be her last NZMWA function, a luncheon for the first women graduates of the Auckland Medical School.[84] Her 1974 appointment diary was already written up with her regular commitments, and her 'spare' time was as crowded as usual. She was working on Zonta's submissions to the Children and Young Persons Act and had accepted an invitation to become a panel member advising on family planning and related matters in the *New Zealand Woman's Weekly* to mark World Population Year.[85] From 8 January she was doing a weekly NZFPA clinic and in early February hosted two sherry parties for overseas visitors at Denestone, one for the Hon. Leota Pita Alailima, a family planner from Samoa, and one for Zena Daysh of the Commonwealth Human Ecology Council. During her final months, Alice had remained, publicly and privately, actively involved in debate surrounding population and ecology issues.[86] At the beginning of February, when asked by her frequent disputant, Pat Dunn, for her comments on recently released statistics that demonstrated a drop of 3500 births over the preceding year, she expressed 'cautious optimism'. She believed there was some hope that 'the babies born will get a standard of health supervision adequate to ensure optimal nutrition and a fair start in life . . . . [and] better opportunities for education at all levels than those born during high birth rate years', but was well aware how variable the birth rate could be and did not think she could claim much credit for any reduction. Population control, Alice argued, was now more important in developed than developing countries. New Zealand must adjust to a stable rather than an expanding economy; she cared too much for children 'to stand by and see them produced just to increase the profit of some business venture'.

> The most optimistic of demographers agrees that this world's resources are finite and the population growth must stop some time. I believe that New Zealanders should take a world view and accept their role as a food producing nation. We are lucky to live in a country that is not already overpopulated. I think we should keep it that way for ever.[87]

Around the same time Alice put the final touches to an article for *Choice* defending NZFPA involvement in the IPPF and the world population programme. The argument was much the same. She saw one of the NZFPA's constitutional objectives, 'to cooperate with other organizations for social welfare at home and abroad', as authorisation for its relationship with the IPPF. She wrote of the interdependence of all people and all countries to sustain the world's resources, the gap between rich and poor nations and contraceptive knowledge as a basic human right. The association was indebted to the IPPF for help in the past; if the NZFPA were to opt out now, another organisation with 'sufficient vision to recognise that our world is getting smaller and its problems can be satisfactorily tackled only by international cooperation' would need to be encouraged.[88] She had probably already written her final President's Message for the magazine. Published posthumously, like the article, it expressed the philosophy that had saved her from the extremes of individualism and on which her mature life had centred: 'The Family Planning Association is concerned first and foremost with human rights but there can be no rights without a recognition of the responsibility to ensure that the exercise of rights for oneself does not limit the rights of others.'[89]

On Sunday 10 February, Alice and Faulkner spent a quiet day at home. The chest pains were coming more frequently but she mentioned this only in a letter to Christine. They went to bed early, though at some time during the night Alice was up, probably writing a book review for the Parents' Centre magazine. She saw patients at the rooms on Monday morning and in the afternoon went to her regular session at Karitane. Her condition deteriorated there but she insisted on driving home. She arrived back at Denestone after five. The house was empty. Patsy, the practice nurse, had left and Faulkner was at the Carlton Club Hotel. When he rang to see if she could pick him up, Alice had already been in touch with Dr Kevin O'Brien, cardiologist at Auckland Hospital, and was waiting for him to arrive to take her in. Faulkner went straight to the hospital, where he was told Alice's condition was stable. She was conscious but said nothing. He returned home, cabled Christine and left a message for Peter. The next morning, as was his habit, he rose early and walked up Mount Eden. When he arrived back at Denestone at 7.20 a.m. Kevin O'Brien was on the doorstep. Alice had suffered a massive coronary during the night. Patsy took Faulkner to see her. She was on oxygen and, speaking with difficulty, said, 'Fun and games here during the night'.[90] They were the last words she spoke to him. Faulkner sat, holding Alice's hand, talking to her, while she drifted into unconsciousness. Uncertain about what he should do, he decided to return home in case Christine was calling from London. When he arrived back at the hospital at 2.15 p.m. Alice was breathing her last. Peter, who had been hunting in the Ruahine Ranges, arrived home that night, and Faulkner went to bed in the early hours of the following morning, the end of 'a long, dreadful day' and the beginning of a lonely widowerhood until his death from cancer in September 1981.[91]

The funeral was delayed until the following Saturday, to give Christine time to fly home. A service at the Anglican Cathedral of the Holy Trinity in Parnell was arranged, to be followed by cremation at Purewa. As the news of Alice's death spread, first through family and hospital and then within the wider community, telegrams, flowers, fruit, letters and cards poured into Denestone. They represented the sympathies and sense of loss of the wide range of people whose lives Alice had touched over almost 60 years. Messages arrived from religious groups, the university, women's groups across the spectrum, a wide variety of health organisations, Hill Top and Diocesan schools, family welfare groups, professional societies, the Health Department, the hospital board, medical practitioners and present and past patients. Older colleagues, including Sammy Ludbrook, Ted Sayers, Eva Fischmann and Douglas Robb, wrote to Faulkner, as did younger professional, paramedical and lay people. NZFPA and IPPF members, family tradespeople and the Stantons' nursemaid from Alice's childhood found they had something in common. There was personal mail for Faulkner, and for Christine and Peter, from schools, ex-pupils, sporting links, relations and friends. Obituaries and less formal tributes appeared in the *Auckland Star*, the *Herald*, Wellington and Christchurch papers, the *NZMJ*, the *Woman's Weekly*, *Thursday*, the *Courier*, the *Parents' Centres Bulletin*, the *IPPF–SEAOR News*, *New Ethicals Patient Management*, the *Asian Population Programme News*, and the *Medical Association Newsletter*. Much of the March issue of *Choice* was devoted to Alice.

The tenor of these tributes was largely in tune with the eulogy delivered by John Rymer, Dean of Auckland, at Alice's packed funeral service. He took as his theme 'And the greatest of these is love', a translation of the final verse of I Corinthians 13: 'And now abideth faith, hope, charity, these three; but the greatest of these is charity'. His text centred on the love of mankind, and referred to Alice's sensitivity to people's needs as individuals, her belief that the family was the cradle of a happy society and her regard for mothers, fathers and children within each family. He touched on Alice's concern 'that women had not yet found their true place in society', and the need of some of them, married or single, for 'a career if they were to know inner happiness', and mentioned the importance of her own happy family life. There was a special tribute for Faulkner, whose role was compared to that of the 'great woman' who was often said to be found behind every 'great man'. The dean spoke of the honesty, courage and tenacity of purpose that surrounded Alice's actions, the need to find 'some tangible expression of our thankfulness . . . not by words but in deeds', even her religious doubts, and ended the eulogy by exhorting everyone in the days ahead, to show 'the love for individual persons which was her consuming passion'.[92] Then, during the final stages of the service, the cathedral organ succumbed to dust and humidity and, to the great discomfort of the organist Peter Godfrey, failed discordantly. Alice's sense of humour had tended to the subtle, the low-key, the quietly subversive. Even John Rymer had to confess, she would have loved it.[93]

Several attempts were made to find 'the tangible expression of our thankfulness' with which to mark Alice's life. In 1975 the NZFPA's Auckland clinic moved to new, larger rooms and was renamed the Alice Bush Centre,[94] and later an Alice Bush Health Education Trust was established to finance New Zealand research and projects in reproductive health and human relationships.[95] Zonta also set up a trust fund to foster postgraduate medical research,[96] and the NZMWA sponsored a paediatric prize at the Auckland Medical School.[97] Other efforts were less successful. Alice's death had coincided with yet another outburst of publicity concerning the need for a new children's hospital in Auckland, stimulating her supporters to suggest that such a hospital should bear her name, a campaign that subsided only when the hospital board formally rejected the idea.[98] A planned memorial wing at the Karitane Hospital fell victim to the institution's closure in the late 1970s.[99] Although her memory remained potent among those who had known her, and her name continued to surface occasionally in the media, the failure of these enterprises and the fact that Alice had not received a formal honour left Faulkner and many of her peers with the abiding sense that she had never received her full due.

For those who knew her best, Alice's name on a clinic sign, or a prize or grant, could not convey either the complexity or the range of her experience. Moulded in her youth to conform, she began from early adulthood to push the boundaries of education, professional achievement, personal satisfaction and public involvement that women had grown to accept, and to open her mind to new ways of achieving these goals. This made her both ordinary and extraordinary in her time, a progressive idealist whose feet remained firmly planted on the ground of practical reality. The resolution of domestic differences with her husband was no less important to her eventual development than any barriers she may have encountered within her profession. After discussing the unusual at specialist conferences, she came home to the everyday illnesses, accidents and unhappinesses of her own household and so understood that, for most people, most of the time, these constituted the major health problems of life. Her public profile may have highlighted her national and international concerns, but local and overseas trips were far less common for her than squeezing the household shopping between working commitments. As Alice ascended the professional ladder, she gained increasing satisfaction from her medical practice but this was no more precious to her than what she found in her personal life. To her, it was a choice of lifestyle which, with personal modifications, all women should be free to make. But her own experience had shown that, in addition to changes in the workplace, it would also mean establishing new priorities on the domestic scene and new kinds of relationships between husband and wife, parents and children. In this she drew on ideas introduced by organisations now so socially acceptable that the extent of their original unpopularity has largely been forgotten. By openly supporting them, she often placed herself outside the mainstream of her society and her profession. This decision called for an unusual strength of character and an unremitting drive which, at various times, drew criticism from both conservative and radical sources. On the other hand, it was the source of her appeal to those who shared her goal of improving the quality of life, not through imposing authoritarian strictures or libertarian ideas of supreme individual rights, but by informed choice backed with supportive programmes and broad educational opportunities. The magnitude of the barriers they faced is apparent in the continuing debate that still surrounds the provision of medical and social services, particularly those concerned with parenting and mental health.

NOTES

Abbreviations

AFB	Alice and Faulkner Bush Papers
AHB	Auckland Hospital Board Archives
AIM	Auckland Institute and Museum
AJHR	*Appendices to the Journals of the House of Representatives*
AKMA	NZMA Auckland Branch Archives
APL	Auckland Public Library
ATL	Alexander Turnbull Library
AUL	Auckland University Library
AUSA	Auckland University Students' Association Archives
AWN	*Auckland Weekly News*
DHS	Diocesan High School Archives
DHSC	*Diocesan High School Chronicle*
HTS	Hill Top School Archives
MC	Meikle Collection
MW	Mary Wood
NA	National Archives, Wellington
NA Auckland	National Archives, Auckland
NCW	National Council of Women Archives
NZFD	*New Zealand Family Doctor*
NZFPA	New Zealand Family Planning Association Archives
NZJH	*New Zealand Journal of History*
NZH	*New Zealand Herald*
NZMJ	*New Zealand Medical Journal*
NZMWA	New Zealand Medical Women's Association Archives
ODT	*Otago Daily Times*
PSNZ	Paediatric Society of New Zealand Papers
Q/S	Question Slips in Meikle Collection

Introduction

1. Alice to Peter, 3 October 1968, from copy made by Faulkner Bush, AFB. Unless otherwise specified, all correspondence is from this source.

1 Becoming a Doctor

1. Alice Bush, quoted in *Auckland Star*, 24 May 1971.
2. Register of Births, Auckland 1914, entry 2027.
3. Deeds Index 5A, Vol. 1, p.602, entry 174 394, Lands Transfer Office. The property at 13 Marine Parade, according to these records, belonged to Francis Leonard Connelly. The Stantons, apparently having never owned it, presumably rented it.
4. Violet Easton, *née* Patterson, (the Stanton's nursery-housemaid) to Phoebe Meikle, 29 July 1977; Q/S

NOTES TO PAGES 6–15

1. Mrs Patricia Rogers, 3 March 1980, Mr Allenby Stanton, 24 December 1981; MC; Taped interview, writer, with Mrs Patricia Rogers and Mrs Aileen Odell, 23 May 1989.
5. Correspondence, Alice to Faulkner, 28 November 1939. The emphasis is Alice's.
6. Typescript, 'The Family – Alice M. Bush', City of Auckland Centenary Lecture Series, delivered AIM, 18 July 1971, NZFPA.
7. Auckland Register of Births, 1884, entry 938.
8. Auckland Register of Deaths 1891, entry 232.
9. Auckland Register of Marriages, 1896, entry 93.
10. Recollections of Stanton family members.
11. Pitt Street Methodist Church Members' Roll, 1906, Methodist Archives, Auckland; for the importance of the class meeting in measuring commitment to the Methodist Church see H.R. Jackson, *Churches and People in Australia and New Zealand 1860–1930*, Wellington, 1987, pp.78–81.
12. E.A. Hames, *100 Years at Pitt Street*, Auckland, 1966, pp.38, 39; Auckland Register of Births, 1884, entry 1289.
13. Marriage Register, Pitt Street Methodist Church, Methodist Archives, Auckland.
14. Memorandum of Transfer, 21 April 1921, No.144853, Land Transfer Office, Auckland.
15. Certificate of Title under the Land Transfer Act, No.155592, Vol.424, Folio 84, 6 November 1925.
16. Alice to Faulkner, 26 May 1940.
17. *The Auckland Provincial Directory, 1932–33*, Pt I, p.185, Pt II, p.2106; Annual Report to Education Department, 1927, HTS.
18. P.V. Boult and Joan Edwards (eds), 'Hill Top School; The First Fifty Years', Auckland, 1965, p.8.
19. 'Headmistress Report, 1927', manuscript, P.V. Boult, HTS; interview notes, Mrs Elizabeth Sullivan and Miss N. Bamford, 15 June 1987. Mrs Sullivan and Miss Bamford were contemporaries of Alice at Diocesan Girls' High School, Auckland.
20. *DHSC*, 1930, pp.8, 21, 32, 34; 1931, pp.2, 3, 16; 1928, pp.4–9.
21. Clippings, Auckland Scrapbook April 1974, pp.202, 288, APL.
22. Alice to Faulkner, 17 May 1944.
23. P.V. Boult, 'Headmistress Report, 1951', HTS.
24. This information is taken mainly from interviews conducted by Phoebe Meikle during the years immediately after Alice's death.
25. Alice to Faulkner, 11 August 1945.
26. Alice to Faulkner, 22 May 1940.
27. *DHSC*, 1930, p.9; both girls had been enrolled as Methodists, see Diocesan School Register, 1904–68, entries 1487, 1557. Aileen's entry (No.2025) in 1937 nominated her religion as Anglican.
28. *AWN*, 29 June 1932, p.71.
29. M. Bassett, 'The 1935 Election and the Kelly Gang', *NZJH*, 28:1, April 1994, p.82.
30. David Smith, 'Bench and Bar: 1928–1950', in R. Cooke (ed.), *Portrait of a Profession*, Wellington, 1969, p.105.
31. *NZH*, 1931. Issues from 31 August to 7 September covered this incident extensively. For a reflective account see J.C. Graham, 'Renewal Found on Mt. Ruapehu', *NZH*, 14 October 1981, clipping, MC; General Register of Deaths 1931, entry 2325.
32. *Craccum* v:10, 17 September 1931, p.3.
33. *AWN*, 6 September 1933, p.27.
34. Alice to 'Meg', 6 August 1933.
35. *Auckland Star*, 24 May 1971.
36. P. Meikle, *Accidental Life*, Auckland, 1994, pp.42–3, 79.
37. Minutes, AKMWA general meeting, 16 April 1970, NZMWA.
38. C. Hercus and G. Bell, *The Otago Medical School Under the First Three Deans*, Edinburgh/London, 1964, p.159.
39. A. Bush, 'Women, Medicine and the Royal College', typescript, nd but probably late 1960s, AFB.
40. Ibid.
41. Alice to Peter, 3 October 1968.
42. D. Montgomerie, '"A Personal Affair between me and Hitler?"', MA thesis, University of Auckland, 1984,

Table 2, p.91. Percentages of married women of all ages in the paid labour force; 1926, 3.5%; 1936, 3.7%; E. Olssen, 'Women, Work and Family; 1880–1926', p.173, in P. Bunkle and B. Hughes (eds), *Women in New Zealand Society*, Auckland, 1980.
43 Q/S A. McM. Stanton, 23 February 1981 to 24 December 1981; MC.
44 Alice to Faulkner, 4 April 1940.
45 Interview notes, Dr R.F. Moody, 9 June 1987.
46 M. Belgrave, 'Medical Men and Lady Doctors', PhD thesis, Victoria University, 1985, pp.i, 62, 69, etc.
47 M. Tennant, 'Natural Directions', in B. Brookes, C. Macdonald, M. Tennant (eds), *Women in History*, Wellington, 1986, pp.90–2; E. Olssen, pp.175–9; R. Fry, *'It's different for daughters'*, Wellington, 1985, pp.79–80, 82–9.
48 D.W. Carmalt Jones, *Annals of the Otago Medical School, 1875–1939*, Wellington, 1945, p.193.
49 Photocopy of Alice's academic record at Otago University, MC.
50 Alice to 'Meg', 6 August 1933.
51 Belgrave, 'Medical Men and Lady Doctors', Table 9.4, p.414.
52 Hercus and Bell, p.53; W.P. Morrell, *The University of Otago: A Centennial History*, Dunedin, 1969, p.244. The one exception was 1936, when the arts faculty, always its nearest rival, briefly established an ascendancy.
53 Hercus and Bell, p.53.
54 Sir William Manchester, interview, 14 May 1987.
55 Dr A.H. Berry, interview, 6 July 1987; Manchester interview; Obituary, D.P. Kennedy, *NZMJ*, February 1973, p.118.
56 Manchester interview.
57 Ida Logan to P. Meikle, May 1982, MC.
58 Recollections of Alice at medical school have been contributed by the following: Dr E.M. Elder, Dr Neil Begg, Dr A.H. Berry, Dr M.L. Talbot, Dr Margaret Gatman, Hon. Mr. Justice Moller, MC. Interviews; Mrs Peggy Gaudin, 28 February 1986, Dr M. Chieffi, 7 July 1987, and Manchester and Berry interviews. Where individual comments are specifically quoted they are footnoted individually.
59 Dr E.M. Elder, Q/S 28 July 1982, MC.
60 Alice to 'Meg', 6 August 1933.
61 *Otago University Review*, 1935, p.66; 1936, photograph opp. p.48, and pp.76, 78.
62 Carmalt Jones, pp.218, 269.
63 *The Digest*, 1934, p.11; 1935, p.7; advertisement, 1935, opp. p.42.
64 *The Digest*, 1934, pp.37–8; 1938, pp.45–6.
65 Correspondence, Dr E.M. Elder, 24 October 1982, MC.
66 E. Baker McLaglan, *Stethoscope and Saddlebags*, Auckland, 1965, p.41.
67 Berry interview.
68 Correspondence, Dr M. Chieffi, 26 July 1987.
69 Q/S Dr Margaret Gatman, 21 January 1983, MC.
70 Alice to Faulkner, 28 May 1940.
71 Correspondence, Dr A.H. Berry, 15 January 1983, MC. Dr Margaret Chieffi could not clearly recall this incident, but she did not think the women would have complained about it because 'we kept a very low profile in those days'. Correspondence, 26 July 1987.
72 *University of Otago Calendar*, 1935, page number not noted, MC; Carmalt Jones, Appendix III, p.271.
73 Correspondence Dr A.H. Berry, 15 January 1983, MC, and interview with Dr Berry, 6 July 1987. Neither Sir William Manchester nor Dr Margaret Chieffi could recall this incident although both thought it possible; existing records begin at the late 1940s. By 1955 students could apply for the position. That year Dr Margaret Cook, the first woman to do so, was appointed. The next woman appointee was Dr Joceylin Williams in 1972. Correspondence, Associate Professor L.R. Robinson, Department of Anatomy, Otago Medical School, 15 July 1987 and 16 November 1987.
74 Berry interview; Morrell, p.139; Belgrave, p.117; Professor J.M. Watt, Q/S 9 April 1978, MC.
75. Correspondence, Nan Berry, May 1984, MC.

76 M. Belgrave, 'A Subtle Containment', *NZJH*, 22:1, April 1988, p.45.

2 Work and War

1 Alice to Faulkner, 15 February 1940.
2 *NZH*, 17 November 1937, p.18.
3 AHB Minute Book, January–December 1937, p.876. All AHB Minute Books covering Alice's lifetime are held at NA Auckland.
4 Class records, Otago Medical School, MC.
5 Q/S Professor J.M. Watt, MC; Manchester interview.
6 Berry interview.
7 *NZH*, 17 November 1937, p.18.
8 Manchester and Chieffi interviews.
9 Interview notes, Dr F. Moody, 9 June 1987; correspondence writer with Dr Calvin Ring, 20 May 1987, and conversation 3 September 1987.
10 AKMWA Minute Book, 1935–46, 22 November 1937, NZMWA.
11 *NZH*, 17 November 1937, p.18.
12 AHB Minute Book, January–December 1937, p.872.
13 AHB Minute Book, July–December 1947, p.571.
14 K. Anderson, 'Beyond the Pioneer Women Doctor', MA thesis, The University of Auckland, 1992, pp.84, 104–7.
15 Hercus and Bell, p.99.
16 AHB Minute Book, January–December 1937, p.882.
17 Manchester interview.
18 Alice to Faulkner, 5 November 1939.
19 Manchester interview.
20 *The Digest*, 1945, pp.81–4. Two women were included on this list: Florence Craig killed at Singapore, and Tessa Craig, a prisoner. These lists apparently contain discrepancies as Hercus and Bell, p.206, put the total number of Otago University Medical Corps members on the 'Roll of Honour' at 682, with 20 killed.
21 Alice to Faulkner, 25 November 1939.
22 N.M. Taylor, *The Home Front*, Wellington, 1986, pp.95, 96, 98.
23 J.B. Lovell-Smith, *The New Zealand Doctor and the Welfare State*, Auckland, 1966, p.101; Taylor, pp.854–5; *NZH*, 16 May 1940, p.8.
24 Correspondence, Sir Edward Sayers, 20 July 1981, MC. Lady Sayers, was interviewed on 13 March 1987, shortly before her death, and confirmed this account.
25 Faulkner to Alice, 6 February 1940.
26 Alice to Faulkner, 29 February 1940.
27 Alice to Faulkner, 15 February 1940.
28 Alice to Faulkner, 14 February 1940.
29 Alice to Faulkner, 23 February 1940.
30 'Financial Aspects of City General Practice Today', 'An Auckland Medical Practitioner Group', *NZMJ*, Vol.52, 1953, pp.201–2, 205, 206.
31 Alice to Faulkner, 27 September 1944.
32 Alice to Faulkner, 7 March 1940, 16 April 1940.
33 Alice to Faulkner, 7–9 March 1940.
34 A. Bush, 'Allergy Over a Quarter Century', *NZMJ*, August 1968, p.101.
35 Douglas Whillans, 'Dr Alice Bush', typescript, 18 October 1981, and Q/S Dr Margaret Gatman, 21 January 1983, MC; interviews, Douglas and Winsome Whillans, 5 February 1986 and Lady Sayers.
36 Alice to Faulkner, 29 February and 25 April 1940.
37 A. Bush, 'Allergy Over a Quarter Century', pp.101–2.
38 *NZMJ*, 1943, Vol.42, p.262; Alice to Faulkner, 28 May in 21–31 May 1944.
39 Alice to Faulkner, 16 September 1944.
40 Alice to Faulkner, 1 December 1944. Part of this extra fee may have been made up of the practical costs of treatment, e.g. laboratory expenses, nevertheless both doctors charged the same amount, which indicates that the proportion of the fee accounting for expertise was judged to be similar.
41 Correspondence, Clair McCurdy, Royal New Zealand Plunket Society, Dunedin, to Peter Miller, Hocken Library, Dunedin, 6 July 1989 and forwarded to writer.
42 Clipping, 'Babies Care Recalled', *NZH*, 12 October 1982, MC.
43 Q/S May 1981, Miss Sydney Lusk, Matron of Karitane Hospital

1939–45, MC; Alice to Faulkner, 7 February 1945.
44 G. Parry, *A Fence at the Top: The First 75 Years of the Plunket Society*, Dunedin, 1982, pp.109, 105–6; Carmalt Jones, p.269; *NZMJ*, 1935, Vol.34, pp.365–6; 1936, Vol 35, pp.64–9; 1938, Vol.37, pp.185–7.
45 Alice to Faulkner, 16 June and 22 July 1940.
46 Alice to Faulkner, 15 February 1940.
47 *NZMJ*, November 1983, pp.944–5.
48 AKMWA Minute Book, 18 September 1945.
49 M. Maxwell, *Women Doctors in New Zealand*, Auckland, 1990, p.17.
50 Alice to Faulkner, 9 August 1940.
51 Alice to Faulkner, 13 June 1940; S. Coney, *Every Girl*, Auckland 1986, p.215; WNSC Annual Reports, 1940, 1941, 1946, and correspondence, Mrs Joyce Jackways, 26 May 1987; interview notes, Mrs June Duffus, 2 June 1987.
52 Taylor, pp.1032–7.
53 Correspondence, Mrs Vera Webster, 19 July 1987; S. Coney, *Every Girl*, p.234 mentions lectures by Alice on venereal disease at Papakura Camp. Faulkner Bush also mentions these (Faulkner's Story, typescript, MC, p.23). National Archives have no record of any official involvement by Alice in such a capacity (correspondence, Sherrah Francis, Reference Archivist, 25 August 1987).
54 A. Bush, Foreword, *Personal Relationships*.
55 Alice to Faulkner, 26 October 1943.
56 J. Tolerton, *Ettie*, Auckland/Harmondsworth, Middlesex, 1992, pp.95, 196.
57 Correspondence, Ethel Law, National General Secretary, YWCA, Wellington, to Librarian, Health Department, 10 May 1944, H1 35/14 25845, NA.
58 'As from One Girl to Another: Youth looks at Promiscuity', (anonymous), *Mirror*, March 1944, pp.15, 47.
59 *Craccum*, 11 April 1945, p.2.
60 Alice to Faulkner, 1 December 1944.
61 D. Robb, *Medical Odyssey*, Auckland, 1968, pp.1–32, 51–5; *Medicine and Health in New Zealand*, Auckland, 1940, pp.17, 120, 81–2.
62 D. Robb, *Medicine and Health in New Zealand*, p.7.
63 A. Bush, et al., *A National Health Service*, Wellington, 1943, pp.54–8.
64 *Ibid.*, pp.27, 13, 24, 39.
65 Alice to Faulkner, 17 September 1943.
66 Alice to Faulkner, 25 September 1944.
67 Alice to Faulkner, 20 April, 15 June, 21 August 1944.
68 Unsigned correspondence (probably Marie Griffin) to Secretary, Wellington Branch Committee, 6 September 1943, NZFPA.
69 Correspondence, Eileen Coyne, Secretary, Auckland Branch, to Mrs Freda Forde, Secretary, NZFPA National Executive, 2 August 1942, NZFPA.
70 Ms, 'List of Doctors', nd but c. 1942–3, NZFPA. Seven of the 21 doctors were located in Auckland.
71 *NZMJ*, Vol.43, 1944, p.102; E.K. Hughes' evidence to Mazengarb Committee, Ms Papers 2384:4, p.851, ATL; Alice to Faulkner, 14 May in 6–17 May 1944.
72 Memo, A.W.S. Thompson to DGH, 12 December 1951, H1 35/12/4 33787 NA.
73 Fischman to Alice, 26 September 1944, AFB.
74 Alice to Faulkner, 11 September in 8–11 September 1944.
75 P. Cody, 'Women Psychiatrists in New Zealand 1900–1990', MA thesis, University of Otago, 1996, pp.38–9, 79–80.
76 Newsletter, March 1945, NZFPA.
77 Alice to Faulkner, 13 December 1944.
78 *NZMJ*, 1943, Vol.42, p.262.
79 *NZMJ*, 1946, Vol.45, pp.57, 59–60.
80 Alice to Faulkner, 30 May in 21–31 May 1944.
81 Alice to Faulkner, 7 June in 7–11 June 1944; for more detail on the background of this debate see D.G. Bolitho, 'The Response of the New Zealand Medical Profession ....', MA thesis, Victoria University, 1979.
82 Alice to Faulkner, 7 and 9 June in 7–11 June 1944.
83 Alice to Faulkner, 22 November 1944.
84 Alice to Faulkner, 1 December 1944.
85 Alice to Faulkner, 27 May 1940.
86 Alice to Faulkner, 3 March 1945.

3 Marriage

1. Alice to Faulkner, 6 March 1940.
2. J.E. Denford, 'Emotional Problems of Doctors Starting General Practice', *NZMJ*, March 1969, p.139.
3. Alice to Faulkner, 11 August 1945. To grasp the full significance of this comment it is helpful to refer to Alice's writings: 'kisses belong properly to that period of courtship the logical termination of which is marriage with all that it implies in privileges and responsibility and they should not be indulged in lightly'. *Personal Relationships*, 1943, p.15.
4. Alice to Faulkner, 11 August 1945.
5. Register General Births 27, No.171, Raglan; *Tauranga Historical Society Journal*, No.36, nd, pp.7–10, *Who's Who in New Zealand*, 1908, p.26 and further information kindly supplied by Jinty Rorke, Special Services Librarian, Tauranga Library, 8 April 1994; Register General of Marriages, 185, No.9.
6. Correspondence, John Crawford, Research Officer History, Ministry of Defence, Wellington, 25 May 1987; J. Cowan, *The Maoris in the Great War*, Auckland, 1926, pp.106–7.
7. Divorce files 1869–1927, No.459, A48/13, NA Auckland; Register General Marriage, 68, Auckland No.291; Register General Births, 95, Ohinemuri No.22749, 21 September 1910.
8. *New Zealand Truth*, 9 October 1930, p.5; Register General of Deaths, entry 3413, 14 September 1930; 'Faulkner's Story', pp.1, 17, and additional material 17 March 1977. These and following contributions attributed to Faulkner as either his story, additional material, or narratives, were written by him following Alice's death specifically for use in a biography and entrusted to Phoebe Meikle.
9. Additional material supplied by Faulkner, 17 March 1977.
10. Faulkner's Story, p.1; interview, Reverend L. Clements, 8 May 1987.
11. Faulkner to Alice, 5–8 September 1939.
12. Faulkner to Alice, 31 October 1939.
13. Alice to Faulkner, 11 September 1943.
14. Alice to Faulkner, 18 December 1939.
15. Alice to Faulkner, 20 November 1939.
16. P. Meikle, *Accidental Life*, pp.258, 264–5.
17. Faulkner to Alice, 13 December 1939.
18. Faulkner to Alice, 10 October 1939.
19. Alice to Faulkner, 11 October 1939.
20. Alice to Faulkner, 21 December 1939.
21. Alice to Faulkner, 9 March 1945. Alice's assessment of the intellectual limitations of Parry is similar to that of Keith Sinclair, who, in *Walter Nash*, p.165, described him as 'a simple soul who would have found mastering so large and complicated a brief [as the Social Security portfolio] rather difficult'.
22. Alice to Faulkner, 15 October 1939.
23. Alice to Faulkner, 15 July 1940.
24. Alice to Faulkner, 12 November 1939.
25. Alice to Faulkner, 21 June 1940.
26. Alice to Faulkner, 24 July 1940.
27. Alice to Faulkner, 20 April 1940.
28. Alice to Faulkner, 1 December, 12 November 1939, 9 June 1940.
29. Alice to Faulkner, 28 November 1939. Also to Faulkner, 9 June 1940, 'I always hope that some day there may come a realisation of the significance and reality of Christ, but perhaps I'm not a receptive person.'
30. Faulkner to Alice, 22 December in 21–22 December 1939.
31. Alice to Faulkner, 23 December 1939.
32. Peggy Gaudin interview, 28 February 1986.
33. Correspondence, Dr Pat Dunn, 17 December 1982, Meikle Collection.
34. *Better Business*, June 1943, pp.39–40, quoted in Montgomerie, p.86. The author of this entertaining piece was a woman, Marie J. Fanning.
35. Faulkner to Alice, 2 March 1940.
36. Faulkner to Alice, 4 March 1940.
37. Alice to Faulkner, 7 March 1940.
38. Alice to Faulkner, 15 March 1940.
39. Alice to Faulkner, 12 February 1940.
40. Alice to Faulkner, 24 July 1941.
41. Alice to Faulkner, 21 June 1940.
42. Faulkner's Story, pp.5–6.
43. Faulkner's Story, p.7; Clements interview, 8 May 1987; Faulkner to Alice, 18 February 1940, refers to a

couple who 'eloped under similar conditions to the ones we proposed'.
44. Alice to Faulkner, 30 May 1940. Alice to Faulkner, 14 July 1944, supports this interpretation, 'There was just this little sneaking feeling that I'd been hurried into it [marriage] prematurely by false pretences.'
45. Faulkner to Alice, 10 November 1939.
46. Faulkner to Alice, 19 June 1940.
47. Alice to Faulkner, 25 April 1940.
48. Alice to Faulkner, 27 May 1940.
49. Alice to Faulkner, 10 June 1940.
50. Alice to Faulkner, 31 May 1940.
51. Faulkner to Alice, 8 June 1940.
52. Faulkner to Alice, 13 June 1940.
53. Faulkner to Alice, 18 June 1940.
54. Faulkner to Alice, 9 April 1944.
55. Faulkner to Alice, 19 September 1943.
56. Alice to Faulkner, 21 April 1944.
57. Alice to Faulkner, 9 February in 8–17 February 1944.
58. Faulkner to Alice, 9 April 1940.
59. K. Sinclair, 'The Lee Sutch Syndrome', *NZHJ*, October 1974, pp.112–3.
60. Alice to Faulkner, 27 March 1940.
61. Faulkner's Story, pp.9–10; *NZH*, 21 August 1940, *AWN*, 21 August 1940, p.18.
62. Alice to Faulkner, 12 July 1940; annotated by Faulkner post 1974.
63. Alice to Faulkner, 17 July 1940.
64. Register of Deaths, Auckland, 1942, entry 2801.
65. Montgomery, pp.89, 143; Taylor, pp.1092–3.
66. Alice to Faulkner, 23 February 1945.
67. Alice to Faulkner, 4 February 1945 and 10 March 1945.
68. Alice to Faulkner, 26 June 1945.
69. Faulkner's Story, p.19.
70. Alice to Faulkner, 14 July 1940.
71. Alice to Faulkner, 7 July 1940.
72. *Telephone Directory, Auckland and District*, 1941, p.7; 1943, p.2.
73. Faulkner to Alice, 25 July 1940.
74. Alice to Faulkner, 11 November 1939.
75. Alice to Faulkner, 23 February 1940.
76. Faulkner to Alice, 21 November 1939.
77. Correspondence, John Crawford, Ministry of Defence, 25 May 1987; personal chronology supplied by F. Bush, 17 March 1977, Faulkner's Story, pp.8–13, 17, 23.
78. Register of Births, Auckland, 1943, entry 3434.

4 Circles are Broken

1. Alice to Faulkner, 12 May in 6–17 May 1944.
2. Alice to Faulkner, 17 September 1943.
3. Alice to Faulkner, 30 November 1943.
4. Alice to Faulkner, 9 December 1943.
5. Faulkner to Alice, 8 September 1943.
6. Alice to Faulkner, 30 November 1943.
7. Alice to Faulkner, 6 October 1944. This was a base salary. Alice also received a share of the profits. At this stage she was obviously paying the nurses out of her own income but early in 1945 Faulkner asked how much she was paying the current children's nurse (not a Karitane) because, 'I count that fee part of my costs out of war emoluments'. Faulkner to Alice, 21 February 1945.
8. Alice to Faulkner, 26 March 1944.
9. Alice to Faulkner, 7 August 1945.
10. Alice to Faulkner, 23 September 1945.
11. Alice to Faulkner, 7 October 1945.
12. Alice to Faulkner, 21 June 1944.
13. Alice to Faulkner, 8 October 1943.
14. Alice to Faulkner, 10 December 1944.
15. Alice to Faulkner, 21 July 1943.
16. Alice to Faulkner, 21 October 1944. Neither the hospital nor the psychiatrist is specified.
17. Alice to Faulkner, 10 July 1945.
18. Faulkner to Alice, 2 August 1945 (No.2).
19. Faulkner to Alice, 11 December 1939, Alice to Faulkner, 13 March 1944.
20. Alice to Faulkner, 20 June 1945.
21. Alice to Faulkner, 21 September 1944.
22. Faulkner to Alice, 18 September 1944.
23. Faulkner to Alice, 18 September 1944.

24 K. Anderson, 'Beyond the Pioneer Woman Doctor', pp.77–97.
25 AHB Minute Book, January–June 1944, pp.237, 250.
26 Alice to Faulkner, 12 May in 6–17 May 1944.
27 Alice to Faulkner, 31 July 1944.
28 AHB Minute Book, June–December 1944, p.955.
29 Alice to Faulkner, 29 September, and Faulkner to Alice, 7 October 1944.
30 Alice to Faulkner, 28 October 1944.
31 Obituary, *NZMJ*, 24 November 1976, pp.415–6.
32 Alice to Faulkner, 15 October 1944. After a month or so Alice and Ludbrook did the Sunday ward round alternately (Alice to Faulkner, 21 November 1944).
33 Alice to Faulkner, 1 December 1944.
34 Alice to Faulkner, 15 November 1944.
35 Hercus and Bell, pp.133–6.
36 Alice to Faulkner, 6 October and 15 November 1944.
37 Alice to Faulkner, 9 June and 6 October 1944.
38 Alice to Faulkner, 2 June, 12 May in 6–17 May, and 6 April 1945. Sammy Ludbrook also encouraged her participation in postgraduate conferences. They gave a paper together on 'Anaemias of Infancy and Childhood, Haemolytic Anaemias and Acholuric Jaundice' at a postgraduate course on blood diseases, 8–10 May 1946, at Green Lane Hospital. (*NZMJ*, 1946, Vol.45, p.137).
39 Alice to Faulkner, 7 June and 19–22 August 1945.
40 *NZMJ*, 1945, Vol.44, p.334.
41 Faulkner to Alice, nd but probably 9 January 1944.
42 Alice to Faulkner, 10 January 1944.
43 Faulkner to Alice, 4 August 1945.
44 Faulkner to Alice, 10 December 1944.
45 Faulkner to Alice, 12 August 1944.
46 Faulkner to Alice, 22 June 1944.
47 Faulkner to Alice, 10 December 1944, and annotation post-1974 on Alice to Faulkner, 20 January 1945.
48 Faulkner to Alice, 4 July 1940.
49 Faulkner to Alice, 1 and 6 August 1945.
50 Faulkner to Alice, 30 July and 1 August 1945.
51 Faulkner to Alice, 30 April, 10 December 1944, 11 February 1945.
52 Faulkner to Alice, 2 June 1945.
53 Faulkner to Alice, 20 and 23 May 1945. This unsettling confusion over troop movements continued until the end of the year.
54 Faulkner to Alice, 18 May 1945.
55 Faulkner to Alice, 9 July 1945.
56 Faulkner to Alice, 2 October 1944, contained a list of 62 issues that she could remove.
57 Alice to Faulkner, 21 May 1944.
58 Alice to Faulkner, 21–31 May 1944. See also 11 June 1944.
59 Alice to Faulkner, 23 June, 4 July, 21 July 1944.
60 Alice to Faulkner, 10 August, 1944, written from Ngawha Springs.
61 Alice to Faulkner, 26 June 1945.
62 Alice to Faulkner, 29 July 1945.
63 Alice to Faulkner, 28 May 1940.
64 Alice to Faulkner, 4 August 1945.
65 Alice to Faulkner, 7 May 1940.
66 Alice to Faulkner, 27 July 1944.
67 *NZWW*, 2 March 1944, p.21.
68 Unsigned correspondence, but probably from Marie Griffin, to the secretary of the Wellington branch committee, 6 September 1943, NZFPA.
69 Faulkner to Alice, 11 February, 1945.
70 Alice to Faulkner, 4 August 1945.
71 Faulkner to Alice, 27 July (No.2) 1945.
72 Faulkner to Alice, 27 July (No.1) 1945.
73 Alice to Faulkner, 3 November (No.1) 1945.
74 Alice to Faulkner, 3 November (No.2), and 4 and 7 November 1945; interview, Lady Sayers, 13 March 1987.
75 Alice to Faulkner, 7 November 1945.
76 Alice to Faulkner, 12 November 1945. Unfortunately, Faulkner's cablegram does not seem to have survived.
77 Alice to Faulkner, 3, 4, 7 November 1945.
78 Alice to Faulkner, 14–20 April 1944.
79 Alice to Faulkner, 12 April in 31 March–12 April 1944.
80 Alice to Faulkner, 12–14 and 24

November 1945.
81 Alice to Faulkner, 12 April in 31 March–12 April 1944.
82 Cody, pp.68, 75, 90, 127, 132.
83 Alice to Faulkner, 5 July 1945.
84 Alice to Faulkner, 7 November 1945.
85 Alice to Faulkner, 24 November 1945.
86 Alice to Faulkner, 12–14 November 1945.
87 Alice to Faulkner, 7, 28 December 1945.
88 Faulkner to Alice, 18 November 1945.
89 Faulkner to Alice, 31 December 1945–1 January 1946.

5 Full Use of Her Talents

1   A. Bush, 'Is Motherhood Enough?', *Men and Women*, National Council of Churches in New Zealand, 1953, p.34.
2   Alice to Faulkner, 13 September 1944.
3   Faulkner to Alice, 7 and 28 April 1945.
4   Alice to Faulkner, 12 May 1945.
5   Alice to Faulkner, 12 August 1945.
6   Faulkner's Story, p.11.
7   Alice to Faulkner, 28 August 1946.
8   Faulkner to Alice, 10 April 1940.
9   Faulkner's Story, pp.43–4, 54.
10 *NZMJ*, 1945, Vol.44, p.205; J.R.M. Thomson, 'The Rehabilitation of Servicemen of World War Two in New Zealand', PhD thesis, Victoria University, 1983, p.193, footnote 55.
11 Faulkner's Story, p.46.
12 Faulkner's Story, p.55.
13 Faulkner's Story, pp.55–6.
14 Faulkner's Story, p.41.
15 Auckland Register of Births, 1947, entry 3328.
16 AHB Minute Book, July–December 1947, pp.1162–3.
17 Alice to Faulkner, 22 November 1947.
18 Faulkner's Story, p.57.
19 Q/S Dr Margaret Gatman, 21 January 1983, MC.
20 Faulkner's Story, p.69.
21 Alice to Mrs F. Pilling, 1 January 1950.
22 H. May, *Minding Children, Managing Men*, Wellington, 1992, is the fullest discussion of this era.
23 May, *Minding Children*, p.11.
24 J. Bowlby, *Child Care and the Growth of Love*, London, 1953, back cover.
25 J. Bowlby, *Maternal Care and Mental Health*, Geneva, 1952, p.6.
26 Bowlby, *Maternal Care*, p.11.
27 Bowlby, *Maternal Care*, p.73.
28 G. Somerset, *I Play and I Grow* (1976 edition), p.60, quoted in A. Else, (ed.), *Women Together*, Wellington, 1993, p.333; see also W.B. Sutch, *The Quest for Security in New Zealand: 1840–1966*, Wellington, 1966, pp.260, 264; M. Dobbie, *The Trouble With Women*, Queen Charlotte Sound, 1990, pp.1–3.
29 Patience Gillies and Marie Griffin, 'Suggestions re Adult Education', NCW Auckland Branch subcommittee recommendations for Conference on Education to be held in Christchurch, August 1944, NZFPA.
30 Bowlby, *Maternal Care*, p.67.
31 A. Bush, typescript, 'Maternal Deprivation in Children', pp.1, 2, AFB.
32 Bush, 'Maternal Deprivation', p.1.
33 Bush, 'Maternal Deprivation', p.10.
34 Bowlby, *Maternal Care*, p.102; Bush, 'Maternal Deprivation', p.3.
35 Bowlby, *Maternal Care*, pp.85–6, 90–1.
36 A. Bush, 'Is Motherhood Enough?', in NCC Women's Committee, *Men and Women*, Christchurch/Dunedin, 1953, p.36.
37 Alice to Faulkner, 14–20 April 1944.
38 Meikle, *Accidental Life*, p.135.
39 Christine Bush to Hon. Martyn Finlay, Min. of Justice, 25 February 1974, AFB.
40 V. Davies, 'Looking for the best daycare centre', *NZWW*, 21 July 1980, p.53, MC.
41 A. Bush, typescript, 'Women, Medicine and the Royal College', AFB.
42 Alice to Peter, 3 October 1968.
43 Faulkner Bush, additional material, 17 March 1977.
44 Phoebe Meikle noticed his 'putting down' of Alice particularly, as did several people she interviewed.

44. Faulkner agreed it did happen and that although Alice did not retaliate or put him down in public she would speak to him later, privately. Information supplied by Faulkner, 9 February 1981.
45. Faulkner's Story, p.108.
46. Alice to Faulkner, posted 12 May 1955.
47. Alice to Faulkner, posted 12 May 1955.
48. Clipping, 'Former Judge Collapses in Street', ann. *NZH*, 10 October 1963, original courtesy Mrs Patricia Rogers, MC; Death Certificate No.94017.
49. Faulkner Bush, Narrative 6, p.14.
50. Faulkner Bush, additional material, 17 March 1977.
51. Faulkner Bush, 27 December 1974, MC.
52. Typescript, address to Medico-Legal Dinner, nd but probably delivered at Tutukaka, Northland, c. 1966, pp.1–2, AFB.
53. This brief impression is compiled from the recollections of visitors to the house and Faulkner's narratives. Most of this material was collected by Phoebe Meikle during the years immediately after Alice's death.
54. Faulkner Bush, Narrative 3, p.29.
55. M. Gunn, eulogy for Faulkner, 1981, MC; interview with Sam Kurtovich, 15 September 1987.
56. Alice to Faulkner, 25 March 1945.
57. Faulkner Bush, additional material, February 1981, MC.
58. J. Phillips, *A Man's Country?*, Auckland, 1987, pp.241–2.
59. Alice to Faulkner, 11 August 1944.
60. Alice to Faulkner, 22 March 1965.
61. Faulkner Bush, 9 February 1981, MC.

6 The Specialist

1. A. Bush, 'Women, Medicine and the Royal College', p.3, AFB.
2. K. Anderson, p.163.
3. N.F. Greenslade, *NZMJ*, February 1973, p.108.
4. Sayers correspondence, 20 July 1981, MC.
5. Alice to Faulkner, 21 January 1944.
6. AHB Minute Book, July–December 1946, pp.715, 716.
7. Notes made by Phoebe Meikle in conversation with Dr David Pyke, August 1978, MC; Pyke correspondence, 18 June 1987.
8. Pyke correspondence, 18 June 1987.
9. Interview, Dr Basil Quin, 14 May 1987.
10. Pyke correspondence, 18 June 1987.
11. Notes in conversation with Dr David Pyke, August 1978, MC; interview, Professor J.M. Watt, 6 June 1988.
12. Alice to Faulkner, 27 November 1947.
13. Bowlby, *Child Care*, 1953, back cover.
14. AHB Minute Book June–September 1967, p.1605.
15. Q/S Dr Margaret Gatman, 21 January 1983, MC; Faulkner's Story, pp.66–8.
16. Watt interview, 6 June 1988. AKMWA Minute Book 1947–53, 18 August 1949.
17. Typescript, BBC Pacific Programme, recorded 15 January 1949, broadcast Monday, 24 January 1949, AFB.
18. AKMWA Minute Book, 1947–53, 18 August 1949.
19. C.J. O'Neill, 'Fertility, Past, Present and Future', in R.J.W. Neville and C.J. O'Neill, *The Population of New Zealand*, Auckland, 1979, pp.132–4.
20. AHB Minute Book, July–December 1949, pp.1331–2.
21. AHB Minute Book, July–December 1949, p.1332.
22. AHB Minute Book, January–June 1950, p.75D.
23. *NZMJ*, Vol.52, 1953, pp.80, 79.
24. AHB Minute Book, January–June 1952, pp.468, 464.
25. AHB Minute Book, January–June 1952, p.1635, July–December 1952, pp.1255, 1257.
26. AHB Minute Book, July–December 1952, p.2212.
27. Minutes of Proceedings, 21 March 1951, 2 June 1954, EB-A 1/75; 1/78; NA Auckland.
28. AHB Minute Book, February–June 1954, p.551.
29. Combined Staff Minute Book, 1936–48, pp.382, 420, A695/3, NA Auckland.

30 Combined Staff Minute Book, 1949–61, p.30, A695/4, NA Auckland.
31 Memorandum, W.E. Henley, Superintendent in Chief, to W.N. Tucker, Hon. Sec., Combined Medical Staff, 30 January 1970, AFB.
32 McKellar interview, 15 May 1987.
33 Typescript, A. Bush, 'What is an Allergy?', nd, AFB; A. Bush, 'Allergy Over a Quarter Century', *NZMJ*, 1968, p.101.
34 A. Bush, 'Allergy Testing in Asthma', *NE Patient Management*, January/February 1974, pp.23–8, AFB.
35 A. Bush, 'A Cause of Discontent', *Timohu*, 2:2, 1971, p.4, MC.
36 A. Bush, 'What is an Allergy?', AFB.
37 E.M. Wood, Typescript, 'Notes for Biography of Alice Bush', August 1981, and 'Notes on Convergence Treatment', *The Ophthalmic Optician*, 10 February 1962, pp.115–8; MC.
38 Teaching slide – Asthma; Correspondence Alice and Dorothy Johnson, Cambridge, 1959; AFB.
39 Typescript, B. Neal to writer, March 1989.
40 Correspondence to Secretary, J. Wattie Canneries, Hastings, c. February 1967 and Mr D.L. Hill, 108 Kupe Street, Orakei, Auckland, 18 November 1970, AFB.
41 'The Unhappy Child', *NZMJ*, February 1962, p.85.
42 Typescript, 'Cross Babies', p.6, nd, but probably early 1970s, AFB.
43 H. May, *Minding Children*, pp.314–8.
44 *Personal Relationships*, end page.
45 Alice to Faulkner, 24 April 1945.
46 Practice correspondence, AFB.
47 Interview, W. Sealy Wood, 19 June 1989.
48 Alice to Faulkner, 3 June 1945.
49 Clipping, 'Healthy to a Degree', *Star*, 8 June 1983; account of conversation, Dr Bartlett Gash and W.B. Lewis, 17 June 1982; MC.
50 Surviving practice records, AFB.
51 Correspondence and transcript of tape, 7 September 1982, Sister C.A. Hanna, MC.
52 Correspondence and transcript of tape, 7 September 1982; interview, Betty Neal, April 1977; MC. interview Betty Neal, 21 February 1989.
53 Clipping, 'BMA Women Delegates Are Enthusiastic', *Star*, 10 February 1953, H-A 10/4/7323, NA Auckland.
54 K. Anderson, pp.156–7.
55 AKMWA Annual Report, 1959.
56 K. Anderson, p.158.
57 AKMWA minutes, 7 June 1951.
58 AKMWA minutes, 15 March 1951.
59 K. Anderson, pp.155, 157–8.
60 AKMWA minutes, 27 July 1950, 15 May 1958.
61 AKMWA minutes, 4 December 1958.
62 AKMWA minutes, 25 June 1953.
63 *NZMJ*, 1947, Vol.46, p.47.
64 Account of meeting, 10 July 1952, p.8, H1 32/12/4 NA.
65 Ibid., p.9.
66 Ibid., pp.8, 7.
67 PSNZ Minute Book I, p.227; NZBMA submissions, p.7, AFB.
68 *NZMJ*, Vol.50, 1951, p.72.
69 W.B. Sutch, *The Responsible Society in New Zealand*, Christchurch, 1971, pp.109–10.
70 A. Mattinson, 'Social Work in Obstetrics', *New Zealand Nursing Journal*, 15 October 1951, p.171.
71 F.J. Cameron, 'Acceptable Standards of Paediatric Nursing Service', *New Zealand Nursing Journal*, 15 October 1953, p.146.
72 Correspondence, Ludbrook to Deputy Medical Superintendent, Auckland Hospital, 21 September 1945, AHB Minute Book, July–December 1945, pp.581–2.
73 Typescript, 'Report on the Proposed Development of the Princess Mary Hospital for Children', nd but probably 1955–6, and copy of minutes, Standing Committee for Administration and Future Hospital Planning, 14 November 1957; AFB.
74 Standing Committee for Administration, 14 November 1957, AFB.
75 Ms and typescript, A. Bush, 'Establishment of General Paediatric Wards in Other Hospitals under the control of the Auckland Hospital Board', nd but 1959, AFB.
76 AHB Minute Book, January–June 1945, p.232; July–December 1945, pp.329–30.
77 Diana Stuart Masters, research essay

in her possession, 'The Change in Attitudes toward Hospital Visiting in Paediatric Areas', pp.2–3.
78 Correspondence from the Pickerells, 3 October 1945, in AHB Minute Book, July–December 1945, p.783.
79 Bowlby, *Maternal Care*, pp.146–8.
80 Bush, 'Maternal Deprivation', p.2, AFB.
81 PSNZ Minute Book I, pp.158–9.
82 *The Welfare of Children in Hospital* (The Platt Report), London, 1959, p.2.
83 AHB Minute Book, February–July 1960, p.3545.
84 PSNZ Minute Book I, p.63.
85 Memo, A.W.S. Thompson to DGH, 12 December 1951, H1 35/12/4, N.A.
86 Typescript, 'Child Guidance – Report of subcommittee to the Paediatric Society of New Zealand', nd, AFB; PSNZ Minute Book I, p.160.
87 Memorandum, T.G. Fox to Dr. A.S. Wallace, MOH, Auckland, 19 January 1956, H1 13/2/4, N.A.
88 *NZMJ*, Vol.57, 1958, p.200.
89 *NZMJ*, 1959, p.806.
90 PSNZ Minute Book I, p.201.
91 Report of NZBMA Mental Health Committee, *NZMJ*, 1959, pp.83–109.
92 *NZMJ*, 1959, p.84.

7 *Education For Life*

1 A. Bush, 'The Family – Yesterday, Today and Tomorrow', in F. Simpson (ed.) *Auckland Yesterday and Tomorrow*, Auckland, 1971, p.22, AFB.
2 'Auckland Yesterday and Tomorrow', p.33.
3 R.H. Caughey, 'The Children's Hospital of the Future', *NZMJ*, 1968, p.120.
4. Alice to Faulkner, 4 September and 12 October 1943.
5. Alice to Faulkner, 17 February 1944.
6. Alice to Faulkner, 9 January 1945.
7. Alice to Faulkner, 21 October 1944.
8. Alice to Faulkner, 24 September 1944.
9. Alice to Faulkner, 11 August 1944.
10. Alice to Faulkner, 24 September 1944.
11. NCC Women's Committee, *Homes and Families*, Christchurch/Dunedin, 1950, p.4.
12. *Homes and Families*, p.32.
13. *Homes and Families*, p.19.
14. Bowlby, *Maternal Care*, p.147.
15. 'Submissions to the Consultative Committee on the Care of Pre-School Children', p.2, AFB.
16. Alice writing as Mary Wood [MW], 'New Deal for Families', *NZFD*, May 1964, p.23. All *NZFD* material is from the Meikle Collection.
17. MW, 'What Little Girls and Boys are Made Of', *NZFD*, January 1963, p.15.
18. 'The Doctor and the Delinquent', *NZMJ*, February 1961, p.61.
19. MW, 'Fathers Really Do Count', *NZFD*, June 1963, pp.25–6.
20. Typescript, 'Measures to reduce the Incidence of Violent Sexual Crimes', outline of address to NCW, nd but c. early 1960s, AFB.
21. 'The Doctor and the Delinquent', p.64.
22. MW, 'It's So Good To Be Alive', *NZFD*, March 1963, p.18.
23. Paper delivered at 'Marriage – A Symposium', RCGP Seminar, 7/8 October 1967, photocopy courtesy Betty Neil: MC.
24. Typescript, review of *Living with Children*, Dr Claire Isbister, Sydney, NSW, nd but c. 1960s, AFB.
25. MW, 'Thinking About Having a Baby', *NZFD*, February 1963, p.14.
26. MW, 'New Deal for Families', *NZFD*, May 1964, p.23.
27. MW, 'What Little Girls and Boys are Made Of', *NZFD*, January 1963, p.15.
28. 'Measuress to Reduce the Incidence of Violent Sexual Crimes', p.3.
29. K. Beuke, Q/S November 1970, MC.
30. Clipping, 'Lifetime of work with sick children', ann. *Auckland Star*, 24 May 1971, AFB.
31. MW, 'What Little Girls and Boys are Made Of', *NZFD*, January 1963, p.17.
32. MW, 'Fathers Really Do Count', *NZFD*, June 1963, p.27.
33. L.W. Leman, Q/S October 1979, MC.
34. MW, 'When To Say No', *NZFD*,

May 1963, p.26.
35. MW, 'Discipline on a Wise and Gentle Pattern', *NZFD*, September 1963, p.27.
36. E. Cole, *Where Did I Come From?*, NZFPA, p.4; *Sex Problems in Marriage I*, NZFPA leaflet, nd but c. later 1940s or 1950s, pp.4, 6.
37. MW, 'World of the Toddler', *NZFD*, April 1963, p.20.
38. MW, 'Time to Take Stock', *NZFD*, August 1963, p.25.
39. MW, 'It's So Good To Be Alive', *NZFD*, March 1963, p.18.
40. MW, 'Fathers Really Do Count', *NZFD*, June 1963, p.25.
41. MW, 'You As Your Children See You', *NZFD*, October 1963, p.24.
42. MW, 'Time to Take Stock', *NZFD*, August 1963, p.25.
43. Clipping, Valerie Davies, 'We must show our children . . .', *NZWW*, nd but post-1974, courtesy Betty Neal.
44. MW, 'You As Your Children See You', *NZFD*, October 1963, p.23.
45. *NZMJ*, February 1961, p.62.
46. Correspondence between Alice and Mrs J. Pond, Matamata, 19 and 22 June 1972, AFB.
47. *NZMJ*, February 1961, p.63.
48. *Report of the Special Committee on Moral Delinquency in Children and Adolescents*, *AJHR* 1954 H-47, [Mazengarb Report], p.7.
49. S.G.M. Glazebrook, 'The Mazengarb Report, 1954; Impotent Victorianism', Research Essay, University of Auckland, February 1978, p.2.
50. Clipping, *Evening Post*, 10 September 1954, MS Papers 2384, Special Committee on Moral Delinquency, Folder 11, ATL.
51. Evidence of Dr E.K. Hughes, September 1954, MS Papers 2384:4, ATL.
52. Mazengarb, pp.7–10.
53. Ibid., pp.41–3.
54. Ibid., p.42.
55. B. Poland, President's Report, Auckland Branch, 31 March 1953, NZFPA.
56. Mrs Amy Slack interview, 11 April 1989; correspondence, J. Forrest, Hon. Sec., Auckland Provincial Council of Parent Teacher Associations to J.R. Marshall, Minister of Health, 22 November 1954, H-1 35/14 25845, NA.
57. *Sex and the Parent*, Pamphlet No.63, New Zealand Department of Health, Wellington, 1955. All the following references may be found in this pamphlet.
58. 'Statement by the Family Planning Association in support of the pamphlets on sex education issued by the Health Department', typescript, nd, NZFPA.
59. Clipping, 'Reply to Criticism of Auckland Sex Pamphlets', *Dominion*, 22 March 1955, H1 35/14 25345, N.A.
60. Correspondence, 17 May 1955, Minister of Health to Hon. Sec., Catholic Women's League and identical text to Sec., New Zealand Inter-Church Council on Public Affairs, H1 35/14 25845, N.A.
61. Clippings, 'Not Enough Sex Pamphlets Parents Claim', *NZH*, and 'Sex instruction pamphlets wanted NOW', *Auckland Star*, 19 October 1955, H1 35/14 25845, N.A.
62. 'Review of Maternal and Child Health', *AJHR* H-31, 1969.
63. Clipping, 'Value of visits to Courts', letter to editor, ann. 12 May 1959, AFB.
64. 'The Unhappy Child', *NZMJ*, February 1962, p.87.
65. Annual Report, Auckland University Students' Association, June 1965, p.28, AUSA Archives, University of Auckland.
66. Typescript, 'The Causes of Sexual Delinquency. The Place of Education in its Prevention', nd, but c. early 1960s, AFB. The general theme followed in this paper is typical of the surviving documents of this period in Alice's papers.
67. Clipping, 'Crowd at Girls' Sex Lecture', AFB; see also YWCA Scrapbook, Ms 1131/99, 1957–June 1970, where the clipping is dated 7 October [1968]; S. Coney, *Every Girl*, p.255.
68. Clipping, 'Letter to the Editor – Family Life Tuition', ann. '*Herald*, 17 May 1967', AFB.
69. Clipping, 'Family Life', D.B. Smith,

Hillsborough, ann. 3 May 1967, ns but probably *NZH*, AFB.
70. Paper delivered at 'Marriage – A Symposium', p.9, AFB.
71. Alice to Faulkner, 25 June 1940.
72. Dobbie, p.5; clipping, *NZH*, 17 September 1958, Auckland Scrapbook June–October 1958, p.88, APL.
73. NZFPA Newsletter, May 1956, p.1, NZFPA.
74. Mrs [Mary] Saker to 'Iris', ann. July 1943, NZFPA. If this date is correct Alice must have been 'mellowed by motherhood' very early since she did not give birth to Lesley until September of that year.
75. Correspondence, Alice to Lex Gray, 14 August 1953, AFB.
76. Alice to Faulkner, 20 April 1944.
77. Alice to Faulkner, 6 December 1944.
78. Auckland Parents' Centres Hospitals Committee Newsletter No.2, December 1958, and 'Course of Relaxation Classes & Lectures Held at Bethany Maternity Hospital', 7 October–16 December 1958, typescript, AFB.
79. Correspondence, Mary Dobbie to Alice Bush, 31 May 1959, and attachment, AFB.
80. Typescript, 'Organisation of Clinic', nd but c. 1950s; National Executive minutes, NZFPA Conference, Lower Hutt, 6 June 1958, p.5, NZFPA.

8 Taking a Stand

1. A. Bush, 'The Doctor and the Delinquent', *NZMJ*, February 1961, p.64.
2. Clipping, 'Quantity, but little quality in New Zealand Marriage', nd, ns, but probably *NZWW*, c. June 1969, p.13, NZFPA.
3. Standing Committee minutes, 25 February, 1957, p.2, NZFPA.
4. K. Sinclair, *A History of the University of Auckland*, Auckland, 1983, pp.274–5; S. Coney, *The Unfortunate Experiment*, Auckland, 1988, p.19.
5. Helen Brew to Christchurch Parents' Centre, quoted in M. Dobbie, *The Trouble With Women*, p.42.
6. Dobbie, p.44.
7. Dobbie, pp.53–4; *NZMJ*, 1959, Vol.58, p.133.
8. Report of Standing Committee meeting, 10 October 1956, p.2, NZFPA.
9. Standing Committee minutes, 6 December 1958; 'Memo for All Branch Secretaries' 26 August 1959; NZFPA.
10. Attached to Zeff to Alice Bush, 21 October 1959, AFB.
11. Correspondence, 16 January and 4 February 1959, AFB.
12. *NZMJ*, Vol.57, 1958, pp.524, 525.
13. *NZMJ*, Vol.54, 1955, pp.159–65.
14. *NZMJ* 1959, Vol.58, p.683.
15. BMA (Auckland Division) Quarterly Minute Book, 2 September 1959, p.29, AKMA.
16. Correspondence, Vivienne Croxford to Alice, 4 October 1959, AFB.
17. *NZMJ*, 1959, Vol.58, pp.813, 814.
18. Standing Committee minutes, 14 March 1959, p.2; 4 July 1959, pp.2–3, NZFPA.
19. Correspondence, V. Croxford to Alice, 4 October 1959, AFB; 'Further Notes for Branches', Standing Committee minutes, 19 October 1959, NZFPA.
20. Correspondence, G. Lowe to P. Zeff, 13 January 1957; Zeff to Lowe, 5 February 1957, NZFPA; V. Croxford to Alice, 4 October 1959, AFB; correspondence, R. Black and M. Topping to Chairman, Auckland Branch, NZFPA, nd but c. September 1959, attached Zeff to Bush, 21 October 1959, AFB; Standing Committee minutes, 3 October 1959, pp.1–2, NZFPA.
21. Phyllis Zeff to Alice, 21 October 1959, AFB.
22. *NZMJ*, Vol.58, 1959, p.809.
23. Belgrave, 'Medical Men and Lady Doctors', pp.82–3.
24. *NZMJ*, Vol.59, 1960, p.114.
25. *NZMJ*, Vol.59, 1960, p.493.
26. Correspondence, Ruth Black to Glenys Lowe, 26 February 1955, NZFPA.
27. Glenys Lowe to Phyllis Zeff and Judy Lunn, 10 March 1960, NZFPA.
28. Cyclostyled letter, nd but c. 1960, AFB.
29. Margaret Topping, Ruth Black,

Sheila Godfrey, Anne Jarvis, *NZMJ*, Vol.59, 1960, pp.262–3; *ibid.*, Helen Barlow, p.306.
30. Topping, Black, Godfrey, Jarvis, *NZMJ*, Vol.59, 1960, pp.262–3.
31. Correspondence, G. Lowe to P. Zeff and J. Lunn, 10 March 1960, NZFPA.
32. Standing Committee minutes, 7 May 1960, p.2, AGM minutes, Auckland Branch Minute Book, 1955–?62, NZFPA.
33. Standing Committee minutes, 7 May 1960, p.2, NZFPA.
34. Typescript, interview Hilda Allum with Judy Lunn, 15 October 1979, and notes taken in conversation, P. Meikle and Judy Lunn, 20 October 1979; MC.
35. Standing Committee minutes, 7 May 1960, p.2, 5, NZFPA.
36. Circular, Auckland Branch Committee to other branches, nd but pre–conference June 1960, NZFPA.
37. Minutes, 1960 Biennial Conference, NZFPA, P1.
38. Minutes, p.6.
39. Minutes, p.5.
40. Minutes, pp.2, 3.
41. A. Bush, Opening Address, NZFPA 8th Biennial Conference minutes, 17–19 June 1966, p.2, AFB.
42. Allum/Lunn and Meikle/Lunn interviews, 15 and 20 October 1979; MC.
43. *NZMJ*, Vol.57, 1958, p.199.
44. Wright St-Clair, *History of the NZMA*, pp.177–8.
45. *NZMJ*, April 1960, p.217; March 1963, p.151.
46. *NZMJ* January 1964, p.47.
47. *NZMJ*, June 1964, p.394.
48. Conference minutes, p.4.
49. Clipping, 'Family Planning Clinics Accepted', ann. *Evening Post*, 20 June 1960, AIM.
50. *NZMJ*, Vol.59, 1960, p.114; Vol.49, 1950, pp.329–30; Vol.55, 1956, p.350.
51. J. Lovell-Smith, *The New Zealand Doctor and the Welfare State*, p.26, quoted in D.G. Bolitho, 'The Introduction of Social Security', *NZHJ*, 18:1, 1984, p.44.
52. Clipping, *Evening Post*, 24 June 1960, NZFPA.
53. AKMWA Minutes, 30 June 1960.
54. NZBMA Auckland Division Quarterly Minute Book, pp.66–7, AKMA.
55. Typescript and carbon copies of 'Notice of Motion', AFB.
56. *NZMJ*, Vol.59, 1960, p.177.
57. Circular-letter, August 1960, AFB.
58. Dobbie, p.60.
59. Correspondence, unsigned, but probably sent by Mary Dobbie, 5 July 1960, AFB.
60. *NZMJ*, Vol.59, October 1960, pp.493–4.
61. Cyclostyled letter, nd but c. October 1960, AFB.
62. Draft letter and list, AFB.
63. *NZMJ*, Vol.60, 1961, pp.60–4.
64. 'Copy of the Report of the Branch Ethical Committee on the Family Planning Association', NZFPA.
65. Minutes, meeting NZFPA and Health Department personnel, 4 December 1972, p.6, AFB.
66. Circular, 'Suggestions for Discussion re clinics between B.M.A. and F.P.A.', March 1961, AFB.
67. Interview, Dr Ruth Black and writer, 7 June 1989; R. Black, 'Years in Family Planning', *Choice*, 12:4, 1974, p.28.
68. *NZMJ*, Vol.60, 1961, p.353.
69. *NZMJ*, Vol.60, 1961, p.492.
70. *NZMJ*, July 1961, pp.352–3.
71. B.M.A. (Auckland Division) Quarterly Meeting Minute Book, pp.94–6, AKMA.
72. Memorandum, D.A. Hunn to Minister of Health, 24 November 1961, H1 35/12/4, NA.
73. Ms and typescript, 'The Role of the Paediatrician in the New Zealand Child Health Clinic', nd but mid-1960s, AFB.
74. A. Bush, review of J.H. Kahn, *Human Growth and the Development of Personality*, *NZMJ*, October 1965, p.608.
75. Clippings, 'Family Planning' 7 July, 'Family Planning' 12 July, 'Planned Families' 25 July 1961, *NZH*; NZFPA.
76. Annual Report 1966–7, AFB.
77. FGC Correspondence and Annual Reports, AFB.
78. Last Will and Testament, 9 February 1968.
79. Clipping, 'Dr Attributes Birth Drop

to Oral Pills', *Dominion*, 1 July 1964, NZFPA.
80. Medical Advisory Committee Report, Biennial Conference minutes, June 1964, p.7, AFB.
81. Conference minutes 1964, p.4.
82. NZFPA 'Medical Report', nd but 1965, p.1, AFB.
83. Clipping, 'Medical Risks', letter to editor, Alice M. Bush, Epsom, ns, ann. 4 October 1964, AFB.
84. May & Baker diaries, AFB.
85. Correspondence, A. Bush to Dr E.G. McQueen, Medical Assessor, Committee on Adverse Drug Reactions, Dunedin, 9 June 1970, AFB.
86. Clippings, 'Fears Over Mini-pill Dispelled By Doctor', nd, ns; '"Pill Only One Factor in Birth-rate Fall', ann. Christchurch *Press*, 24 September 1964; 'More Maori Infants in Fatal Accidents', *Press*, 18 February 1967; 'Illogical Tests For Useful Drugs', ann. *Star*, 27 January and *Herald*, 26 January 1967; AFB; 'Birth Control By Injection is More Popular', ann. *Herald*, 22 April 1972, NZFPA; 'President's Message', *Choice* 7:4, November 1969, p.5.
87. Correspondence, 1964, AFB.
88. Correspondence, 1969, 1970, AFB.
89. *NZMJ*, September 1966, p.619.
90. Undated Mss and May and Baker diary, 6 July 1966, AFB.
91. Clipping, 'Some Girls Should Be Given Pill', ann. *Press*, 18 February 1967, AFB.
92. Clipping, 'Abortion – how live an issue in N.Z. today?', *Auckland Star*, . 20 June 1970, NZFPA.
93. Clipping, 'Doctor, Professor give ideas on contraception', *South Auckland Courier*, Eastern edition, 13 October 1971, NZFPA.
94. Section 2 of the Police Offences Act (1954), NZFPA.
95. *Choice*, 8:4, December 1970, p.13.
96. *NZMJ*, July 1973, p.39.
97. *Choice*, May 1973, pp.27–9, and submissions, NZFPA.

9 Going to the Needy

1. A. Bush, 'President's Report to Biennial Conference 1964', *Choice* 2:2, August 1964.
2. I. Pool, 'Population Growth and Urbanisation', in E. Schwimmer (ed.), *The Maori People in the Nineteen-Sixties*, Auckland, 1968, p.189.
3. Standing Committee Minutes, 29 October 1957, p.2, NZFPA.
4. R.J. Rose, 'Maori-European Contrast in Infant, Child and Maternal Mortality', p.13, Medical Statistics Branch, Health Department, nd but c. early 1960s, H1 194/1, NA.
5. Rose, pp.15–16.
6. Rose, p.16.
7. 'President's Message', *Choice*, 2:1, April 1964.
8. Clipping, 'Should these people marry?', ns, ann. 24 April 1971, AFB.
9. *Choice*, November 1971, pp.5–6.
10. Copy of correspondence, Hon. Duncan MacIntyre, Minister of Maori Affairs, to Dr R.R. Lycette, Havelock North, 11 February 1970, AFB.
11. Correspondence, Alice to Dr Lycette, Hastings, 29 June 1970. AFB.
12. Conference minutes, p.1, NZFPA.
13. Standing Committee Minutes, 4 September 1962, pp.1, 2, NZFPA.
14. Standing Committee Minutes, 5 November 1962, p.1, NZFPA; 'Report of Preliminary Discussions – Second Tai Rawhiti (Ruatoria) Maori Leadership Conference 1962', p.4, AFB; clipping, 'New Zealand', *News of Population and Birth Control*, No.119, November 1963, (report dated 14 September 1963), NZFPA.
15. Minutes, 7th Annual Conference, Napier, April 1959, p.8, MWWL Ms Papers 1396:4, ATL.
16. 'Report of Preliminary Discussions – Second Tai Rawhiti (Ruatoria) Maori Leadership Conference 1962, pp.4–5, AFB.
17. *Choice*, 2:2, August 1964.
18. Standing Committee Minutes, 1 October 1962, p.1, NZFPA.
19. Memo, B.W. Christmas, MOH Auckland, to DGH, Wellington, 28 May 1962, H-A 10/54/9813, NA Auckland.
20. Clipping, '"Pill" Only One Factor in

Birth-Rate Fall', ann. Christchurch *Press*, 24 September 1964, AFB.
21. 'President's Message', *Choice*, 2:2, August 1964.
22. 'President's Message for Christmas and the New Year', *Choice*, 9:4, November 1971, p.5.
23. J. Bassett, 'Contraception as a Woman's Issue', Women and the Law Seminar Paper, University of Auckland, 1979, p.10.
24. Medical Advisory Committee Report, 26 June 1964, p.6, attached to Conference Minutes, AFB.
25. Correspondence, D.N. McKay to Alice, 26 August 1964, and attached memo to Minister of Education, NZFPA.
26. Clipping, 'Maori Needs', Alice M. Bush, ann. *Herald*, 6 July 1964, AFB.
27. Correspondence, Hanan to Alice, 18 August 1964, AFB.
28. Faulkner's Story, p.163.
29. Correspondence, A. Bush to Mr B.W. Souter, Asst Secretary, Department of Maori Affairs, Auckland, 20 August 1964, AFB.
30. Newsletters, Vol. III, No.9, October 1964, p.3, MWWL Collection, Ms Papers 1396:8, ATL.
31. 'For a Better Understanding of the Maori', p.3, AFB.
32. *Ibid.*, p.4.
33. Typescript, A. Bush, 'Talk to Maori Health Committee – Family Spacing', 2 December 1964, p.1, AFB.
34. *Ibid.*, p.1.
35. *Ibid.*, p.3.
36. *Ibid.*, p.5.
37. 'Family Planning Absent Where It Is Most Needed', *ODT*, 8 September, 1969, AFB; see also J. and J. Ritchie, 'Children' in E. Schwimmer (ed.), *The Maori People in the Nineteen-Sixties*, p.324.
38. 'Talk to Maori Health Committee', p.3.
39. *Ibid.*, p.4.
40. Minutes, Maori Health Committee, 2 December 1964, p.2, H-A 14/9154, NA Auckland.
41. Auckland Division NZBMA Minute Book, pp.198–9, AKMA.
42. *NZMJ*, January 1965, p.44; Memo, H.B. Turbott, DGH to Minister of Health, 14 December 1964, H1 13/20/3, NA Wellington.
43. Conference remits, 1965, p.3, MWWL Ms Papers 1396:5, ATL.
44. *Choice*, 2:4, February 1965, p.3.
45. This continuing correspondence may be found in H1 13/20/3, NA.
46. Correspondence, Minister of Health to Secretary, NCW, 9 November 1966; Prime Minister to Minister of Health regarding FUW questionnaire, 28 September 1966, and response, 7 October 1966, H1 13/20/3, NA.
47. Clipping, 'Women Send Queries to Party Candidates', *ODT*, 22 November 1966, H1 13/20/3, NA.
48. Written 4 November 1966, published 8 November 1966, ns but probably *Star*, AFB.
49. Memo, D.P. Kennedy, DGH, to Minister of Health, 1 December 1966, H1 13/20/3.
50. Circular Memorandum No.1966/315, D.P. Kennedy, DGH, 22 December 1966, H13/20/3 NA.
51. NCW National Minute Book, June 1967, p.15; correspondence, Mrs J.J. Herd, National Secretary, NCW, to Minister of Health, 18 July 1967, H 13/20/3.
52. Kennedy to Dr Molly Woodroffe, 20 September 1967, H 13/20/3, NA.
53. Correspondence, T.D. Patterson, District Health Office, Gisborne, to DGH, Wellington, 15 December 1964, H1 194/1/30140, NA.
54. *Choice*, 6:1, February 1968.
55. Standing Committee minutes, 14 October 1969, p.2; 2 December 1969, pp.1–3; President's Report, Auckland Branch, 1969, p.1, NZFPA.
56. Clippings, 'Birth Control Ban Penalises Maoris', ann. *NZH*, 15 October 1969, 'No to birth control advice', *Waikato Times*, 15 October 1969, H1 13/20/3, NA; 'Association follows a basic right', *Auckland Star*, 18 October 1969, NZFPA; 'Birth Control Policy Slated', *Waikato Times*, 4 November 1969, H1 13/20/3, NA.
57. Clipping, 'Family Disability', 2 May 1970, ns, AFB.
58. Clipping, 'Will Not [?Help] Maoris',

ns, ann. 26 May 1970, AFB.
59. Clipping, letter to editor, 'Family Spacing', ns, ann. 12 June 1970, AFB.
60. *NCW Quarterly*, February 1971, p.21, MC.
61. J.T. France, 'The Theoretical Basis of Catholic Methods of Family Planning – The Rhythm Method', cyclostyled paper, nd but c. early 1970s, AFB.
62. *Choice*, 2:1, April 1964.
63. *Choice*, 3:2, May 1965, p.1.
64. *Choice*, 3:2, May 1965, p.5.
65. Correspondence, Sir Colville Deverell, Secretary-General, IPPF, to Secretary NZFPA, nd but c. April 1965–January 1966, NZFPA.
66. *Choice*, 6:3, August 1968, p.7; clipping, 'The Pope and the Pill', *Press*, 30 July 1968, NZFPA.
67. *Choice*, 6:3, August 1968, pp.11–13.
68. Correspondence to Alice, 16 February 1965, AFB.
69. Correspondence, J.S. Hopkirk, Secretary, Hawke's Bay Division, NZBMA, to Alice, 7 April 1965; Alice to Faulkner, received 3 October 1968, and annotated by Faulkner post 1974, AFB.
70. Clippings: 'Doctors Discuss Pill', *Press*, 22 August 1968; 'Doctors and Bishop Discuss Pill Ruling', *Press*, ann. August 1968; 'Ruling Restricts Catholic Doctors', *Zealandia*, 22 August 1968, p.1; 'More Practical Help for Married Couples', *Ibid.*, NZFPA.
71. Clipping, 'Doctors Discuss Pill', *Press*, 22 August 1968, NZFPA.
72. *Choice*, 6:3, August 1968, pp.12, 13.
73. Clipping, 'Effect of Encyclical "Out of Proportion"', 5 November 1968, *Press*, AFB.
74. E. Olssen, 'Truby King and the Plunket Society. An Analysis of a Prescriptive Ideology', *NZJH*, 15:1, April 1981.
75. *NZMJ*, February 1966, p.133.
76. NZFPA Standing Committee minutes, 8 June 1971, p.4; 6 July 1971, p.3; *Choice*, 9:3, August 1971, p.12; NZFPA Standing Committee minutes, 3 August 1971, p.2.
77. *Plunket News*, April 1972, pp.11–15, AFB.
78. Clipping, 'Family Planning and Plunket', 7 December 1972, *Auckland Star*, AFB; see also *Plunket News*, February 1973, p.37.
79. Correspondence to National President, Plunket Society, 7 November 1972, AFB.
80. Circular/Memo No.1971/80, 8 April 1971, H-A 10/54/9813, NA Auckland.
81. 'Report of Meeting....', 7 December 1970, AFB.
82. 'Functions and Responsibilities: Family Health Branch, August 1971', H-A 10/54, NA Auckland.
83. Circular Memo 1971/217, 30 September 1971; 'Department's Position Restated', press release received 4 October 1971, H-A 10/54 9813, NA Auckland.
84. 'Extension of New Zealand's Family Planning Service', attached to correspondence, Minister of Health to Dominion Secretary, NZFPA, 14 December 1971, AFB.
85. Standing Committee minutes, 14 December 1971, p.1; Correspondence, Alice to Joan Mackay, 27 December 1971, AFB.
86. Clipping, 'Birth control clinic network gets go-ahead', ann. *Sunday Herald*, 19 December 1971, NZFPA.
87. 'President's Message for Christmas and the New Year, *Choice*, November 1971, p.5.

10 Widening Horizons

1. A. Bush, 'President's Message', *Choice*, 4:3, August 1966, pp.16–17.
2. *Choice*, 2:4, February 1965, p.6.
3. Correspondence, E. Simpson, MOH, Rarotonga, Cook Islands, to MOH, Auckland, 22 May 1961; B.W. Christmas, MOH, Auckland, to Simpson, 9 June 1961, H-A 10/54 9813, NA Auckland.
4. Newsletter, M. Griffin, nd but c. November 1956, p.1; report, Standing Committee Meeting, 1 July 1957, p.2; typescript, 'Report of Survey into the need for family planning in the Pacific Islands of Fiji, Tonga, Niue and Eastern and Western Samoa', August 1957; newsletter, Phyllis Zeff, October

1958; NZFPA.
5. AHB Minute Book, May–September 1962, pp.1937, 1956.
6. 'Report on Visit to Rarotonga on behalf of NZFPA', Ms by Alice in writing pad annotated by Faulkner, 'Rarotonga July/August, 1962', AFB.
7. Standing Committee minutes, 1 October 1962, NZFPA.
8. *Choice* 2:2, August 1964.
9. Standing Committee minutes, 4 November 1963, p.1.
10. A. Bush, 'President's Message', *Choice* 2:2, August 1964; Standing Committee Minutes, 2 or 3 February 1964, p.1; Minutes, 7th Biennial Conference, 26–28 June 1964, p.4; NZFPA.
11. Typescript, 'President's Report', 1964, pp.2, 1, NZFPA.
12. Alice to Faulkner, 21 February 1964, AFB; 'President's Message', *Choice*, 2:2, August 1964.
13. Alice to Faulkner, nd and 1 March 1964.
14. Alice to Faulkner, 1 March 1964.
15. Alice to Faulkner, nd.
16. 'President's Message', *Choice*, 2:2, August 1964.
17. Standing Committee minutes, 4 November 1963, p.1, NZFPA.
18. *Choice*, 2:2, August 1964.
19. *Choice* 3:4, November 1965, p.8.
20. A. Bush, 'Statement to the Committee of the Whole on Education for Agricultural Development', *Choice*, 3:3, August 1965, pp.12–13.
21. *Choice* 3:4, November 1965, p.8.
22. Standing Committee minutes, 10 August 1965, p.2.
23. Cc. correspondence, Ong Kah Kok, Deputy Director (Field), People's Association, to P.S. Lendrum, High Commissioner for New Zealand, Singapore, 27 September 1965 and enclosure Ong Kah Kok to A. Grey, Department of Education, Epsom, Auckland, 27 September 1965, AFB.
24. *Choice*, 3:4, November 1965, p.9.
25. 'Review of the Social Situation in the ECAFE Region', ECAFE 21st Session, 16–19 March 1965, Wellington, 14 January 1965, AFB.
26. A. Bush, 'Statement on the Effect of Population Growth on the Economic Situation in the ECAFE Region', delivered 30 July 1965, AFB.
27. Clipping, 'Death Control', letter to editor, ns, ann. 18 April 1973. The phrase was attributed to Alan Guttmacher of IPPF in a paper, 'Developing a Christian Viewpoint of Responsible Parenthood', delivered at the 1964 conference, AFB.
28. A. Bush, 'Statement on the Effect . . .', pp.1–2, AFB.
29. 'Censorship – Planned or Unplanned?', *Choice* 3:2, May 1965, p.5; 'Review of the Social Situation . . .', pp.4–14, AFB.
30. Clipping, 'Doctor welcomes birth control aid', ann. *Star*, 30 March 1965, AFB.
31. Mss Alice to *NZH*, 2 April 1965, AFB; clipping, ann. *NZH* 6 April 1965, AFB.
32. Correspondence, Dr Erich Geiringer to Alice, 7 January 1965, AFB.
33. Geiringer correspondence, 15 November 1989.
34. Correspondence, Alice to Geiringer, 12 January 1965, AFB; 'Appeal for Population Control', Newsletter No.1, ann. 1 August 1966, AFB.
35. Sir Edmund Hillary correspondence, 29 November 1989.
36. Material in AFB.
37. 'Appeal for Population Control', Newsletter No.1, ann. 1 August 1966, H1 13/20/3, NA.
38. Vols 4:1, February 1966, p.1; 4:3 August 1966, p.7; 5:2, May 1967, p.1.
39. Correspondence, Alice to Geiringer, 22 April 1966, AFB.
40. Geiringer correspondence, 15 November 1989.
41. *Choice*, 4:1, February 1966, p.3.
42. *Choice*, 3:3, August 1965, p.11.
43. Standing Committee minutes, 13 July 1965, p.1, NZFPA.
44. *Choice*, 3:3, August 1965, p.11.
45. 'From the President's Biennial Report to Conference, June 1966', *Choice*, p.9.
46. Standing Committee minutes, 13 July 1965, p.1.
47. Standing Committee minutes, 10 August 1965, p.1.
48. 1966 Annual Report – Planned

263 NOTES TO PAGES 180–188

Parenthood – World Population, ann. 'Standing Committee', p.12, AFB.
49. Alice to Faulkner, 3 May and 6 May, 1966, AFB.
50. Alice to Faulkner, 12 and 15 May 1966, AFB.
51. Medical Committee Minutes, SEAOR, IPPF, Sunday 22 May 1966, AFB.
52. SEAOR of IPPF Regional Council Meeting Minutes, Monday 23 May 1966, Appendix 1, p.2, AFB.
53. *Choice*, 4:2, May 1966, p.9.
54. Standing Committee minutes, 8 February 1966, p.1.
55. Circular-letter, E. Biddle, Dominion Secretary, to branch presidents and secretaries, 11 February 1966, NZFPA.
56. Correspondence: Alice to Holyoake, 13 December 1965, H 13/20/3; to Hon. D.N. McKay, Min. of Health, 30 May 1966; to Dr Douglas Kennedy, DGH, 31 May 1966; NZFPA.
57. Invitation and acceptance lists, NZFPA.
58. Correspondence, R.G. McElroy to Alice, 16 March 1966, NZFPA.
59. Correspondence, D.C. Williams on behalf of Lady Fergusson, to Mrs E. Biddle, Dominion Sec., 18 March 1966, NZFPA.
60. *Choice*, 4:3, August 1966, pp.3, 16.
61. Correspondence, Prime Minister, to Sec. Gen. UN, New York, 16 November 1967, H 13/20/3.
62. Press statement: 'New Zealand Endorses World Leaders' Statement on Population', 16 November 1967, H13/20/3; *Choice*, 6:1, February 1968.
63. UN Doc. A/CONF. 32/41, Resolution 18. See (1969) *American Journal of International Law*, Vol.63, pp.678–9, 674–7, cited in B. Brown and R. Lawson, 'The Law Relating to Family Planning in New Zealand', Research Paper, Faculty of Law, University of Auckland, March 1972, p.1, NZFPA.
64. I. Stanton, 'Bandung, June 1969,' Standing Committee Minutes, 8 July 1969, p.3.
65. *Choice*, 7:3, August 1969, pp.23–4.

66. Standing Committee minutes, 2 December 1969, p.1, and 3 February 1970, p.1.
67. *Choice*, 9:1, February 1971, p.17.
68. Standing Committee minutes, 6 April 1971, NZFPA.
69. *Choice*, 8:4, December 1970, p.17.
70. A. Bush, Ms, nd, ann. WAFB 'Found in case used for Baguio Conf[erence] Mar[ch] '71', AFB.
71. Standing Committee Minutes, 6 April 1971, NZFPA.
72. Clipping, ann. *NZH*, 18 January 1972, AFB.
73. Clipping, *Auckland Star*, 12 February 1972, p.14, AFB.
74. Clipping, ann. *NZH*, 17 February 1972, NZFPA.
75. Clipping, ann. *NZH*, 1972, NZFPA.
76. Clipping, 'Needs of 1971', ann. 5 January 1971, ns, AFB.
77. *Choice*, 9:4, p.6.
78. Clipping, 'No Virtue In Having a Baby By Chance', ann. *Nelson Mail*, 19 September 1972, AFB.
79. Correspondence, Shirley Rowe to Alice, 12 March 1971, and 'Summary of Decisions Taken by the National Council of Women', July 1973, p.16; clipping, 'Pakistani Crisis', letter to editor, ns, ann. 16 June 1971, AFB.
80. *Choice*, 9:3, August 1971, p.24.
81. Standing Committee minutes, 3 August 1971, p.2, NZFPA.
82. Typescript, 'Press Statement – Released 26.8.71 – New Zealand Grant for Population Activities', AFB; this was later reproduced in *Choice* 9:4, November 1971, p.8.
83. Standing Committee minutes, 6 July 1971, p.1.
84. Standing Committee minutes, 9 November 1971, p.3.
85. *Choice*, 10:2, May 1972, p.21.
86. Minutes, Special Meeting of Standing Committee, 25 May 1972, AFB.
87. *Choice*, 10:4, November 1972, p.15.
88. Clipping, ann. *Herald*, 8 September 1973, AFB.

11 New Feminism: New Medicine

1. Typescript, 'The Family – Alice M. Bush', City of Auckland Centenary

1. Lecture Series, 1971, p.17, NZFPA.
2. AKMWA Minute Book 1966–74, p.75, NZMWA.
3. *NZMJ* March 1969, pp.174–5.
4. J. Leeson and J. Gray, *Women and Medicine*, London, 1978, pp.35–6; P. Day, *Women Doctors: Choices and Constraints in Policies for Medical Manpower*, London, 1982, pp.20–1; NZMWA Minutes, 1966–74, p.143.
5. *NZMJ*, April 1973, pp.219–29.
6. *NZMJ* April 1973, pp.258–9.
7. AKMWA Minute Book, p.244, NZMWA.
8. AHB Minute Book, October–December 1961, p.3517.
9. Typescript, A. Bush, 'Annual Report Paediatric Department', nd but placed by Dr Alison Hunter as c.1964, AFB.
10. Alice to Faulkner, 18 August 1971.
11. Typescript, 'Women, Medicine and the Royal College', AFB.
12. *Choice*, 8:2, May 1970, pp.20–3, 33; 9:2, May 1971, pp.19–24.
13. RCSS 35/6/257; 35/6/250; 35/6/244; 35/6/237; NA.
14. Correspondence, L.G.H. Sinclair to Secretary RCCSS, 17 December 1970; LFFCS Submissions, pp.4–5; AFB.
15. 'Zonta Club of Auckland – Submission to the Royal Commission on Social Security', Phase III, AFB.
16. Correspondence, Alice to Secretary, Auckland Division, NZBMA, 29 May 1970 and draft of submissions to Phase III, RCSS, ann. 1970, AFB.
17. Betty Holt to Phoebe Meikle, 27 May 1976, MC.
18. Cherry Raymond, Zonta tape, 30 March 1978, MC.
19. Marcia Russell, Valerie Davies, Colleen King, *Choice*, 12:1; Cherry Raymond, Zonta Tape, MC.
20. Correspondence, Alice to Deirdre Milne, Secretary, NOW, Auckland, 19 June 1972, AFB.
21. Correspondence, Mrs B. Read to Alice, 29 September 1967, Alice to Mrs Read, 16 October 1967; AFB.
22. 'Room for Upgrading in Status – but . . . .', *Auckland Star*, 27 August 1970.
23. Photocopied clipping, 'Lifetime of work with sick children', ann. *Auckland Star*, 24 May 1971, AFB.
24. H. May, *Minding Children, Managing Men*, pp.230–1.
25. Photocopy, NZMA Newsletter, II:6, May Day 1966, courtesy of Dr Erich Geiringer.
26. Typescript, 'The Family – Alice M. Bush', pp.15–16, 1, NZFPA.
27. Typescript, as above, pp.9–12; 3.
28. P. Bunkle, in S. Coney (ed.), *United Women's Convention 1973 Report*, Auckland, 1973, p.16.
29. A. Bush, 'Is Motherhood Enough?', p.35.
30. Annual Report, NZMWA, 1969, p.2.
31. Clipping, 'Women's Talents', ann. 24 April 1970, ns, AFB.
32. N.C. Begg, *The Child and His Family*, Christchurch, 1974, pp.20–1.
33. *NZMJ*, February 1961, p.61.
34. Typescript, 'The Family – Alice M. Bush', 1971, p.16, NZFPA.
35. A. Bush, 'The First Year – Mother and Child', *NE Patient Management*, August/September 1973, pp.9–15, AFB.
36. Ms notes, A. Bush, on draft submissions, AFB.
37. Typescript, AFB; see also 'The Family – Alice M. Bush', pp.22–3, NZFPA.
38. A. Bush, 'The First Year – Mother and Child', *NE Patient Management*, August/September 1973, AFB.
39. Correspondence, L.G.H. Sinclair to Dr B.W. Christmas, MOH, Auckland, 25 May 1966, H-A 13/9851, NA Auckland.
40. Correspondence, Peter Lewis to Alice, 20 February 1967, AFB.
41. Case Work Report for year ending 31 October 1969, Mrs D.M. Dunlop, Social Worker, LFFCS, AFB.
42. Clipping, *Thursday*, 8 June 1972, AFB.
43. Faulkner Bush, Narrative 9, p.58.
44. Correspondence, K. Robson, Registrar, RCP, London, to Alice Bush, 30 April 1970, AFB.
45. *College Commentary*, RCP London, July 1970, 4:4, pp.59–65, AFB.
46. B. Holt, Cyclostyled Typescript, 'Passing Parade of Women', p.15, AUL.
47. Cody, pp.10–11.

48. Combined Medical Staff Minute Book, 1962–70, minutes 17 May 1967 and following, NA Auckland.
49. Corrected draft copy of notes taken on 24 July 1963 by D.R. Goodfellow, Medical Superintendent of Auckland Hospital, on Alice's behalf, Goodfellow to Alice, nd, AFB.
50. Alice to Chairman, 17 September 1963, AFB.
51. Typescript, 'A Statement of Concern', nd but c. 1966, AFB.
52. Photocopy, Henley to Medical Superintendent, Auckland Hospital, 25 May 1966, AFB.
53. Paediatric Staff minutes, 13 June 1966, p.1, photocopied memorandum, Henley to Goodfellow, 23 September 1965; AFB.
54. Correspondence, Alice to J. Costello, Secretary, Paediatric Staff, Auckland Hospital, 30 May 1966, photocopy, AFB.
55. Auckland Parents' Centre Newsletter, June 1966, AFB.
56. *NZH*, 15 July 1966, p.4.
57. Correspondence, Alice to 'Pat' (T.H.C) Caughey, 15 July 1966, AFB.
58. T.H.C. Caughey to Alice, 19 July 1966, AFB.
59. Circular-letter, 18 July 1966, AFB.
60. Correspondence, Henley to Alice, 29 July 1966, AFB.
61. Paediatric Staff minutes, 1 August 1966, p.2, AFB.
62. Paediatric Staff minutes, 1 August 1966, AFB.
63. Paediatric Staff minutes, 5 December 1966, p.1, AFB.
64. 'Ways in which Zonta might help the Children's Hospital', attached to Alice to Mrs B. Simmons, Hon. Sec., Zonta Club of Auckland, 7 December 1966, AFB.
65. Alice to Henley, 19 January 1970, AFB.
66. Henley to Alice, 28 January 1970, AFB.
67. Minute Book II, p.105, PSNZ.
68. Clipping, 'Rotary Plan for $400,000 Gift', ann. *NZH*, 22 June 1971, PSNZ.
69. Interview, Professor R.B. Elliott, 26 October 1989; S. Ludbrook, 'Paediatrics in New Zealand', *NZMJ*, May 1972, p.262.
70. Notes made by Phoebe Meikle in conversation with Alison Hunter, 24 June 1979, MC.
71. Ms 'Zonta – Recommendations towards a reconstruction of Health Care Services', AFB.
72. Clipping, 'Malnutrition in N. Z. Babies', *Press*, 9 September 1969, AFB.
73. *NZMJ*, July 1965, p.397.
74. Paediatric Staff minutes, 1 August 1966, p.2, AFB.
75. Correspondence, Helen Evans Reid to Phoebe Meikle, 25 May 1979, MC.
76. Correspondence, Alice to Dr C.P. Anyon, Lower Hutt, 11 June 1969, AFB.
77. Correspondence, Alice to North, 10 January 1969, AFB.
78. A. Bush, 'Allergy Over a Quarter Century', *NZMJ*, August 1968, p.101.
79. Clipping: 'Health Plan for Youth', ann. *Central Leader*, 8 October 1968; correspondence, M.C. Ensor, Returning Officer, to A. Bush, 22 October 1968, AFB.
80. AKMWA Minute Book, 1966–74, p.54, NZMWA.
81. Correspondence, Alice to North, 10 January 1969, AFB.

12 Reproductive Politics

1. A. Bush, 'Abortion: A Personal View', ALRANZ, August 1971, p.3, AFB.
2. Correspondence, Alice to Secretary, Students' Association, University of Canterbury, Christchurch, 8 June 1970, AFB.
3. Correspondence, Alice to the Editors, *The Little Red Schoolbook*, 1 May 1972, AFB.
4. Correspondence, Alister Taylor to Alice, 19 June 1972, AFB.
5. Correspondence, Alice to Alister Taylor, 9 August 1972, AFB.
6. Correspondence, Alan C. Webster to Alice, 18 August 1972, AFB.
7. Correspondence, Alice to Deirdre Milne, NOW, Auckland, 19 June

1972, AFB.
8. Alice to Faulkner, 30 May 1940.
9. Faulkner to Alice, 4 June 1940.
10. Alice to Faulkner, 8 June 1940.
11. Faulkner to Alice, 10 June 1940.
12. Alice to Faulkner, 2 March 1944.
13. *Craccum*, 27 March 1944, p.3.
14. 'Our Population Problems', *NZWW*, 14 September 1944, pp.18–19.
15. Faulkner to Alice, 25 May 1944, and ann. WAFB post-1974.
16. Occasional references in practice correspondence, AFB.
17. Correspondence, Olive Johnson to Jean Dawson, 5 July 1938, Birth Reg. Ms Papers 1388:2, ATL.
18. Clipping, 'Family Planning', *Evening Post*, 4 July 1964, NZFPA.
19. Report of IPPF Conference, Europe, Near East, Africa, in *Choice*, 2:3, November 1964, p.11.
20. Correspondence, Alice to Mrs M. Pearson, IPPF, London, 16 June 1969, AFB.
21. Clipping, 'Finding diseased embryo seen as boon to parents', ann. *Star*, 17 December 1971, AFB.
22. Clipping, *Press*, 9 September 1969, AFB.
23. Correspondence to Alice, 1 October 1969, AFB.
24. Standing Committee minutes, 4 November 1969, p.2.
25. President's Report, Auckland Branch, 1969, p.2, NZFPA.
26. AKMWA minutes, 10 September, 1970, NZMWA.
27. Clipping, 'Abortion Laws Unfair In Doctor's View', ann. *Herald*, 22 September 1970, AFB.
28. Minutes, 10th Biennial Conference, 25–27 September 1970, pp.4, 6, AFB.
29. Correspondence, Carol Shand to Alice, 17 November 1971, AFB.
30. Alice to Carol Shand, 6 December 1971, AFB.
31. *NZMJ*, October 1968, p.257.
32. Quoted in M. Pryor, *The Right to Live*, Auckland 1986, p.17.
33. Clipping, 'Abortion – how live an issue in NZ today?', *Auckland Star*, 20 June 1970, NZFPA.
34. APC Newsletter, No.1, August 1966, p.2.
35. Alice to R.N. Howie, 30 November 1970, PSNZ.
36. Correspondence, Howie to Bush, 8 December 1970, PSNZ.
37. ALRANZ leaflet, NZFPA.
38. 'A Personal View', p.2.
39. 'A Personal View', p.3.
40. 'A Personal View', p.4.
41. 'A Personal View', p.3.
42. Correspondence, Bishop E.A. Gowing to Alice, 4 June 1970, AFB.
43. Clipping, 'Lifetime of work with sick children', *Star*, 24 May 1971, AFB.
44. Q/S Margaret Gatman, 21 January 1983, MC.
45. Clipping, 'Unwanted child not a nation builder', *South Auckland Courier*, 1 September 1971, NZFPA.
46. Clipping, 'Birth Control Issue – Now a Concern of the State', ann. *NZH*, 18 November 1971, AFB.
47. *NZMJ*, December 1971, p.411.
48. *Zealandia*, 7 May 1972, p.1, NZFPA.
49. Clipping, 'Is Population Pollution or Progress?', ns, c. January 1972, AFB.
50. Clipping, letter to editor, *NZH*, 24 January 1972, AFB.
51. Clippings, 'Experts Disagree on Polynesian Family Planning', ann. *Star*, 9 November 1971, 'Tapu Topic for Maoridom', *NZH*, 9 November 1971, AFB; 'No Tapu on family planning', *NZH*, 10 November 1971, p.14.
52. J. Metge, *New Growth From Old*, Wellington, 1995, p.22.
53. Ms, letter to editor, *NZH*, nd, AFB.
54. *Choice*, 7:1, February 1969, p.3.
55. *Craccum*, 18 March 1971, p.13.
56. P. Fenwick, 'The New Zealand Family Planning Association ...', MA thesis, University of Canterbury, pp.146, 238, 254–6.
57. Draft letter to be sent by NZFPA to Mrs Swingler, IPPF, London, nd but October/November 1969, AFB.
58. Correspondence, J. Wurzer, Boehringer Ingelheim, Christchurch, to Mary Taylor, Auckland Asthma Society, 5 March 1971, AFB.
59. Clipping, 'Effect Of Encyclical "Out Of Proportion"', ann. *Press*, 5 November 1968, NZFPA.
60. Correspondence, Alice to Mrs Joyce Johns, Administrative Asst. to

NOTES TO PAGES 222–229

Secretary-General, IPPF Central Office, London, nd but ann. 1970, AFB.
61. 'Report for IPPF SEAOR Council Meetings, March 28–30 1965', p.2, AFB.
62. Correspondence, Alice to Judy Heaps, NZFPA Christchurch, 6 June 1969, AFB.
63. Standing Committee minutes, attachment, 14 October 1969, and minutes 4 November, p.2, and 2 December 1969, p.1; Standing Committee minutes, 3 February 1970, p.1, NZFPA.
64. Draft letter to Mrs Swingler, as above; photocopy, R.J. Seddon et al., '"Micro-dose" Chlormadinone Acetate', Clinical Proceedings, IPPF SEAOR Congress, nd but post-1972, NZFPA.
65. Fenwick, thesis, pp.92–4.
66. Clipping, 'Cook Islands', letter to editor, ns, ann. 3 January 1972, AFB.
67. 'Report of Meeting . . . 7 December 1970', AFB.
68. Medical Advisory Committee minutes, attached to conference minutes, November 1968, p.7, AFB.
69. Correspondence from president, Hamilton branch, 18 September 1968, and Mrs J. Heaps, Christchurch, 6 June 1969; AFB.
70. Typescript, 'Meeting of the NZFPA Doctors. Held at Auckland on November 6th & 7th 1971', p.1, NZFPA; *Choice*, November 1968, p.3.
71. *Choice*, 10:4, November 1972, p.15.
72. Conference minutes, 1972, pp.7–8.
73. *Choice*, 10:4, November 1972, p.1.
74. Faulkner Bush Narrative 9, c. 1979, p.58, Narrative 8, pp.11–12, MC.
75. Fenwick thesis, pp.47, 57–2, 185–6.
76. *Choice*, 11:1, February 1973, p.31.
77. *Choice*, 11:1, February 1973, p.31; 11:2, May 1973, pp.30, 31, 22.

13 *The Quality of Life*

1. Correspondence, Alice to R.H. Smythe, Managing Director, New Zealand Forest Products, 10 June 1969, AFB.
2. Faulkner's Story, p.206.
3. Faulkner's Story and other information supplied by him; MC; entries in Alice's appointment diaries and other ephemera; AFB.
4. Faulkner's Story, pp.182–4.
5. *NZMJ*, vol 49, 1950, p.586–7.
6. Correspondence: to St James Assoc. of Presbyterian Women, Pukekohe, 14 April 1970; Pukekohe St Andrews Young Wives Group, 24 April 1970; Muscular Dystrophy Association of New Zealand Inc., 2 June 1971; Northern Wairoa Women's Club, Dargaville, 7 April 1971; Mr S. Hoare, Royal Oak, Auckland, 4 June 1971; AFB.
7. Correspondence, Alice to Stuart Macaskill, Upper Hutt, 15 April 1970, AFB.
8. Correspondence, Alice to Mary Taylor, 23 September 1970, AFB.
9. Faulkner's Story, pp.205, 232.
10. Clipping, 'Therapeutic Conferences – Angina Pectoris II', *BMJ* 6 March 1971, pp.545–6, AFB.
11. Correspondence to Treasurer, Auckland Hospital Board, 15 June 1970, AFB.
12. Correspondence, Alice to Rosemary Wheeler, 19 June 1972, AFB.
13. Mary Wood, 'Explosion on the Home Front', *NZFD*, February 1964, p.21.
14. Dr Ian Hassall, Q/S and correspondence, c.1981, MC; interview, Sister June Milne, 20 April 1989; Faulkner's Story, p.232.
15. *Choice*, 11:2, May 1973, p.11.
16. Correspondence, Alice to Dr David Scott, 5 June 1973, AFB.
17. Mary Taylor, Q/S, 30 September 1980, MC.
18. Cherry Raymond, Zonta tape, 30 March 1978, MC.
19. Correspondence, Alice to Dr F. Moody, Superintendent-in-Chief, AHB, 25 June 1973, AFB.
20. Memo from Medical Superintendent, Auckland Hospital, 29 December 1973, quoted 25 February 1974, Staffing & Appointments Committee Book 1973–74, A695/104, NA Auckland.
21. Correspondence, Betty Neal to Faulkner, 8 June 1975, AFB.
22. Alice to Peter, 3 October 1968;

Additional material from Faulkner, 17 March 1977.
23. Typescript: Summary of paper given by Alice Bush attached to Minutes of meeting of Committee for the Co-operation of Men and Women in the [Anglican] Church, Hamilton, 16 July 1965; Minutes, Connexional Commission on Family Life, Trinity College, Auckland, 29 July 1967; AFB.
24. Faulkner Bush, Narrative 4, p.29.
25. Typescript, 'The Family . . .', p.5, NZFPA.
26. 'Abortion: A Personal View, p.2, AFB.
27. Clipping, 'Public upset at way doctors use powers', ann. *Star*, 29 October 1971, AFB.
28. Clipping, 13 November 1971, p.9, AFB.
29. Alice, Mss notes, nd but c. November 1971; correspondence, G.T. Upton, Editor-in-chief, New Zealand Newspapers Limited to Alice, 16 November 1971, copies to Auckland Hospital Board, Dr R.J. Methven, Marinoto Clinic, Professor C. Lewis, Dean, Auckland Medical School, Mr S. Tong; correspondence, G.T. Upton to Alice, 16 November 1971, Alice to Dr Shirley Tonkin, 18 November 1971; clipping, 'Apology to Dr Bush, ann. *8 O'Clock*, 29 November, 1971, AFB.
30. Alice to Faulkner, 8 April 1940.
31. Clippings, 'Capping week charity', ns but probably Christchurch paper, c. 8 April 1972; 'G.P.'s Wary Over Clinics', ann. *NZH*, 19 January 1973; NZFPA.
32. Clipping, 'Unwanted Child Not Nation Builder', *South Auckland Courier*, eastern edition, 1 September 1971, p.12, NZFPA.
33. *Choice*, 11:1, February 1973, p.9.
34. Clipping, 'We need those clinics, women insist', ann. *NZH*, 7 March 1973, NZFPA.
35. Clippings, 'Don't give up on family doctor women told', ns, ann. 14 March 1973 and response from Ruth Black on behalf of NZFPA Medical Advisory Committee, NZFPA.
36. Auckland Branch, minutes of doctors' meeting in association with general staff meeting, 9 April; NZFPA 'Medical Ethics', duplicated typescript, 13 June 1973, AFB.
37. Clipping, 'Family Planning Aims Explained at local Gathering', ann. 2 October 1973, NZFPA.
38. Clipping, '"Spacing" Aim of Family Planning', ann. *Christchurch Star*, 9 September 1969.
39. *Thursday*, 6 September 1973, p.35.
40. Correspondence, Alice to Angela Jelicich-Ranford, 18 April, 1973, AFB.
41. *Choice*, 12:1, March 1974, p.15.
42. NZFPA Standing Committee minutes, 14 August 1973, p.1.
43. Clipping, 'New Outlook Vital for Survival of Mankind', ann. *Courier*, 23 August 1973, AFB.
44. Clipping, 'Postscript', ann. *Sunday Herald*, 5 August 1973, AFB.
45. *Choice* 11:2, May 1973, p.5.
46. NZFPA Standing Committee minutes, 11 September 1973, p.2.
47. *Choice*, 11:1, February 1973, p.19.
48. Minutes, Advisory Board Meeting, 1 March 1973, p.2, AFB.
49. *NZMJ*, August 1970, p.143; the first reference for vasectomy in her papers is dated 7 August 1961, AFB.
50. Correspondence, Alice to Mrs M. Becroft, Hon. Sec., Muscular Dystrophy Assoc., 2 June 1971, AFB.
51. Correspondence, Alice to Bernard Brown, University of Auckland Law School, 13 June 1972.
52. Alice to Faulkner, 1 March 1973.
53. Minutes, Advisory Board Meeting, 1 March 1973, p.2, attached to memo from Marcia G. Arnold, Coordinator, ICAVS, to Alice, 15 March 1973, AFB.
54. Alice to Faulkner, 12 March 1973.
55. Clements interview, 20 September 1989.
56. Minutes of Abortion Consultation, 27–8 February 1973, AFB.
57. Alice to Faulkner, 28 February 1973.
58. Clipping, 'More Baby Bashing Feared!', ann. *Sunday News*, 25 March 1973, AFB.
59. P. Bunkle, 'A Woman's Right to Choose', *2nd Opinion*, Auckland, 1988, pp.10–11; S. Coney, in A. Else (ed.), 'Health Organisations', *Women*

Together, p.250.
60. *NZMJ*, 24 April 1974, pp.862, 864.
61. Clipping, 'Family Planning Aims Explained at Local Gathering', ann. *Courier*, 2 October 1973, NZFPA.
62. Clipping, '"Abortions for $300" at private hospital', *Press*, 14 August 1973, Scrapbook 9, Wayne Facer Collection, NZFPA, courtesy Charlotte Parkes.
63. Clipping, 'Abortion', ns, ann. 27 August 1973, AFB.
64. Correspondence to Alice from the Hon. P. Amos, 12 September 1973; N. King, 17 August 1973; R. Tizard, 11 September 1973, AFB.
65. MSS, Draft letter to Hon. Norman King, Minister of Social Welfare, from Alice, nd but c. August 1973, AFB.
66. Correspondence, Alice to Dianne [sic] Shanahan, NZBC, Wellington, 12 June 1972; AGM minutes, PSNZ, 1971, p.23; AFB.
67. Faulkner's Story, p.234.
68. Clipping, 'Sparkling with Frost', ann. *Thursday*, 13 September 1973, AFB.
69. Clipping, 'You don't have to be a parent', *Courier*, 14 March 1974, p.14, AFB.
70. *Choice*, 11:3, September 1973, p.11.
71. Correspondence, Alice to Dr P. Eisdell Moore, Auckland, 10 November 1970, AFB; Faulkner's Story, p.222.
72. Faulkner's Story, p.227.
73. Faulkner's Story, pp.234, 235.
74. Auckland Branch NZFPA report, December 1972–73, p.1, AFB.
75. Typescript, Mrs D. Bennett, Northbridge, Auckland, 10 July 1974, MC.
76. Convention Report, p.8.
77. Convention Report, p.4.
78. Typescript, 'Manu Rere – Bird in Flight', p.3, NZFPA.
79. Convention Report, pp.66–7.
80. Maxwell, *Women Doctors in New Zealand*, pp.87–8.
81. Clipping, 'The Quiet Women Who Work for Others', *NZH*, ann. 13 November 1973, AFB.
82. Faulkner Bush, Narrative 5, p.17. Ruth Black also recalled this attitude on Alice's part, interview, 7 June 1989.
83. NZFPA Standing Committee minutes, 13 November 1973, p.3.
84. Correspondence, D.I. Houghton to Faulkner, 20 February 1974, AFB.
85. *NZWW*, 18 February 1974, p.19.
86. Correspondence, Peter Cardinal McKeefrey, Archbishop of NZ, to Alice, 17 September 1973, AFB.
87. Correspondence, Dunn to Alice, 21 January 1974; Alice to Dunn, 4 February 1974, AFB.
88. *Choice*, 12:3, pp.5, 7, 8.
89. *Choice*, 12:1, p.7.
90. Faulkner's Story, p.240.
91. Faulkner's Story, p.241. The entire account of Alice's death is taken from here, pp.239–41, and a typescript of further material provided by Faulkner, '1973–4 AMB's Heart Attack and Death', MC.
92. J. Rymer, 'Dr Alice Bush – "And the greatest of these is love"', 16 February 1974, typescript courtesy of Betty Neal.
93. Correspondence, Peter Godfrey to Faulkner, 16 February 1974, AFB; correspondence, Joan Wharton, 21 April 1982, MC.
94. *Choice*, 13:4, p.25.
95. Clipping, *Western Leader*, 27 November 1986.
96. Clipping, *NZH*, 15 May 1974, AFB.
97. Maxwell, *Women Doctors in New Zealand*, pp.43, 45, 54.
98. Clippings, *Star*, 13 January 1975; *NZH*, 14 January 1975, AFB.
99. Clipping, ann. *Star*, 31 October 1974, AFB.

SELECTED BIBLIOGRAPHY

1 *Archives*

NATIONAL ARCHIVES (AUCKLAND)
Auckland Hospital Board Records and Minute Books.
Divorce Proceedings Records.
Health Department Records.
Probate Records.

NATIONAL ARCHIVES (WELLINGTON)
Health Department Records.
Royal Commission of Inquiry into Social Security in New Zealand 1969 Records.
Witness Statements, Select Committee on Dominion Population, 1946. Evidence prepared by the Family Planning Association of New Zealand to Present before the Parliamentary Select Committee on Dominion Population, April, 1946, Le 1/1946/3.

ALEXANDER TURNBULL LIBRARY
Maori Women's Welfare League Collection, Ms Papers 1396.
New Zealand Special Committee on Moral Delinquency in Children and Adolescents, 1953–54, Ms Papers 2384.
Sex Hygiene and Birth Regulation Society Collection, Ms Papers 1388.

AUCKLAND INSTITUTE AND MUSEUM
Women's Archives.
YWCA Archives.

MISCELLANEOUS ARCHIVES
Alice and Faulkner Bush Papers; correspondence held by the Bush family and supplementary material by the late Phoebe Meikle, Auckland.
Auckland College and Grammar School Archives, Auckland Grammar School.
Auckland Scrapbooks, Auckland Central Public Library.
Auckland University Students' Association Archives, University of Auckland.
Diocesan High School Archives, Diocesan High School, Auckland.
Hill Top School Archives, Hill Top School, Blockhouse Bay, Auckland.
King's College; photocopied school records, courtesy of the headmaster, King's College, Auckland.
Land Transfer Office Records, Auckland.
Meikle Collection, the property of the late Phoebe Meikle, Auckland.
Methodist Church Archives, Auckland.
National Council of Women Archives, NCW Headquarters, Wellington.
New Zealand Family Planning Association Archives, Auckland Branch Library.
New Zealand Medical Association (Auckland Division) Minute Books of Quarterly

271   SELECTED BIBLIOGRAPHY

Meetings, February 1959–April 1985, and Annual General Meeting Minutes, December 1963–1987, NZMA Auckland Division Office, Marion Davis Library, Auckland Hospital.
New Zealand Medical Women's Association Archives.
Paediatric Society of New Zealand Papers, held by current executive.
Prince Albert College Papers, St John's College Library, Auckland.
Registers of Births, Deaths and Marriages.
WNSC Memorabilia. The Sherwin Family Scrapbook, supplied by Mrs Joyce Jackways, Auckland, and newspaper clippings supplied by Mrs Betty Morris.

2   Official Publications

Appendices to the Journals of the House of Representatives:
Report of the Committee of Inquiry into the Various Aspects of the Problem of Abortion in New Zealand, H-31A, 1937.
Report of the Dominion Population Committee, I-17, 1946.
Report of the Special Committee on Moral Delinquency in Children and Adolescents, H-47, 1954.
Report of the Royal Commission of Inquiry into Social Security in New Zealand, H-53, Vol. IV, 1972.
Review of Maternal and Child Health, H-31, 1969.
Report of the Consultative Committee on Hospital Reform, Government Printer, Wellington, 1953.

3   Newspapers and Periodicals

Auckland Star
Auckland Weekly News
British Medical Journal
Choice
Craccum
Diocesan High School Chronicle
Mirror
New Zealand Herald
New Zealand Journal of Family Planning
New Zealand Medical Journal
New Zealand Methodist Times
New Zealand Truth
New Zealand Woman's Weekly
Otago University Review
The Digest
The Lancet
The Medical Journal of Australia
The New Zealand Nursing Journal
Western Leader

4   Published Works

Abrams, R., *'Send us a Lady Physician': Women Doctors in America, 1835–1920*, New York, 1985.
Aitken, J., *A Woman's Place?: A Study of the Changing Role of Women in New Zealand*, Auckland, 1975.
Antler, J., 'Feminism as Life-Process: The Life and Career of Lucy Sprague Mitchell.' *Feminist Studies*, 7, No.1, Spring, 1981, pp.134–57.

Auckland and District Telephone Directory, 1941, 1943.
Banks, J.A., *Prosperity and Parenthood*, London, 1954.
Barrett, J., *Cancer & Cure: A Doctor's Story*, London, 1976.
Barrington, R. and Gray, A., *The Smith Women*, Wellington, 1981.
Bassett, M., 'The 1935 Election and the "Kelly Gang": An American Observation', *NZJH*, Vol.28, No.1, April 1994, pp.80-5.
Begg, N.C., *The Child and His Family*, Christchurch, 1974, (1st ed., 1970, revised 1972).
Belgrave, M., 'A Subtle Containment: Women in New Zealand Medicine, 1893-1941', *NZJH*, April 1988, Vol.22, No.1, pp.44-55.
Bell, E. Moberly, *Storming the Citadel*, London, 1953.
Bevan-Brown, M., *Nerves, Nerviness & Neurosis*, Lighthouse Series, No.2, Christchurch 1945.
Binney, J. and Chaplin, G., *Nga Morehu: The Survivors*, Auckland, 1986.
Bolitho, D.G., 'Some Financial and Medico-Political Aspects of the New Zealand Medical Profession's Reaction to the Introduction of Social Security', *NZJH*, Vol.18, No.1, April 1984, pp.34-49.
Bowlby, J., *Maternal Care and Mental Health*, Geneva, 1952.
Bowlby, J., *Child Care and the Growth of Love*, London, 1953.
Bowman, M.A., and Allen, D.I., *Stress and Women Physicians*, New York, 1985.
Bretos, C.T., *Women in the Medical Profession*, University of NSW, 1980.
Brookes, B., *Abortion in England, 1900-67*, London, 1988.
Brookes, B., 'Housewives' Depression: The Debate over Abortion and Birth Control in the 1930s', *NZJH*, Vol.15, No.2, October 1981, pp.115-34.
Brookes, B., Macdonald, C., Tennant, M. (eds), *Women in History*, Wellington, 1986.
Bryder, L. (ed.), *A Healthy Country: Essays on the Social History of Medicine in New Zealand*, Wellington, 1991.
Bryson, E., *Look Back in Wonder*, Dundee, 1965.
Buist, Father J.D., *New Zealand Faces Disaster: Birth Control, Abortion and Other Evils*, Wellington, 1943.
Bunkle, P., *Second Opinion: The Politics of Women's Health in New Zealand*, Auckland, 1988.
Bunkle, P. and Hughes, B., *Women in New Zealand Society*, Auckland, 1980.
Bush, A., *Personal Relationships*, Auckland, 1944.
Bush, A. et al., *A National Health Service*, Wellington, 1943.
Cole, E., *Where Did I Come From?*, Family Planning Association, c.1942.
Coney, S., *Every Girl*, Auckland, 1986.
Coney, S., *Standing in the Sunshine: A History of New Zealand Women Since They Won the Vote*, Auckland, 1993.
Coney, S. and Bunkle, P., *The Unfortunate Experiment*, Auckland, 1988.
Coney, S. (ed.), *United Women's Convention 1973 Report*, Auckland, 1973.
Contraception, Sterilisation and Abortion in New Zealand: Report of the Royal Commission of Inquiry, Government Printer, Wellington, 1977.
Cook, E. *Sex "Education"*, Lighthouse Series, No.6, Christchurch, 1945.
Cook, E. and Bevan-Brown, M., *The Psychology of Childbirth*, Lighthouse Series, No.9, Christchurch, 1947.
Cook, R. (ed.), *Portrait of a Profession: Centennial Book of the New Zealand Law Society*, Wellington, 1969.
Cowan, J., *The Maoris in the Great War*, Auckland, 1926.
Dalziel, R., *Focus on the Family: The Auckland Home and Family Society, 1893-1993*, Auckland, 1993.
Davis, P., *Health and Health Care in New Zealand*, Auckland, 1981.
Dawson, M. and Radi, H. (eds), *Against the Odds*, Sydney, 1984.
Day, P., *Women Doctors: Choices and Constraints in Policies for Medical Manpower*, London, 1982.
Dobbie, M., *The Trouble with Women: The Story of Parents' Centre New Zealand*, Queen Charlotte Sound, 1990.
Dominion Settlement and Population Association, *New Zealand Must Populate or Perish*, Wellington, c.1944.
Ebbett, E., *Victoria's Daughters*, Wellington, 1981.

SELECTED BIBLIOGRAPHY

Ebbett, E., *When the Boys were Away*, Wellington, 1984.
Edmond, L. (ed.), *Women in Wartime*, Wellington, 1986.
Else, A., *A Question of Adoption: Closed Stranger Adoption in New Zealand 1944–1974*, Wellington, 1991.
Else, A. (ed.), *Women Together: A History of Women's Organisations in New Zealand/Nga Ropu Wahine o te Motu*, Wellington, 1993.
Epstein, C.F., *Woman's Place: Options and Limits in Professional Careers*, Berkley, Los Angeles and London, 1970.
Fett, I., 'The Future of Women in Australian Medicine', Special Supplement, *The Medical Journal of Australia*, November 1976, pp.33–9.
Fry, R., *'It's different for daughters': A History of the Curriculum for Girls in New Zealand Schools, 1900–1975*, Wellington, 1985.
Fry, R., *Out of the Silence: Methodist Women of Aotearoa, 1822–1925*, Christchurch, 1987.
Gatlin, R., *American Women Since 1945*, Jackson, USA, 1987.
Gerson, K., *Hard Choices: How Women Decide about Work, Career, and Motherhood*, Berkeley, 1985.
Gilson, M., 'Population Growth in Post-war New Zealand', in *Social Process in New Zealand*, J. Foster (ed.), Auckland, 1969, pp.29–48.
Gilson, M., 'Women in Employment', in *Social Process in New Zealand*, J. Foster (ed.), Auckland, 1969, pp.183–97.
Gordon, D., *Backblocks Baby Doctor*, London, 1955.
Gordon, D., *Doctor Down Under*, London, 1957.
Gordon, L., *Woman's Body, Woman's Right*, New York, 1976.
Grimshaw, P. and Strahan, L. (eds), *The Half-open Door*, Sydney, 1984.
Hames, E.A., *100 Years at Pitt Street*, Auckland, 1966.
Hanson, E., *The Politics of Social Security*, Auckland, 1980.
Hardyment, C., *Dream Babies: Three Centuries of Good Advice on Child Care*, New York, 1983.
Health Department Sex Education Series: *Sex and the Parent; Sex and the Young Child; Sex: The Adolescent and Sex: The Parents Role; Sex and the Adolescent Boy; Sex and the Adolescent Girl*; Wellington, 1955.
Heins, M. et al., 'Attitudes of Women and Men Physicians', *American Journal of Public Health*, November 1979, pp.1132–9.
Hercus, C. and Bell, G., *The Otago Medical School Under the First Three Deans*, Edinburgh/London, 1964.
Heslop, B., et al., 'Women in Medicine in New Zealand', *NZMJ*, Vol.77, April 1973, pp.219–29.
Holt, B., Herd, J., Horsman, D., *Women in Council: A History of the National Council of Women*, Wellington, 1980.
Houston, H.S. (ed.), *Marriage and the Family in New Zealand*, Wellington, 1970.
Hughes, B., 'Early Women Doctors in New Zealand', in *Papers of Women Studies Association Inaugural Conference, University of Waikato, August 1978*, Hamilton, 1978.
Jackson, H.R., *Churches and People in Australia and New Zealand, 1860–1930*, Wellington, 1987.
Jones, D.W. Carmalt, *Annals of the Otago Medical School, 1875–1939*, Wellington, 1945.
Kennedy, D.M., *Birth Control in America*, New Haven, 1970.
Koopman-Boyden, P. (ed.), *Families in New Zealand Society*, Wellington, 1978.
Koopman-Boyden, P., and Scott, C., *The Family and Government Policy in New Zealand*, Sydney/London/Boston, 1984.
Latimer, R.J. (ed.), *Health Administration in New Zealand*, Wellington, 1969.
Leathard, A., *The Fight for Family Planning*, London/Basingstoke, 1980.
Leeson, J., and Gray, J., *Women and Medicine*, London, 1978.
Lineham, P.J., *New Zealanders and the Methodist Evangel*, Auckland, 1983.
Lopate, C., *Women in Medicine*, Baltimore, 1968.
Lorber, J., *Women Physicians: Careers, Status and Power*, New York, 1984.
Lovell-Smith, J.B., *The New Zealand Doctor and the Welfare State*, Auckland, 1966.
Manson, C. and Manson, C., *Dr Agnes Bennett*, London, 1960.
Marieskind, H.I., *Women in the Health System*, St Louis, 1980.

Markell, R., Pomerlea, C., Fenichel, C. (eds), *In Her Own Words: Oral Histories of Women Physicians*, Connecticut, 1982.
Masters, D.S., 'The Children's Hospitals of Auckland', *Auckland Hospital Registered Nurses Club Newsletter*, March and July 1992.
Max, L., *Children: Endangered Species?*, Auckland, 1990.
Maxwell, M., *Women Doctors in New Zealand: An Historical Perspective*, Auckland, 1990.
May, H., *Minding Children, Managing Men: Conflict and Compromise in the Lives of Postwar Pakeha Women*, Wellington, 1992.
McKinlay, Robin, *The Care of Children in New Zealand Hospitals*, Dunedin, 1982.
McKinney, J.B., *Official History of New Zealand in the Second World War 1939–45: Medical Units*, Wellington, 1952.
McLaglan, E.B., *Stethoscope and Saddlebags*, Auckland, 1965.
Meikle, P., *Accidental Life*, Auckland, 1994.
Metge, J., *New Growth from Old: The Whanau in the Modern World*, Wellington, 1995.
Middleton, S. (ed.), *Women and Education in Aotearoa*, Wellington, 1988.
Morrell, W.P., *The University of Otago, A Centennial History*, Dunedin, 1969.
Murchie, E., *Rapuora: Health and Maori Women*, Wellington, 1984.
Nadelson, T. and Eisenberg, L., 'The Successful Professional Woman: On Being Married to One', *The American Journal of Psychiatry*, October, 1977, pp.1071–6.
National Council of Churches in New Zealand, *Men and Women*, Christchurch/Dunedin, 1953.
National Council of Churches in New Zealand, Women's Committee, *Homes and Families*, Christchurch/Dunedin, 1950.
Neville, R.J.W. and O'Neill, C.J. (eds), *The Population of New Zealand: Interdisciplinary Perspectives*, Auckland, 1979.
NZFPA, *Sex Problems in Marriage I*, nd but c. 1950s.
New Zealand Five Million Club (Report of the Birth Rate Committee), *After the First 100 Years*, Wellington, 1939.
Oliver, W.H. (ed.), *The Oxford History of New Zealand*, Wellington, 1981.
Olssen, E., 'Truby King and the Plunket Society: An Analysis of a Prescriptive Ideology', *NZJH*, Vol.15, No.1, April 1981, pp.3–23.
Parry, G., *A Fence at the Top: The First 75 Years of the Plunket Society*, Dunedin, 1977.
Phillips, J.O.C., *A Man's Country? The Image of the Pakeha Male*, Auckland, 1987.
Preston, F., *Lady Doctor, Vintage Model*, Wellington, 1974.
Progressive Publishing Company, *Venereal Disease: The Shadow Over New Zealand*, Wellington, 1942.
Pryor, M., *The Right to Live: The Abortion Battle of New Zealand*, Auckland, 1986.
Reed, J., *The Birth Control Movement and American Society: From Private Vice to Public Virtue*, Princeton, 1978.
Ritchie, J. and J., *Growing up in New Zealand*, Sydney, 1978.
Robb, D., *Medical Odyssey0*, Auckland, 1968.
Robb, D., *Medicine and Health in New Zealand*, Auckland, 1940.
Scarr, S., *Mother Care/Other Care*, New York, 1984.
Scholefield, G.H., *Who's Who in New Zealand and the Western Pacific*, Masterton, 1908.
Scholefield, G.H. (ed.), *Who's Who in New Zealand, 1925*, Masterton, 1924.
Schwimmer, E. (ed.), *The Maori People in the Nineteen-Sixties*, Auckland, 1968
Sinclair, K., *Walter Nash*, Auckland, 1976.
Sinclair, K., *A History of the University of Auckland*, Auckland, 1983.
Sinclair, K., 'The Lee-Sutch Syndrome', *NZJH*, Vol.8, No.2, October 1974, pp.95–117.
Smith, P.L.M., *Maternity in Dispute*, Wellington, 1986.
Summers, A., 'A Home from Home – Women's Philanthropic Work in the Nineteenth Century', in Burman, S. (ed.), *Fit Work for Women*, New York, 1979.
Sutch, W.B., *The Quest for Security in New Zealand: 1840–1966*, Wellington, 1966.
Sutch, W.B., *The Responsible Society in New Zealand*, Christchurch, 1971.
Taylor, N.M., *The Home Front: The New Zealand People at War*, Vols I and II, Wellington, 1986.

275   SELECTED BIBLIOGRAPHY

The Auckland Provincial Directory, 1932–33, pt I and pt II
The Welfare of Children in Hospital, Report of the Committee on the Welfare of Children in Hospital, Ministry of Health [The Platt Report], United Kingdom, Her Majesty's Stationery Office, London, 1959.
Tolerton, J., *Ettie: A Life of Ettie Rout*, Auckland/Harmondsworth, Middlesex, England, 1992.
Trembath, K.A., *Ad Augusta: A Centennial History of Auckland Grammar School, 1869–1969*, Auckland, 1969.
Vicinus, M. (ed.), *A Widening Sphere: Changing roles of Victorian women*, Bloomington, 1977.
Watson, J.E., 'Marriages of Women Teachers', *New Zealand Journal of Educational Studies*, Vol.1, No.2, 1966, pp.149–60.
Weeks, J., *Sex, Politics and Society*, Essex, 1981.
Wright, Helena, *The Sex Factor in Marriage*, 3rd ed., 1941, London (1st ed., 1930).
Wright, Helena, *More About the Sex Factor in Marriage*, London, 1959 (1st ed., 1947).
Wright-St Clair, R.E., *A History of the New Zealand Medical Association*, Wellington, 1987.
Yohalem, A.M., *The Careers of Professional Women: Commitment and Conflict*, New York, 1979.

5   Unpublished Works

Anderson, Kathleen, 'Beyond the Pioneer Woman Doctor: A Study of Women Doctors in Auckland, 1900–1960', MA thesis, University of Auckland, March 1992.
Bassett, J.O., 'Contraception as a Woman's Issue', Women and the Law Seminar Paper, 1979, University of Auckland.
Bassett, J.O., 'Great Expectations: The Children and Young Persons Act 1974–1982', Dissertation for LLB (Hons), University of Auckland, March 1983.
Belgrave, M., 'Medical Men and lady Doctors', PhD thesis, Victoria University of Wellington, 1985.
Bishop, S., '"Married with Children": Perceptions of New Zealand Women's Lives in the 1950s.', BA Hons research essay, University of Otago, 1991.
Bolitho, D.G., 'The Response of the New Zealand Medical Profession to the Introduction of Social Security', MA thesis, Victoria University of Wellington, 1979.
Bourke, J., 'Catholic Fertility in Australia and New Zealand, 1880–1939', MA thesis, University of Auckland, 1985.
Burgin, A.M., 'Women in Public Life and Politics in New Zealand', MA thesis, Victoria University of Wellington, 1967.
Chandler, H.M., 'Mary Manson Dreaver – Political Woman', MA research essay, University of Auckland, 1984.
Cody, Paula, 'Women Psychiatrists in New Zealand 1900–1990', MA thesis, University of Otago, August 1966.
Conference Papers, Federation of New Zealand Parents' Centres Conference, 15–17 February 1963, Palmerston North University College.
Dobbie, M., 'History of the New Zealand Family Planning Association', c.1981, typescript held at the National Office, NZFPA, Auckland.
Edwards, V., 'New Children's Hospitals of the Past', paper presented to the Auckland Medical Historical Society, 18 August 1988.
Fenwick, P., 'The New Zealand Family Planning Association: Its Growth and Development', MA thesis, University of Canterbury, 1977.
Fleming, P., 'Eugenics in New Zealand, 1900–1940', MA thesis, Massey University, 1981.
Fougere, G., 'Exit, Voice and the Decay of the Welfare State Provision of Hospital Care', MA thesis, University of Canterbury, 1974.
Glazebrook, S.G.M., 'The Mazengarb Report, 1954: Impotent Victorianism', MA research essay, University of Auckland, 1978.
Golding, K.D., 'Popular Concepts of the New Zealand Woman's Role and Self-Image Between the First World War and the Great Depression', MA research essay,

University of Auckland, 1978.
Griffiths, S., 'Feminism and the Ideology of Motherhood', MA thesis, University of Otago, 1984.
Holt, B., 'Passing Parade of Women', a pageant presented by the Auckland Branch of NCW to celebrate the 82nd anniversary of Suffrage Day, 19 September, 1975, International Women's Year, University of Auckland Library.
James, B.L., 'The Maori Women's Welfare League: From Social Movement to Voluntary Association', MSSc thesis, University of Waikato, 1977.
Jones, J.I., 'Towards a Dual System', MA research essay, University of Auckland, 1979.
Masters, D.S., 'The Change in Attitudes Toward Hospital Visiting in Paediatric Areas', privately held, c.1975.
McKinlay, R., 'Where Would We Be Without Them? Motherhood and Self-definition in New Zealand', PhD thesis, Victoria University of Wellington, 1986.
Montgomerie, D.A., '"A Personal Affair between me and Hitler?", Public Attitudes to Women's Paid Work in New Zealand during World War Two', MA thesis, University of Auckland, 1986.
Simpson, A.J., 'The New Zealand Medical Lobby: A Study in Conflict', MA thesis, University of Canterbury, 1968.
Thomson, J.R.M., 'The Rehabilitation of Servicemen of World War Two in New Zealand, 1940–54', PhD thesis, Victoria University of Wellington, 1983.
van Rooyen, J.C., 'Women in Medicine', Occasional Paper, Department of Health, Wellington, 1978.
Woods, M.A., 'The Emotional Needs of Young Children in Hospital', MA thesis, University of Auckland, 1975.

6 Correspondence

Ms B. Booth, Assistant Archivist, Hocken Library, University of Otago, 13 August 1987.
Dr M. Chieffi, Wellington, 26 July 1987.
J. Crawford, Research Officer, History, Ministry of Defence, Wellington, 25 May 1987.
Ms Sherrah Francis, National Archives, Wellington.
Dr Erich Geiringer, Wellington, 15 November 1989.
Sir Edmund Hillary, Auckland, 29 November 1989.
Professor B. Heslop, Department of Surgery, University of Otago Medical School, 18 August 1987.
Mrs Joyce Jackways, Auckland, 26 May 1987.
Mrs R.K. Logan, Dunedin, 24 June 1987, 6 July 1987.
Dr Dorothy Potter, Masterton, 27 June 1987.
Dr David Pyke, Registrar, RCP, London, 18 June 1987.
Dr C. Ring, Auckland, 20 May 1987.
Associate Professor L.R. Robinson, Department of Anatomy, University of Otago Medical School, 15 July 1987, 16 November 1987.
Mrs D.F. Rogers, Warkworth, 14 June 1987.
Mrs Jinty Rorke, Special Services Librarian, Tauranga Library, 8 April 1994.
Dr J.M. Tweed, Honorary Archivist (New Zealand), RACP, Wellington, 24 July 1987.
Professor J.M. Watt, Auckland, 12 June 1988.
Mrs V.M. Webster, Tauranga, 19 July 1987.
Professor Margaret Wilson, School of Law, University of Waikato, 2 March 1994.

7 Interviews

Miss Nancy Bamford, Auckland, 15 June 1987.
Dr D.M.O. Becroft, Auckland, 15 November 1994.
Dr A.H. Berry, Wellington, 6 July 1987.

Dr R. Black, Auckland, 7 June 1989.
Dr K. Bowden, Ngunguru, 25 September 1989.
Dr M. Chieffi, Wellington, 7 July 1987.
Dr E. Cole, Auckland, 14 June 1988.
Reverend L.F. Clements, Auckland, 8 May 1987, 20 September 1989.
Mrs M. Dobbie, Auckland, 12 September 1987.
Mrs June Duffus, Auckland, 2 June 1987.
Professor R.B. Elliott, Auckland, 26 October 1989.
Mrs E. Ellis-Pegler, Auckland, 6 December 1988.
Dr T.G. Fox, Auckland, 11 July 1988.
Mr and Mrs H. Gaudin, Auckland, 28 February 1986.
Dr A.O.M. Gilmour, Auckland, 24 July 1987.
Dr M. Hardy, Auckland, 8 March 1989.
Dr A. Hunter, Auckland, 5 December 1988, 1 May 1989.
Mr. S. Kurtovich, Auckland, 15 September 1987.
Mr. G. Maitland, Auckland, 1 November 1988.
Sir William Manchester, Auckland, 14 May 1987.
Mrs D. Stuart Masters, Auckland, 13 February 1989.
Dr J.D. Matthews, Auckland, 2 June 1988.
Miss L. McKellar, Auckland, 15 May 1989.
Ms P. Meikle, Auckland, 21 May 1988.
Dr R.J. Methven, Auckland, 21 February, 1989.
Sister J. Milne, Auckland, 20 April 1989.
Dr R.F. Moody, Auckland, 9 June 1987.
Ms Betty Neal, Auckland, 21 February 1989.
Mrs A. Odell, Auckland, 23 May 1989.
Dr B. Quin, Auckland, 14 May 1987.
Dr C. Ring, Auckland, 3 September 1987.
Mrs D.F. Rogers, Auckland, 23 May 1989.
Lady Sayers, Auckland, 13 March 1987.
Mrs A.V.C. Slack, Auckland, 11 April 1989.
Mr. and Mrs A. McM. Stanton, Auckland, 11 April 1989.
Mrs E. Sullivan, Auckland, 15 June 1987.
Mr. E. Sun, Auckland, 1 November 1988.
Dr C.E. Watson, Auckland, 6 June 1988.
Professor J.M. Watt, Auckland, 6 June 1988.
Mr. and Mrs D. Whillans, Auckland, 5 February 1986.
Mr. and Mrs W. S. Wood, Auckland, 19 June 1989.
Dr M. Woodroffe, Auckland, 28 April 1989.

INDEX

Abortion, 151, 189, 208-219, 229, 233-5, 237
Abortion Law Reform Association of New Zealand (ALRANZ), 213, 216, 232, 234, 237
Alice Bush Centre, 242
Alice Bush Health Education Trust, 242
Allergy Clinic (at Auckland and later at Green Lane Hospitals), 101, 228
Allergies, 103-105, 198, 204-6
A National Health Service (1943), 35, 37, 54
Appeal for Population Control (APC), 178, 180, 215
Asthma Society, 222, 227
Auckland Clinical Society, 38, 227
Auckland Grammar School, 6, 8
Auckland Hospital, 23, 25, 27, 30, 63-4, 100, 111, 191, 201, 204, 228, 240
Auckland Hospital Board, 23, 24, 64, 100, 199, 200, 205, 241, 242
Auckland Medical School, 190, 199, 202, 203, 227, 236, 238, 242
Auckland Parents' Hospitals Committee (later Parents' Centre, Auckland), 132
Auckland Postgraduate Committee (1940s), 38
Auckland University College (later the University of Auckland), 6, 7, 11, 15, 55, 57, 128, 232
Auckland War Memorial Museum, 29
Auckland Young People's Club, 33

Baguio (Philippines), 183
Baker, Dr Eleanor, 20
Bangkok (Thailand), 156, 172-4, 175-6, 177
Bari (Italy), 63, 67
Begg, Dr (later Sir) Neil, 109, 113, 142, 145, 166, 195-6
Bennett, Elsie, 32
Berry, Dr A. H. (Nan), 19, 20-22, 23, 24, 26

Bertram, James, 12
Bevan Brown, Dr Maurice, 85
Biddle, Ethel, 175
Black, Dr Ruth, 138, 139, 146, 151, 160, 175, 183, 192
Bonham, Professor Dennis, 179, 181, 235
Boult, Phyllis, 9, 10, 31
Bowlby, John (*see also* 'maternal deprivation' and *Maternal Care and Mental Health*), 84, 112, 189
Brighton (England), 232
Bryant, D.J., 202
Brych, Milan, 103
Burns, Sir Charles, 113, 114
Bush, Alice (*née* Stanton),
 abortion, 207, 208-219, 234-5
 alignment with postwar family welfare groups, 84-6, 115-7, 130-49
 asthma and allergies, 29, 99, 103-5, 198, 204-6, 227
 attitude to Bowlby, 84, 86-7, 112-4
 attitude to social obligations, 10, 12, 14, 16-17, 47, 78, 109-110, 130-3, 240, 241
 attitude to war, 26, 27, 31-2, 58
 attitude to women in medicine, 14, 20-22, 30, 31, 107-8
 belief in educational process, 47, 115, 120, 128, 160, 231-2
 birth of children, 59, 81, 83
 choice of, and preparation for, medical career, 13, 15-22
 continuing family loyalty, 51, 79, 93-4
 courtship and marriage, 41-56
 DCH, 99
 development of religious doubts, 47-8, 75, 229, 234
 early education, 9-10
 early life and close family ties, 5-6, 8, 11, 12, 16
 early religious influences, 7, 11, 14, 17, 33
 family planning, 36-7, 88, 146, 149-

169, 198, 203, 231, 233
feminism, 20, 51-2, 71-2, 87-90, 96, 116, 192-6, 208-9, 221-4, 234, 241
FRACP, 92-3
full commitment to career, 62-6, 71-3, 97-8, 101
graduation 23
hospital appointments, 30, 63-64, 65, 98, 100-102, 111
health, 225, 227, 228-30, 235
interest in mental health as counterbalance to loss of religious faith, 75-6, 229
international population and conservation movements, 170-187, 223, 232-3, 239
last illness, death and funeral, 240-242
locum for Dr Edward Sayers, 27-8
marriage and career, 41, 48-50, 57, 67-70, 82, 91-2, 94-6
mature personality, 94, 105-6, 224-5
medical politics (*see also* Medical Study Group), 34-36, 38-40, 52-54, 109-110, 134-47, 203-6, 230-231
mental health, 37-38, 84, 85, 99, 112-4, 116-7, 137
motherhood and career, 60-62, 74-6, 80, 81, 82-3, 84, 87-91
MRACP, 77
MRCP, 80-83, 98-9
need for intellectual stimulation, 44-5
paediatrics, 30, 98-102, 106-7, 110-2
parenting theories, 116-125
personality as young woman, 18, 25-6, 41-2
political views, 45-47
problems obtaining resident post, 23-5
reactions to death, 241-243
recreation, 26, 94
religion as authorisation for social action, 48, 75, 88, 162-3, 173
residency at New Plymouth Hospital, 25-6
sexuality and sex education, 32-34, 84, 116-7, 122, 125-130
stress of lifestyle, 69-70, 218-9
youthful personality, 9-10
Bush, Christine Mary (later Moorhouse, daughter), 83, 90-1, 171, 226, 233, 237, 238, 240, 241
Bush, Faulkner (W.A.F.),
attitude to Alice's career, 49, 52-3, 56, 60, 63, 64-5, 67-8, 73, 76, 78-9, 81-2, 91-2, 93-6
attitude to women, 67
courtship, 44-56

death, 240
decision to take up law, 55
depression, 68-69
experience and influence of Depression, 43, 45-6, 52
family background, 42-3
first meeting with Alice, 42
interests, 94-95
later life, 219, 225, 226-7, 228, 238-242
personality, 43-44
political views, 52, 55
postwar rehabilitation, 79-80, 82
reaction to Lesley's death, 76
return to New Zealand, 76-77
teaching career, 43, 80-1, 82, 91
war service, 43, 57-9, 60, 66-9, 73
wedding, 55-6
Bush, George Arthur (Faulkner's father), 42
Bush, Lesley Elizabeth (daughter), 59, 60-2, 66, 70, 73-74, 83, 91, 95
Bush, Muriel (*née* Dempsey, later Hamilton, Faulkner's mother), 42, 79
Bush, Peter Joseph (son), 81, 81-2, 91, 226, 238, 240, 241

Carey, Professor Harvey, 133, 134-5, 138, 139, 140, 142, 147, 179
Casey, (later Dame) Stella, 163-4
Caughey, Dr Ronald, 66, 102, 199, 202
Caughey, T.H.C. (later Sir Harcourt), 200
Child Health Clinic, 109, 112-3, 130, 136, 147-8, 153, 156, 159, 228
Children and Young Persons Act (1974), 197, 238
Choice, 148, 160, 165, 169, 173, 174, 176, 178, 179, 181, 183, 185, 186, 221, 223, 224, 225, 230, 231, 239, 241
Clements, Rev. Les, 43, 233
Cole, Dr Elizabeth, 30, 36, 131
Cole, Mr James McMurray, 40
Collins-Williams, Dr Cecil, 204
Combined [Medical] Staff Committee (Auckland Hospital Board), 101-2, 111, 204
Consultative Committee on Pre-School Health Services (1959), 109, 118
Contraception (*see also* New Zealand Family Planning Association), 36, 85, 88, 131, 135, 146, 149-151, 163-66, 168, 189, 208, 212, 224, 228, 230, 233, 237
Cook, Dr Enid, 85
Cornere, Brian, 227
Cotter, Thomas, 6, 7

280 INDEX

Craccum, 12, 210
Cranwell, Lucy, 29
Craven, Dr J.W., 23
Croxford, Dr Vivienne, 136, 138, 140

Davidge, Dr Elsie, 108, 168
Davies, Valerie, 91
Deem, Dr Helen, 30, 109
Deep Creek (beach house), 7-8, 51, 56, 226
Denestone (family home), 7, 9, 12, 24, 56, 79, 94, 107, 168, 179, 181, 187, 226, 227, 238, 240, 241
Depression (1930s), 11, 13, 35, 43, 100
Deverell, Sir Colville, 175, 181
Diocesan High School Chronicle, 13
Diocesan School for Girls, 9, 16, 67, 241
Diploma in Child Health (DCH), 99
Doctorate in medicine (MD), 65, 73
Dreaver, Mrs Mary, 25
Dunn, Dr Patrick, 215, 219-220, 239

Economic Commission for Asia and the Far East (ECAFE), 164, 176-7
Education of girls, 13, 15
Elliott, Professor R.B. (Bob), 203
Ellis, Havelock, 84

Family Guidance Centre (Auckland), 38, 85, 130, 148, 192
Family Planning Association (British), 132, 142, 181
Farmer, Dr Keitha, 191
Federation of Labour ('Red Feds'), 34
Federation of Parent-Teacher Associations, 126-7
Federation of University Women, 108, 161
Feminism, 13, 33, 72, 87-8, 107, 188-190, 207, 208-9, 221-224, 237-8
Fischmann, Eva, 37, 38, 113, 241
Fox, Dr T.G. (Grahame), 102, 113
Freud, Sigmund, 37, 84
Friedan, Betty, 193
Frost, David, 236
Furkert, Mr F.P., 74

Gatman, Dr Margaret, 83
Gaudin, Mr Howard, 35
Geiringer, Dr Erich, 178, 214, 215
Geneva (Switzerland), 233
Gowing, Rt Rev. Eric, 218
Gowland, Professor W.P., 21
Gray, Lex, 176
Great Ormond Street Childrens' Hospital (London), 99

Green Lane Hospital, 64, 227, 234
Griffin, Marie, 238
Gunson, Dr E.B., 25
Guttmacher, Dr Alan, 179

Halls, Dr Theodora, 99
Hanan, Ralph, 157
Hanna, Sister C.A., 107
Hamilton, Alfred (Faulkner's stepfather), 43
Hardy, Dr Morag, 203
Hawkins, Dorothy, 32
Health Department, 23, 33, 107, 109, 112-4, 126-8, 130, 134, 136, 157, 160-2, 163, 168, 192, 200, 219, 220, 221, 223, 230, 241
Henley, Wilton, 199, 200, 201-2, 218
Hill Top School (also known for a short time as Stanton Junior College), 9-10, 32, 241
Hillary, Sir Edmund, 178
Holt, Betty, 193
Holyoake, Keith, 181, 182
Homes and Families (1950), 117-118
Hospital for Sick Children (Toronto), 204
Hughes, Dr Elizabeth (or 'Kate'), 30-31, 35, 36, 37, 64, 66, 108, 126, 195
Hunn, J.K., 155
Hunn Report, 157
Hunter, Dr Alison, 191, 203
Hunton, Dr Rex, 236
Hurrey, Mavis, 192, 232

International Planned Parenthood Federation (IPPF), 141, 170-187, 212, 232, 233, 237, 239, 241
International Project of the Association for Voluntary Sterilization, 233
International Women's Year (1975), 198
Isaacs, Susan, 85, 117

Jackson (later Chieffi), Dr Margaret, 19, 20-22, 23, 24, 26
Jamieson, Dr J.P.S., 143, 144, 145-6, 150
Jelicich-Ranford, Angela, 231

Karitane Hospital (Auckland), 30, 65, 118-9, 122, 153, 167, 228, 240, 242
Karitane nurses, 30, 60-1, 80, 116
Kennedy, Dr Douglas, 161, 168
King, Colleen, 163, 237
King, Sir Frederick Truby, 30
King, Norman, 235
Kirk, Norman, 232
Kuala Lumpur, 233

Labour governments, 34, 99, 230, 232
Lady Fergusson Family Counselling Service (LFFCS), 192, 197
Latter, Dr Rosalind, 99
Lawson, Ida (cousin), 18
Lawson, Professor Richard (married to maternal aunt), 18
Lee, John A., 55, 73
Lewis, Dr Peter, 197
Liley, Dr, later Sir William, 215, 218, 234
Littlewood, Mary, 225
Lowe, Glenys, 135, 139, 146, 180, 223, 224
Ludbrook, Dr Samuel, 30, 64, 65, 100, 102, 108, 110, 111, 199, 241
Lunn, Judy, 139, 141, 180

Macdonald, Dr Fraser, 194
MacIntyre, Duncan, 154
McKay, D.N., 157
MacKay, Dr Joan, 168
McKellar, Lola, 80, 82, 102, 106
McMaster, Dr Archibald (Archie), (maternal uncle), 13
McMaster family (maternal antecedents), 5, 7
McMaster, Marjorie (later Stanton), 7
McMaster, Thomas (maternal grandfather), 7
Maori people, 152-164, 180, 197, 220, 223
Maori Health Committee, 157, 158-60
Maori Education Foundation, 175, 176
Maori Women's Welfare League (MWWL), 155, 158, 160, 220
Marriage Guidance, 85, 145
Maternal Care and Mental Health (1952), later published as *Child Care and the Growth of Love* (1953), 84, 86-7, 118
'Maternal deprivation' (Alice's review of Bowlby's work), 84, 86-7, 112
Matthews, Dr J.D. (Jack), 102
'Mazengarb' Committee and Report, *see* Special Committee on Moral Delinquency in Children and Adolescents
Medical Association of New Zealand (MANZ formerly NZBMA), 192, 193, 212, 241
Medical Practitioners' Act (1950), 25
Medical Research Foundation, 205
Medical Study Group (1940s - *see also A National Health Service*), 34, 35, 37, 38, 39, 46, 54, 110, 138
Medical Women's Association (NZMA and AKMWA), 13, 24, 31, 99, 107-8, 191, 195, 205, 214, 238, 242
Medico-Legal Society, 94, 197

Meggett, Ron, 192
Meikle, Phoebe, 70, 90
Men and Women (1953), 87
Mental health, 37, 75-6, 84-85, 88, 112-4, 116-7, 130, 137, 148, 224, 235, 242
Mental Health Association, 130, 132, 148
Methodist religion, 6, 14, 17, 28, 33
Methven, Dr R.J., 147
Milne, Deirdre, 209
Mirror (magazine), 33
Moir, Dr Phyllis, 30

Nannestad, Dr Elizabeth, 30
National Council of Churches in New Zealand, 87, 117, 156, 172, 174
National Council of Women (NCW), 108, 161, 185, 192, 193, 198, 219, 237
National governments, 99, 157, 161
National Organisation of Women (NOW), 192, 193-4, 198, 209, 237
National Women's Hospital, 100, 102, 133, 179, 181, 202, 219, 222
Neal, Betty, 107, 229
Nelson (later Schuchard), Dr Beatrice, 19, 24
New Education Fellowship, 85, 117
New Plymouth Hospital, 25-26
New Zealand Branch of the British Medical Association (NZBMA), *see also* Medical Association of New Zealand (MANZ); 34, 39, 40, 53, 101, 108, 109, 113-4, 130, 132, 145, 160, 161, 165, 166; and NZFPA and Parents' Centres, 134-47, 150, 221
New Zealand Educational Institute, 129
New Zealand Family Doctor (1960s), 121
New Zealand Family Planning Association (NZFPA), 36, 37, 72, 85, 116, 127, 128, 129-30, 131, 132, 134-150, 152-163, 163-66, 167-169, 170-187, 192, 210, 211-2, 213-4, 219, 220-225, 229, 230, 231, 232, 234, 237, 238, 239, 241, 242
New Zealand Herald, 11, 69, 129, 148, 157, 177, 184, 200, 201, 230, 238, 241
New Zealand Medical Journal (*NZMJ*), 38, 66, 114, 124, 137, 145, 151, 167, 190, 202, 205, 215, 229, 241
Nicholson, Doris, 238
North, Professor Derek, 205

Odell, Aileen (*née* Stanton, sister), 66
Odell, Alan (brother-in-law), 66
Organ transplantation, 193, 204-6
Otago Medical School, 13, 14, 16, 17-22,

24, 29, 110, 197
Otago Medical School, Auckland Branch Faculty, 101
Otago University, 17

Pacific Islands' people, 155, 163, 171-2, 220, 223
Paediatrics, 99, 100, 110-112, 116, 136, 199-203, 204
Paediatric Society of New Zealand, 107, 108-9, 110, 112-3, 126, 130, 168, 192, 202, 215, 218
Panapa, Bishop Wiremu, 155
Parenting, 115-125, 242
Parents' Centres, 85, 127, 130, 131, 132, 134-8, 142, 144-5, 147, 148, 200, 219, 237, 240, 241
Parry, W. (Bill), 46
Personal Relationships (1944), 32-4, 105
Phillips, Dr Leo, 102
Pickerill, Drs H.P. and C.M., 112
Pinkerton, Dr Grace, 143
Pitt Street Church, 6
Platts-Mills, Dr Adah, 60, 70
Play Centres, 85, 145, 175, 219
Plunket Society (see Royal New Zealand Plunket Society)
Police Offences Act (1954), 151, 228
Porritt, Sir Arthur, 19
Princess Mary Hospital (also Princess Mary Block or Princess Mary), 100, 102, 110-112, 153, 191, 199, 200, 201, 203, 204, 205, 228
Progressive Book Club, 36
Psychiatric Society (1940s), 37, 38, 116
Public Health Nurses, 156, 160, 167, 235

Quin, Dr Basil, 30

Rarotonga, 171-172, 180
Rawlings Scholarship, 6
Registered Nurses' Association, 29
Red Roofs Salvation Army Hospital, Dunedin, 21
Rehabilitation schemes (World War Two), 80
Robb, Sir Douglas, 34-5, 36, 38, 54, 69, 142, 241
Robinson, Thelma, 158
Rogers, Dacre Fox (brother-in-law), 56
Rogers, Patricia (née Stanton, sister), 56, 57
Roman Catholic Church, 128, 164-6, 209, 210, 211, 215, 219
Rose (later Tallerman), Dr Alice Campbell, 99

Royal Australasian College of Physicians (RACP), 65-6, 73, 76, 77, 92-3
Royal College of Physicians (London), 30, 80, 198, 215
Royal Commission of Inquiry into Social Security (1972), 192, 203
Royal New Zealand Plunket Society, 30, 85, 109, 119, 142, 166-7
Russia (see also Soviet Union), 19

Sage, Ruiha, 158
Sandford, Miss H.K., 9
Sayers, Dr (later Sir) Edward, 27, 62, 65, 66, 72, 74, 80, 241
Sayers, Jean (later Lady), 74
School Medical Service, 14,
Sexuality and sex education (see also Bush, Alice, and *Personal Relationships*), 32, 34, 85-6, 122, 125-130, 207-8, 224, 237
Shand, Dr Carol, 214
Singapore, 175, 176, 178, 180
Social Security Act (1938), 34, 38-40
Society for the Protection of Home and Family, 197
Society for the Protection of the Unborn Child (SPUC), 215, 218, 219, 234
Soviet Union (see also Russia), 43
Special Committee on Moral Delinquency in Children and Adolescents ('Mazengarb', 1950s) and report, 125-6, 151
Speech Therapy Assocation, 219
Stallworthy, Dr K.R., 113
Stanton, Aileen (sister, later Odell), 5, 9, 11, 57, 74
Stanton, Alfred (paternal grandfather), 6
Stanton, Alice see Bush, Alice
Stanton, Allenby (brother), 5, 57, 140
Stanton, Elizabeth ('Aunty Betty', paternal aunt), 79
Stanton, Fanny (née Stephenson, paternal grandmother), 6
Stanton, Isabel (sister-in-law, née Macky), 179, 182, 213, 216
Stanton, Joseph (father, later Sir Joseph), acceptance of Alice's marriage, 56, 79
continuing close relationship with Alice, 92-4
courtship and marriage, 7
early life and education, 6
effects of Depression, 11
effects of Warwick's death, 12
health, 13, 15
knighthood and death, 93

legal career and rise in social status, 7-8, 140
religion, 6-7
reservations about Faulkner, 51, 55
support for Alice's medical career, 15-16, 24-25, 27
Stanton Junior College (*see* Hill Top School), 10
Stanton, Marjorie (mother, *née* McMaster), 5, 7, 12, 25, 28, 55, 56
Stanton, Patricia (sister, later Rogers), 5, 9, 11, 12, 56
Stanton, Warwick (brother), 5, 11-12
Star (Auckland), 177
St Margaret's Hostel, 19
Student Christian Movement, 7, 18
Summerskill, Dr Edith (later Baroness), 72, 88, 149
Swinburn, Bobbie, 231

Tavistock Clinic (London), 84, 99
Taylor, Alister, 208
Taylor, Mary, 227
Temperance movement, 6-7
The Digest (Otago Medical School magazine), 19, 26
The Little Red Schoolbook, 208
Thompson, Dr A.W.S., 112, 113
Thompson, Dr Margaret, 30
Thursday, 198
Tizard, R.J., 230

United Nations, 175, 177, 182, 186, 232
United Women's Convention (1973), 237

University of Canterbury Students' Association, 207

Watt, Dr (later Professor) James, 113, 142, 145
Webster, Alan, 208
Werry, Professor John, 227
Whillans, Douglas, 29
Woman's National Abortion Action Campaign (WONAAC), 234
World Council of Churches, 233
World Population Year (1974), 232, 238
World War Two, 26-9, 31-2, 34, 37, 57-9, 63, 66-9, 77, 100, 152
Women in the paid workforce, 7, 15, 25, 33, 49, 56, 83-4, 86-91,
Women doctors, 13, 14-15, 19-21, 23-25, 27, 28, 30, 33, 37, 41, 63, 75, 97, 99, 107-8, 115, 125, 189-192
Women's National Service Corps (WNSC), 31-32
'Wood, Mary' (Alice Bush), 121-4
World Health Organisation (WHO), 84, 110, 114, 183

Young Women's Christian Association (YWCA), 32, 129

Zeff, Phyllis, 135, 137, 139, 140, 141, 142
Zeisler, Peggy, 187, 232
Zero Population Growth Society, 184, 232
Zonta, 192, 193, 197, 201, 203, 236, 237, 238, 242